Aerosols and the Lung

Aerosols and the Lung: Clinical and Experimental Aspects

Edited by
Stewart W. Clarke, MD, FRCP
Consultant Physician, Senior Lecturer and Head of Department of Thoracic Medicine, Sub-Dean for Admissions, The Royal Free Hospital and School of Medicine, London

and

Demetri Pavia, MSc, PhD, FInstP
Principal Scientific Officer, Department of Thoracic Medicine;
Honorary Lecturer, Academic Department of Medicine, The Royal Free Hospital and School of Medicine, London

Butterworths
London Boston Durban Singapore Sydney Toronto Wellington

First published 1984

British Library Cataloguing in Publication Data

Aerosols and the lung.
1. Lungs—Diseases 2. Aerosols—
Physiological effect
I. Clarke, Stewart W. II. Pavia, Demetri
616.2′4 RC756

ISBN 0–407–00265–0

Library of Congress Cataloging in Publication Data
Main entry under title:

Aerosols and the lung.

Includes bibliographical references and index.
1. Lungs—Diseases. 2. Aerosols. 3. Pulmonary function tests. 4. Lungs. I. Clarke, Stewart W.
II. Pavia, Demetri.
RC756.A33 1984 616.2′4 84-3151
ISBN 0–407–00265–0

Typeset by Scribe Design, Gillingham, Kent
Printed by Thetford Press Ltd
and bound by Anchor Brendon Ltd

Preface

This book was conceived out of the editors' longstanding interest in the lung defences coupled with the radioaerosol means of assessing their efficiency. This interest grew to embrace all aspects of aerosols and the lung, including aerosol use in clinical medicine.

The logic behind the book's structure is as follows: knowledge of the physical properties of aerosols is required to assess their inhalation into the lung; information about how to produce an aerosol suitable for inhaling is equally important; determining aerosol deposition within the lung requires a basis of lung anatomy and physiology; and the estimation of lung clearance requires knowledge of cilia, lung secretions and mucociliary action.

In clinical diagnosis, radioaerosols can be used for ventilation imaging, detecting airway disease and estimating airway calibre. They provide the best means of measuring mucociliary clearance, which may be affected by a variety of physiological, pathological, pharmacological and environmental agents. Sputum clearance by cough and chest physiotherapy may be assessed as may alveolar clearance with the syndromes of 'leaky lung'.

Therapeutic aerosols are used increasingly in the treatment of asthma and chronic obstructive airways disease, whether they be aerosol bronchodilators, anticholinergics, cromoglycate, steroids, mucolytics, or, as in cystic fibrosis, antibiotics.

Aerosol challenge, an important aspect in the diagnosis of occupational asthma, is another expanding field. Of course, inhaled dust aerosols have long been known to cause disease, but further information has been gained about this topic from the current interest in aerosols.

All these aspects of aerosols and the lung are gathered together in this book, and we hope that the result is useful and informative. Certainly, we have found the exercise of compiling this book to be so, and our interest in the field remains unabated.

Contributors

John E. Agnew, BA, MSc, PhD
Principal Physicist, Department of Medical Physics;
Honorary Lecturer, Academic Department of Medical Physics, The Royal Free Hospital and School of Medicine, London, England

P. Sherwood Burge, MB, BS, MSc, MRCP, MFOM, DIH
Consultant Physician, East Birmingham and Solihull Hospitals;
Honorary Senior Lecturer, Department of Occupational Health, University of Birmingham, West Midlands, England

Stewart W. Clarke, MD, FRCP
Consultant Physician, Senior Lecturer and Head of Department of Thoracic Medicine, Sub-Dean for Admissions, The Royal Free Hospital and School of Medicine, London, England

Robert B. Douglas, BSc, MTech, PhD, MInstP
Senior Lecturer in Applied Physiology, TUC Centenary Institute of Occupational Health, London School of Hygiene and Tropical Medicine, London University, London, England

J. Gareth Jones, MD, FRCP, FFARCS
Member of the Scientific Staff of the MRC, Clinical Research Centre;
Honorary Consultant Anaesthetist, Northwick Park Hospital, Harrow, Middlesex, England

Maria Teresa Lopez-Vidriero, MD, PhD
Research Fellow and Honorary Lecturer, Department of Thoracic Medicine, The Royal Free Hospital and School of Medicine, London, England

Stephen P. Newman, MA, MSc, PhD, MInstP
Principal Physicist, Department of Thoracic Medicine;
Honorary Lecturer, Academic Department of Medical Physics, The Royal Free Hospital and School of Medicine, London, England

Demetri Pavia, MSc, PhD, FInstP
Principal Scientific Officer, Department of Thoracic Medicine;
Honorary Lecturer, Academic Department of Medicine, The Royal Free Hospital and School of Medicine, London, England

Philip P. Sutton, BSc, MB, BS, MRCP(UK)
Senior Registrar in Respiratory Medicine, Aberdeen Hospitals, Aberdeen, Scotland

Contents

Abbreviations and symbols

C	concentration
$C_{2.0}$	tracheobronchial clearance of deposited radioaerosol at 2.0 h
$C_{6.0}$	tracheobronchial clearance of deposited radioaerosol at 6.0 h
CBF	ciliary beat frequency
CF	chemotactic factor
COAD/COLD/COPD	chronic obstructive airways/lung/pulmonary disease
COV	coefficient of variation
CP	chest physiotherapy
CV	closing volume
d	particle diameter
D	tube/obstacle diameter
DLCO/TLCO	diffusion/transfer in lung of CO
DTPA	diethylenetriamine pentaacetic acid
F	inhalation flow rate
FEV_1	forced expiratory volume in 1 s
FET	forced expiration technique
FRC	functional residual capacity
FVC	forced vital capacity
g	gravitational constant
G^*	mechanical impedance (of mucus)
G'	storage modulus (elasticity of mucus)
G''	loss modulus (of mucus)
G_{AW}	airway conductance
GMD	geometric mean diameter
GSD	geometric standard deviation
Hz	hertz
IPPB	intermittent positive pressure breathing
L	length of tube
LMC	lung mucociliary clearance
m	mass of a particle
M	molar
MAF	macrophage activating factor

MDI	metered dose inhaler
$MEF_{50-75\%}$	forced expiratory flow rate in the third quarter of FVC
MEFV	maximal expiratory flow volume
MHC	major histocompatibility complex
MIF	macrophage migration inhibition factor
MMAD	mass median aerodynamic diameter
MMD	mass median diameter
MMFR	maximum mid-expiratory flow rate
MSAF	mean small airways function
MW	molecular weight
NCF	neutrophil chemotactic factor
PAS	periodic acid schiff
PD	postural drainage
PD_{20}	dose of histamine/methacholine causing a 20 per cent fall in FEV_1 from baseline
PEFR	peak expiratory flow rate
PEFV	partial expiratory flow volume
PMF	progressive massive fibrosis
PN	percussion
PVC	polyvinylchloride
r	radius of curvature of airflow streamlines
R	disc radius
$R_{2.0}$	tracheobronchial retention of deposited radioaerosol at 2.0 h
$R_{6.0}$	tracheobronchial retention of deposited radioaerosol at 6.0 h
R_{AW}	airway resistance
RMM	remnant magnetic moment
RV	residual volume
SD	standard deviation
SRS-A	slow reacting substance of anaphylaxis
Stk	Stokes' number
SQUID	superconducting quantum interference device
T	surface tension
T_{50}	time taken to clear 50 per cent of tracheobronchial deposition
TC	T cell—cytolytic function
TGV	thoracic gas volume
TH	T cell—helper function
TLC	total lung capacity
TLV	threshold limit value
TMV	tracheal mucus velocity
TS	T cell—suppressor function
U	velocity of an aerosol particle or airflow
$\dot{V}$	airflow
$\dot{V}_{max}25$	flow rate at 25 per cent of VC from a MEFV curve
$\dot{V}_{max}50$	flow rate at 50 per cent of VC from a MEFV curve
V_D	anatomical dead space (volume)
v_g	settling velocity
V_L	lung volume

$V_{T/TV}$	tidal volume
VC	vital capacity
VIP	vasoactive intestinal peptide
$\dot{V}/\dot{Q}$	ventilation perfusion ratio

Greek symbols

β	angle of a tube relative to the horizontal
Δ	limiting trajectory displacement
η	air viscosity
λ	mean free path
μ	viscosity fluid
ρ	density
ω	angular velocity

Chapter 1

Anatomy and physiology of the human lung: aspects relevant to aerosols

Stewart W. Clarke

Introduction

Aerosols are widely used in the lung for therapeutic (Lourenço and Cotromanes, 1982, a and b) diagnostic (Wagner, 1976) and experimental (Pavia *et al.*, 1980) purposes. The order in which these uses are listed is deliberate, reflecting the fact that aerosol therapy has been recommended for centuries in asthma (Ellul-Micallef, 1976) while their use in diagnostic (e.g. pulmonary embolism) and experimental (e.g. mucociliary clearance) work has blossomed in the past decade or two.

However, in the past insufficient attention has been paid to the problems of actually inhaling the aerosol particles, although breathing dust particles (Muir, 1972) has been widely studied in an industrial context (e.g. pneumoconiosis). The two aspects are not necessarily identical. Inhaled particles are filtered out of the airstream by the aerodynamic defences of the upper airways (above the larynx), which ensure that only a small proportion (<10 per cent) reach the bronchial tree (Proctor, 1977a and b). This amount occurs when inhalation conditions and aerosol size are optimal with a mass median aerodynamic diameter (MMAD) of $\simeq$2–5 μm. In the lower airways (below the larynx) flow conditions partly determined by the branching nature of the bronchial tree ensure that many particles will deposit centrally and arguably not at the appropriate desired site, even after penetrating the larynx.

In order to understand the fundamental importance of aerosol deposition within the tracheobronchial tree, knowledge of airway and lung anatomy is important as is a certain amount of physiology. Thus this chapter will attempt to focus on these aspects, which receive a further mention in several of the ensuing chapters.

Anatomy of the upper and lower airways (Proctor, 1977a and b)

The respiratory tract can be divided into upper and lower parts by the lower border of the cricoid cartilage. The upper airways not only conduct air but also take part in swallowing, air conditioning (warming and humidification), smell and speech. Additionally, many inhaled particles will be filtered from the main airstream by impaction in the nose and oropharynx. The lower airways, including the trachea

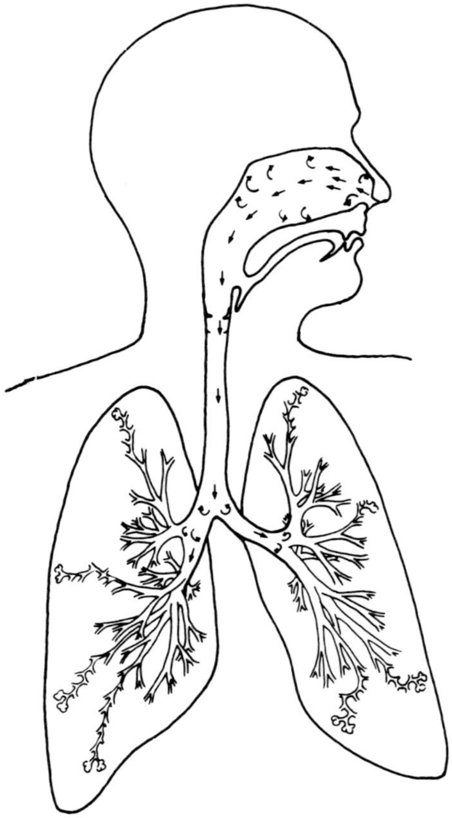

Figure 1.1 Schematic diagram illustrating flow through the upper and lower airways

and bronchial tree, conduct air to and from the alveoli for gas exchange (*Figure 1.1*).

The nose (Douek, 1979)

The nose develops from the cranial portion of the primitive foregut of the embryo. The anterior nares (nostrils) lead from the outside to the beginning of the ciliated mucosa at the anterior ends of the nasal septum and turbinates. This region has the smallest total cross-sectional area in the respiratory tract. The main channel extends backwards 6–8 cm to the posterior ends of the turbinates and septum. The cavity is divided by the septum, and the lateral walls comprise the folds of the inferior, middle and superior turbinates which divide the airway into the corresponding inferior, middle and superior meati.

The entrance or vestibule is lined by skin with sebaceous glands and contains long strong hairs which also help to filter the airstream. Elsewhere, the mucus membrane of the nasal cavity is ciliated, highly vascular and rich in mucus glands and goblet cells, with underlying clumps of lymphoid tissue, being inseparably applied to the periosteum. The olfactory portion containing bipolar nerve cells comprises the upper part of the superior meatus lying on the cribriform plate.

The nasopharynx lies 12–14 cm from the external nares where the septum ends and where there is a transition from columnar ciliated to squamous epithelium extending to the larynx. The adenoids lie in the posterior nasopharyngeal wall, their surface being partially ciliated. Functionally, the nasopharynx ends at the lower border of the soft palate.

The upper airway has several key functions:

1. It permits a change in the direction of airflow to and from the trachea in a smooth, curvilinear way.
2. It involves a change in cross-sectional area, being narrow at the trachea, wider in the meati and nasopharynx and narrow again in the larynx, which helps to control and filter the airflow.
3. It transmits a relatively narrow airstream, chiefly through the middle meatus.
4. It provides a large surface area over the turbinates for heating and humidification.
5. It is lined by nasal mucosa which has the capacity to vary the patency of the airway, its blood flow and secretions considerably.

Other functions include olfaction, vocal resonance with speech and nasal reflexes.

Airflow

The inspiratory airstream converges 1.5–2.5 cm from the external nares, then bends at an angle of 60–130 degrees to pass mainly along the middle meatus (with a small stream along the inferior meatus), gradually bending by about 90 degrees in the nasopharynx to enter the larynx and trachea directly. During a quiet breath with the peak of inspiration, say, $0.5\,\ell\,s^{-1}$ there may be some turbulence in the mainstream. During expiration, however, the airstream flows more evenly over the surface of the main nasal passage.

The nose accounts for about 50 per cent of the total respiratory resistance. Almost all of this occurs in the first 2–3 cm of the total 12–14 cm length. Thus, the anterior constriction provides the major airflow resistance though congestion of the main passage may increase resistance there by up to fivefold. The degree of congestion, primarily under autonomic nervous control, varies with ambient air temperature (cold air at 7°C congests), posture (lying down leads to congestion on the dependent side) and disease, while exertion dilates. Ventilation switches to the oropharyngeal airway when there is nasal obstruction and also during exercise and phonation.

Inspiratory collapse of the anterior nares usually limits flow. However, the nares are relatively rigid with a fibrous and cartilaginous framework so that they may resist a range of pressures from 0.6 to 20 cmH_2O during quiet and maximal inspiration.

During expiration, a similar nasal route for flow is traversed apart from there being a large central eddy in the nose.

Clearance

Nasal secretions are swept backwards by mucociliary action to the nasopharynx and thence swallowed. The clearance rate is on average about $6\,mm\,min^{-1}$ with a wide range. From a small region at the anterior end of the inferior turbinate, mucus is swept forward to the anterior nares, there to be blown or wiped away.

Air temperature

With an ambient air temperature of 23°C, by mid-nasal passage the temperature of inspired air will rise to about 30°C and 33°C in the nasopharynx with a relative humidity of 100 per cent at each site. Even with ambient extremes between −20°C to +55°C equilibration is good. During expiration some of the heat and water is returned to the nose as the air cools.

Inhaled particles

The high linear velocity of the airstream as it narrows and bends in the anterior nares entraps particles of 5–10 μm aerodynamic diameter. Within the size range 2–5 μm diameter, some particles will penetrate the lungs and impact there. Smaller particles especially those which are submicronic may be breathed in and out. Particles deposited in the nasopharynx are cleared and swallowed rapidly.

Thus the nose subserves important functions, acting as an adaptable air passage without excessive airflow resistance, as a heater and humidifier and as a filter for particles.

The larynx

The larynx lies at the upper end of the trachea opposite the 3rd–6th cervical vertebrae in adult males and slightly higher in females and children. In men, the laryngeal dimensions are about 4.4 cm length × 4.3 cm across × 3.5 cm in anterior-posterior extent, being somewhat smaller in women. The cavity of the larynx extends from the pharynx to the commencement of the trachea and the lower border of the cricoid cartilage. The inlet of the larynx is directed backwards and slightly upwards being bounded superiorly and anteriorly by the upper cage of the epiglottis and on each side by the aryepiglottic folds extending from the lateral edge of the epiglottis to the arytenoids. The lower part of the cavity contains the vocal cords covered by closely attached stratified squamous epithelium.

The larynx has several functions:

1. It acts as the respiratory channel and airflow regulator.
2. It exerts a circulatory function in promoting venous return, e.g. Valsalva manoeuvre.
3. It acts as a sphincter in fixation of the thorax during cough and expectoration and with protective closure on swallowing and vomiting.
4. It is a receptive field for reflexes, e.g. cough reflex.
5. It is involved in phonation and speech.

Within the larynx and glottis the cross-sectional area which of course is variable is less than at any other level in the upper airways. This contributes significantly to airway resistance and the onset of turbulence, secondary eddies and the inertial impaction of particles. During normal quiet respiration the cords are relaxed and held halfway between adduction and full abduction. The cords usually abduct slightly during inspiration and adduct during expiration, these movements being more marked as breathing increases in depth so that during vigorous exercise the cords are virtually fully abducted and flow resistance is minimal.

In patients with airflow obstruction the 'glottis chink' was found to be narrowed during quiet breathing, particularly on expiration and remaining so on maximal exhalation whereas in patients with an $FEV_1 > 80$ per cent predicted, the glottis opened to an inspiratory width. This suggests the glottis may play an important part in controlling airflow in such patients (Higgenbottam and Payne, 1982). By the same token, it may influence the retention of inhaled aerosol.

There are three laryngeal sphincters:

1. The aryepiglottic folds which close on deglutition and vomiting and thus prevent inhalation of food or vomit.
2. The false vocal cords which close rapidly and briefly during cough or slowly and voluntarily as in thoracic fixation during micturition, defaecation, parturition and vomiting. They act as a second line of defence.
3. The true vocal cords have a flat upper surface and a curved surface concave downwards which act as an efficient sphincter against incoming air but not against outgoing airflow.

These sphincters may act separately or together.

The lower airways—development and anatomy

The respiratory system develops from a midline diverticulum in the foregut called the laryngotracheal groove, appearing in 25 day old embryos. The bronchial tree is developed by the 16th week of intrauterine life; alveoli develop after birth, increasing in number until the age of eight years, and in size with growth of the chest until growth of the chest wall is finished. Blood vessels are remodelled and increased, certainly while new alveoli are forming and probably until growth of the chest is complete. The number of alveoli in the lungs increase from about 24×10^6 at birth to 280×10^6 at age eight years after which the number remains virtually constant (Polgar and Weng, 1979).

The trachea is D-shaped with 16–20 cartilaginous rings, 3–4 mm wide and posterior longitudinal smooth muscle, extending from the larynx to the bifurcation (carina). The average adult length is 11 cm (range 9–15 cm) with a lateral diameter of 20 mm and anteroposterior of 15 mm. The diameters increase during inspiration and decrease during expiration, particularly that involving the membranous posterior wall of the trachea and main bronchi. The carina is usually sharp and mobile on deep breathing or coughing, and lies 25–27 cm from the upper incisors. The mucosa is pseudostratified, ciliated columnar with numerous goblet cells resting on a broad basement membrane with mucus glands containing mucus and serous elements lying in the submucosa and contributing to the mucus 'blanket' overlying the cilia.

Nomenclature of the bronchial tree

There is still some debate over the nomenclature of the bronchial tree. In Britain that described by Foster-Carter (1963) is still used in the main. However, with the advent of flexible fibreoptic bronchoscopy which permits visualization to subsegmental levels and beyond, the Japanese have formulated a new numerical system (Ikeda, 1974).

TABLE 1.1. Large airway dimensions and branching angles (with respect to parent airway). Data from Horsfield model 2

Arbitrary identification number	*Airway*	*Diameter* (mm)	*Length* (mm)	*% of tracheal flow*		*Branching angle* (deg)
0	Trachea	16.0	100.0	100		
10	R. main bronchus	11.1	22.0	54.5		35
1	L. main bronchus	12.0	50.0	45.5		73
11	Lobar bronchus	7.3	15.6	21.7	} 54.5	63
13	Lobar bronchus	8.9	26.0	32.8		15
15	Lobar bronchus	6.4	8.0	23.2	*	15
2	Lobar bronchus	7.5	16.0	20.5	} 45.5	48
6	Lobar bronchus	8.0	11.0	24.9		44

*Airway 15 is distal to 13
Reference: Horsfield *et al.* (1971)

The trachea divides into right and left main bronchi which themselves give off three lobar bronchi on the right (upper, middle and lower lobes) and two on the left (upper and lingula and lower). Both main and lower lobe bronchi lie outside the lung substance and may be termed the 'large bronchi' (*Table 1.1*) being 7–12 mm in diameter (Horsfield, 1974). The lower bronchi divide into about 20 bronchopulmonary segment bronchi—the 'medium bronchi' 4–7 mm in diameter. Bronchioles have no cartilage in their walls and are 0.5–0.8 mm in diameter. The terminal bronchiole which is the last on any pathway not to bear alveoli, is at the limit of the *conducting airways*, the structures distal to it constituting an 'acinus'.

The cartilaginous rings buttress the tracheobronchial tree, their C-shape persisting to the origin of the apical lower bronchus on each side and being located mainly in the extrapulmonary airways on each side where the walls need to be relatively rigid whereas intrapulmonary airways receive some support from the surrounding lung parenchyma. In these latter airways the cartilage is discontinuous and, therefore, becomes progressively less, being absent from bronchioles less than 0.8 mm in diameter. Circular and diagonal muscle fibres normally surround the ligaments inside the cartilage, contracting, constricting and shortening the airway. Lymphoid tissue is found in the mucosa often in solitary nodules and particularly at points of bifurcation.

While referring to the dimensions of the adult tracheobronchial tree two descriptions are often cited. Weibel (1963) in his model A measured the airway dimensions of an average adult lung with a volume of 4800 cm^3 at about three-quarters maximal inflation. Horsfield *et al.* (1971) measured a similar specimen and subsequently reported various aspects thereof, including branching angles which is important for airflow and aerosol impaction. While Weibel used a symmetrical branching order from trachea 0 numbering distally, Horsfield numbered in the reverse way, the trachea being order 31, and stressing asymmetry. Comparing their dimensions Weibel vs. Horsfield the trachea is 120 mm vs. 100 mm in length, 18.0 mm vs. 16.0 mm in diameter, the main bronchi 48.0 mm vs. 36.0 mm in length and 12.0 mm each in diameter.

In life the tracheobronchial tree varies depending on lung inflation and breathing manoeuvre (e.g. forced inspiration or expiration, cough, etc.), both in airway diameters, lengths and branching angles. Furthermore, the right and left bronchial trees are asymmetrical reflecting the differing lung volume (right 55 per cent, left 45 per cent) and position of the heart to the left of the mid-line. Consequently

Horsfield notes the main bronchi are 22.0 mm (right) and 50.0 mm (left) long respectively. He notes a branching angle of 35 degrees between the trachea and right main bronchus and 73 degrees on the left. Further information is given in *Table 1.1*. In smaller animals it may be noted that the mean angle of branching of daughter branches increases from 30 degrees in 3.0—4.0 mm parent branches to 50 degrees in 0.7–0.9 mm parent branches.

The Horsfield system of airway numbering from the periphery to the centre (trachea) has some merit, particularly since it allows for different transit pathways—a terminal bronchiole for instance will have a low number irrespective of the length of the transit path, which will be short in the perihilar and long in the apical and basal regions. However, it is difficult to apply to the intact human lung *in vivo*.

The terminal bronchiole divides into about three generations of respiratory bronchioles, which are about 0.5 mm in diameter, their first part being lined by ciliated pseudocolumnar epithelium, without goblet cells, changing to non-ciliated low cuboidal epithelium thereafter. The respiratory bronchioles divide further into about four generations of alveolar ducts (Horsfield, 1974) from which open numerous alveolar sacs. Some alveoli arise from the respiratory bronchioles but not from the side adjacent to the pulmonary artery branch. Airway branching is principally by dichotomy with occasional trichotomy.

The ultrastructure of the lung is very delicate. The alveolar-capillary membrane is composed of three layers, epitheliod (about 0.1 μm thick), basement membrane plus interstitial substance, and capillary endothelium, giving a total thickness of 0.7–0.8 μm. The continuity of the alveolar walls is interrupted by the pores of Kohn which may allow collateral ventilation and the migration of phagocytes. The cells lining the alveoli are the type I and II pneumocytes. Clara cells found in the terminal bronchioles probably secrete surfactant. The alveolar surface area averages 143 m^2 (range 100–190 m^2) while the capillary surface is 120–150 m^2 (about 80 per cent of the alveolar surface area) suggesting a fairly congruent match. The blood capillary volume is 150–200 mℓ (Weibel, 1979).

Lung models

The morphometric data of Weibel (1963) has been used to predict aerosol deposition (Lippmann, 1977). Similarly, the data of Horsfield *et al.* (1971) have been used by Yeates and Aspin (1978) to predict the frequency distribution of pathway lengths in the lungs, fluid flow in the airways and mucociliary clearance. Gerrity *et al.* (1981) used the same model to assess the distribution of deposited particles, using a realistic distribution of ventilation. Others (Yu *et al.*, 1979) have used combined morphometric data to determine the total and regional deposition of inhaled aerosols taking into account variability in airway dimensions. Finally Yeh and Schum (1980) included branching angles and angles of inclination to gravity in their lung model for aerosol deposition.

Patterns of flow down the tracheobronchial tree

During breathing the whole of the tidal volume passes through the nose or mouth, pharynx and larynx. There the velocity of flow is high and the flow is not wholly laminar, with secondary eddies forming and turbulence at higher flow rates such as in forced expiration or during exercise. At the tracheal bifurcation further secondary eddies are formed while the velocity falls progressively thereafter as the cross-sectional area of the main bronchi and their subsequent divisions increases in a bell-shaped fashion (*Figure 1.3*). In the terminal ventilatory units the linear velocity of the inspired gas falls to a fraction of a $mm\,s^{-1}$. Weibel (1963) and Horsfield *et al.* (1971) pointed out the following:

1. A large part of the airways resistance lies in the upper respiratory tract.
2. Since flow is not entirely laminar but complicated by secondary eddies, calculations of pressure drop and resistance relying solely on Poiseuille's equation may be in error.
3. The resistance of the peripheral airways will be only a small part of the total.

It is worth mentioning here that from Poiseuille's equation

$$\Delta P = 8\dot{V}\mu l/\pi r^4 g^*$$

if the radius of the bronchial tube is halved the resistance is increased sixteenfold. With turbulent flow gas density becomes a factor and the Fanning equation is applicable

$$\Delta P = fl\rho\dot{V}^2/\pi^2 r^5 g^*$$

Most resistance occurs in airways of 2–5 mm diameter (Weibel order 1–8 or Horsfield 9–13). Inspired gas (and in particular oxygen) moves by three processes in the lung:

1. Convective flow in the conducting airways.
2. Molecular diffusion in the respiratory airways.
3. Molecular diffusion in the tissue phase across the alveolar-capillary membrane.

There is of course some overlap throughout. The interaction between convective flow and simultaneous molecular diffusion is known as Taylor dispersion. In humans breathing quietly, tracheal flow is mainly laminar though on inspiration some turbulence may occur at the larynx gradually dying out distally. Secondary vortices are generated on bifurcations and eddies may occur on bends or surface irregularities. Each of these factors will cause gas mixing and counteract Taylor dispersion.

Flow in the intermediate conducting airways is laminar, though individual bronchi are too short to allow fully developed laminar flow with a parabolic profile.

In the small conducting and respiratory airways forward flow velocity becomes low and axial diffusion becomes dominant. It is important to note that the terminal bronchiole divides so frequently that the summed cross-sectional area increases from 80 cm^2 to 10^4 cm^2 in the distal ducts over a length of about 7 mm. In this region molecular diffusion plays an important part (Horsfield, 1980).

Tissue diffusion through the alveolar-capillary membrane is the final step; the surfactant layer (5–20 nm thick), the tissue of the alveolar wall, the plasma in the capillary (5–10 nm thick) and the red cell wall must all be passed. The oxygen molecule must reach the alveolar wall, go into solution, diffuse through the tissues and combine with haemoglobin. Any increase in surfactant layer, in the alveolar-capillary membrane thickness, or in capillary size (dilatation) will reduce gas transfer.

*Where ΔP is pressure drop, $\dot{V}$ is airflow, μ is viscosity, l is tube length, r is radius, g is the gravitational force, f is a friction factor, ρ is air density.

Pulmonary circulation

The main pulmonary artery ($\simeq$18 mm diameter) arises from the right ventricle and within 2 cm branches to form the right and left main branches visible at the lung hilum on chest X-ray. From each main branch large vessels carrying blood to the twenty main segments, ten in each lung arise. As these vessels diminish in size, the smooth muscle diminishes and in vessels <100 μm there is an endothelial lining and elastic laminum alone. The vessels in the alveolar network are about 7 μm in diameter comprising endothelial cells alone supported by the mesh of elastic and collagen fibres in the alveolar wall. The endothelial thickness is 0.3–2.0 μm. The pulmonary vessels branch sooner than the bronchial airways. Each alveolar wall is rich in blood vessels although there may appear to be one precapillary per alveolus numerically the blood supply appears to come from at least six different precapillaries (Horsfield, 1974).

The pulmonary blood volume is about 500 ml, of this 150 ml is in alveolar vessels (about 30 per cent as opposed to 95 per cent of gas in the alveoli) with 120 ml in the pulmonary artery and 230 ml in the pulmonary veins. The pulmonary circulation is a low pressure system, mean pulmonary artery pressure being 15 mmHg with alveolar vessels $\simeq$0.3 μm thick carrying a pressure of 5–10 mmHg. Most of the pressure drop ($\simeq$6 mmHg) would appear to occur in the pulmonary artery before the precapillary region. The red cells probably take between 0.5 and 8.0 seconds to traverse the alveolar precapillary (Cumming and Semple, 1980).

The pulmonary bronchial arterial systems (Daly and Hebb, 1966)

The pulmonary artery accompanies the bronchi closely as far as the respiratory bronchioles. There it gives off one branch to each alveolar duct which divides into several small arteries supplying capillaries to the alveolar sacs in which the duct terminates. Branches supplying capillaries to the lateral alveoli also arise at the level of the alveolar duct. Here there is a confluence of pulmonary and bronchial capillaries.

The pulmonary veins arise from alveolar ducts and respiratory bronchiolar capillaries (the last two being supplied by pulmonary and bronchial arteries), and bronchial capillaries supplying pleura.

The bronchial arteries arise from the aorta (62 per cent), the first right intercostal artery (23 per cent) and elsewhere in the remainder. They supply the bronchi, pleura, walls of the pulmonary blood vessels, bronchial glands and interstitial substance of the lung. Two or three branches of the bronchial artery accompany each of the larger bronchi giving off one branch to each subdivision. Anastomosing branches connect the arterial trunks with each other, forming a plexus with an elongated and irregular mesh. Distinct bronchial arteries tend to disappear after the level of the smaller and respiratory bronchioles with alveoli. Their terminal mesh anastomoses with the pulmonary capillaries to form a common network in the region of the respiratory bronchioles. Beyond, blood supply is from the pulmonary artery only.

The bronchial venous drainage includes contributions from the following:

1. The bronchial veins draining the first one or two bronchial divisions, via the superior azygos vein into the right atrium or less so the pulmonary veins into the left atrium.

TABLE 1.2. Weibel (1963) data linked to a functional airway classification, and blood supply. The pulmonary artery does not supply but runs parallel to the tracheobronchial tree, perfusing arterioles and pulmonary capillaries whose main function is gas exchange. The sites of potential anastomoses between the bronchial and pulmonary circulations are described in the text

Generation Number	*Diameter* (cm)	*Total cross-sectional area* (cm^2)	*Classification of airways*			*Blood supply*	
0	1.8	2.54			Trachea		
1	1.22	2.33					
2	0.83	2.13			Bronchi		
3	0.56	2.00		Large airways (>2 mm)			Elastic pulmonary arteries
4	0.45	2.48					
5	0.35	3.11					
6	0.28	3.96	Conductive zone		Small bronchi	Bronchial circulation	
7	0.23	5.10					
8	0.186	6.95					
9	0.154	9.56					
10	0.130	13.4					Muscular pulmonary arteries
11	0.109	19.6		Small airways (<2 mm)			
12	0.095	28.8					
13	0.082	44.5					
14	0.074	69.4			Bronchioles		
15	0.066	113.					
16	0.060	180.					
17	0.054	300.		Respiratory bronchioles			
18	0.050	534.	Transitory zone				
19	0.047	944.				Arterioles	
20	0.045	1600.		Alveolar ducts and sacs			
21	0.043	3220.					
22	0.041	5880.					
23	0.041	11800.					
			Respiratory zone			Pulmonary capillary bed	

2. The bronchopulmonary veins draining the third order and small bronchi into the pulmonary veins.
3. Pulmonary venules proper draining oxygenated blood into the left atrium.

An attempt has been made to relate airway number, dimensions and classification with the bronchial and pulmonary circulations (*Table 1.2*) to accentuate possible anastomoses where soluble aerosol uptake and mucociliary clearance may be confused.

Lung physiology

The physiological factors which determine aerosol deposition in the lung (Pavia *et al.*, 1977) include: (1) lung volumes, (2) flow rates, (3) airflow obstruction either in large (>2 mm) or small (<2 mm) airways, and (4) regional ventilation determined by gravity (Chamberlain *et al.*, 1983) and local ventilation which may be affected by selective obstruction by bronchial inflammation and mucus strands or plugs for instance. Any soluble aerosol reaching the alveolar region may be absorbed into the pulmonary circulation, whereas soluble particles depositing proximally but adjacent to the alveolar region may be absorbed into the bronchial circulation—the watershed between the two is not clearly defined *in vivo* (*see Table 1.3*). Aerosol uptake through the alveolar-capillary membrane will be dependent on the prevailing local ventilation perfusion ($\dot{V}/\dot{Q}$) balance. The monograph on experimental methods in respiratory medicine edited by Howell and Tattersfield (1981) gives a particularly clear and up-to-date view of means whereby lung physiology may be assessed.

Lung volumes

These are shown in *Figure 1.2*. Basically they are determined by the balance of compliance (lung and chest wall) and resistance (lung, chest wall and airflow) the product of which is the time constant which determines the equality of ventilation throughout the lung.

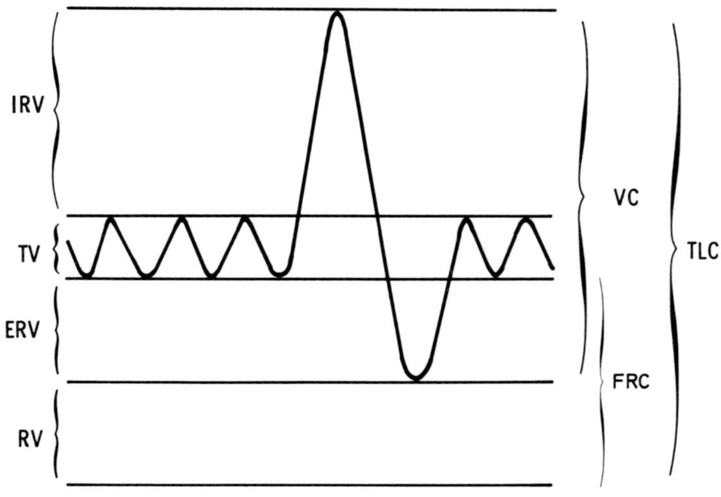

Figure 1.2 Schematic spirogram indicating lung volumes

Simple quasi-static volumes (Freedman, 1981)

The measurement of lung volumes are of value in lung aerosol studies. In particular the vital capacity (VC) may need measuring and checking to see there is no change between studies. Any change may reflect technical artefact, inadequate effort or change in lung compliance or airway resistance, very likely the latter.

Vital capacity (VC)

This is the greatest voluntary expiration following the deepest inspiration. It is a slow breath as opposed to a fast or forced breath though in normal subjects this volume may be virtually the same—with airways disease such as asthma, chronic bronchitis and emphysema, airways closure and gas trapping creates a discrepancy.

The reading may vary due to instrumental factors, observed variation and the effect of smoking, drugs, posture and disease. In normal subjects the coefficient of variation is up to 2.5 per cent. The VC is taken as the mean of three measurements differing by less than 200 ml (although some suggest 500 ml in disease). There is a small diurnal variation in normal subjects which is increased in patients with airways obstruction with troughs in the morning and peaks at night.

Complex (static) lung volumes

Total lung capacity and subdivisions

The absolute lung volumes are measured most accurately in the constant-volume, whole-body plethysmograph or body box (Dubois *et al.*, 1956), clear details of which are given by Howell and Tattersfield (1981), further description being outside the range of this text. However, the reproducibility is not good and the coefficient of variation for individual reading lies between 10 and 20 per cent with a wide range. The method may be useful in time-course and dose-response studies, the quantitative assessment of bronchial β adrenoreceptor blockade and the investigation of physiological differences between normal subjects and patients. No preceding inspiration or forced expiration is required, both of which may themselves affect bronchomotor tone.

Volume displacement or pressure-flow plethysmographs may be used for specific purposes (e.g. measuring volume changes during forced expiration). Variability of readings is about 12 per cent of the mean for thoracic gas volume (TGV).

Gas dilution or washout methods may be multiple or single breath. With the multiple breath either the 'closed circuit helium dilution' technique may be used or that of 'nitrogen washout'. Both methods have their single breath equivalent.

With all these techniques the volume measured is that communicating with the airway and ventilating so that lung cysts and bullae for example will not be measured, whereas they would be included in the plethysmographic estimation. Furthermore, the single breath methods give erroneous results particularly in the presence of airways obstruction, and therefore may only be useful in the study of fairly normal populations. Finally, the multiple breath method may be prone to error with airways obstruction, since gas equibrilation or washout may be unduly long leading to an underestimation of lung volume.

Dynamic lung volumes and flow rates

The forced expired volume in one second (FEV_1) following deepest inspiration is recorded as volume versus time either with a wet or dry spirometer. The best of three congruent readings is taken and converted from ATPS to BTPS, usually an addition of about 10 per cent.

The peak expiratory flow rate (PEFR) is usually measured with a Wright peak flow meter. Again, the best of three congruent readings is taken without correction. Both FEV_1 and PEFR are reliable measures of airway function, applicable both to laboratory and field study.

The PEFR probably disturbs the airways less than the FEV_1 and therefore particles, mucus and airway reactivity may be less prone to test-induced change.

Large and small airways function

In trying to assess aerosol deposition in the tracheobronchial tree it may be convenient to attempt the measurement of large and small airways function separately. Clearly this separation is not absolute, nor are the tests which can be used.

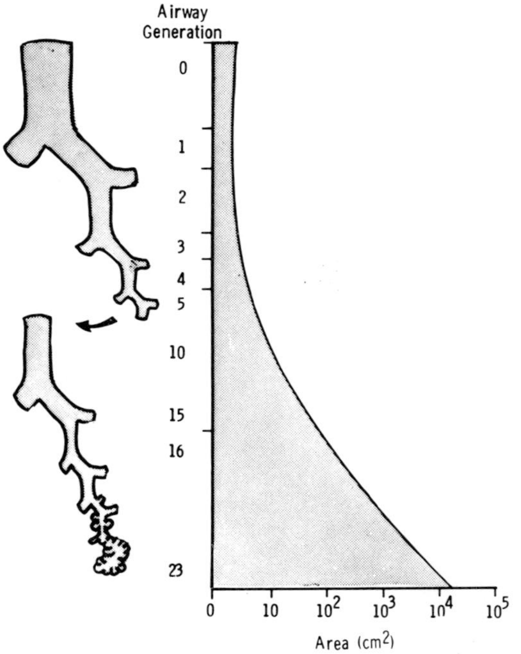

Figure 1.3 Diagram indicating the marked increase in cross-sectional area of the small airways as opposed to the large

It is known that considerable obstruction may be present in small airways (<2 mm in diameter) with little effect on airway resistance and conventional spirometric tests. As discussed earlier this is because most airflow resistance lies proximally between the carina and lobular bronchi, where the cross-sectional area is small by comparison with the enormous increase seen distally (*Figure 1.3*).

Resistance in large and small airways

During a forced vital capacity expiration (FVC), dynamic compression of airways occurs in segmental or lobar bronchi immediately distal to the equal pressure point (EPP, when pressure is equal inside and outside the bronchial wall) in normal man, following which downstream resistance is relatively unimportant. The compressed segment acts like a sluice and maximum flow is determined by the resistance of upstream intrapulmonary airways, by the elastic recoil of the lungs and by the collapsibility of the airways. This situation occurs over the lower two thirds of the forced expiration where maximum flow rates are independent of effort and therefore reflect the behaviour of the intrapulmonary (small) rather than large airways.

For obstruction in large airways (>2 mm) the best tests are the PEFR and maximal expiratory flow-volume curve (MEFV) at high lung volumes (e.g. $\dot{V}_{max}$ 25 per cent), airway resistance (R_{AW}) and its reciprocal airway conductance (G_{AW})—the last two measured in the body box. For obstruction in small airways (<2 mm) the best tests are lung volumes, MEFV over the lower two thirds of lung volumes (e.g. $\dot{V}_{max}$ 50 per cent, $\dot{V}_{max}$ 25 per cent), closing volume (CV), nitrogen washout, gas exchange, frequency dependence of compliance and MEFV repeated after a breath of helium and oxygen (this mixture changes gas density which will only affect turbulent flow in the large and not the small airways, thereby contributing nothing to the MEFV over the lower two thirds of lung volume, depending on the sites of the EPP and flow-limiting segments). Of these, two are worthy of further mention, namely MEFV and closing volume measurements.

MEFV curve (Pride, 1981)

The maximum expiratory flow volume curve (*Figure 1.4*) where the peak is effort-dependent is a reflection of both small and large airways function. This test requires a fast responding flow measuring system, linear to $\simeq 12\,\ell\,s^{-1}$, three reproducible curves and differences in VC of <5 per cent together with a rapidly responding direct-writing recorder. $\dot{V}_{max}$ 50 per cent and $\dot{V}_{max}$ 75 per cent are thought to reflect obstruction in small airways. However, these instantaneous measurements are susceptible to small changes in residual volume since flow is changing rapidly.

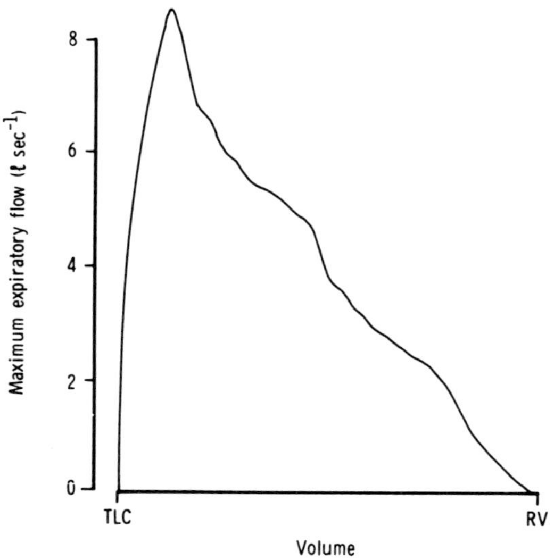

Figure 1.4 Maximum expiratory flow volume curve (MEFV)

These two indices of small airways function have poor reproducibility within individual, probably reflecting changes in RV and particularly so with readings from the lower limb of the MEFV curve (e.g. $\dot{V}_{max}$ 75 per cent) where trace noise may be significant. Gas compression artefact may also contribute to this problem.

Partial expiratory flow-volume (PEFV) curves from about 50 per cent VC avoid changes in bronchomotor tone following a full inflation, which may be a problem in some asthmatics. They may be used to detect bronchoconstrictor and bronchodilator responses in normal subjects also and are less tiring for the subject.

Closing volume (CV)

This test may utilize a resident gas such as nitrogen in the lung which when diluted with a vital capacity breath of oxygen will give a characteristic expired nitrogen volume trace (*Figure 1.5*), the terminal rise over the lower quarter or so of the vital capacity being termed the 'closing volume', where lower zone airways derecruit and 'close'. Disease of small airways will increase CV.

The CV shares the poor reproducibility of the MEFV curve being affected by small changes in VC and expiratory flow rate; also in 10 per cent of subjects the curves show no clear phase IV (Buist, 1981). However, tests of small airways

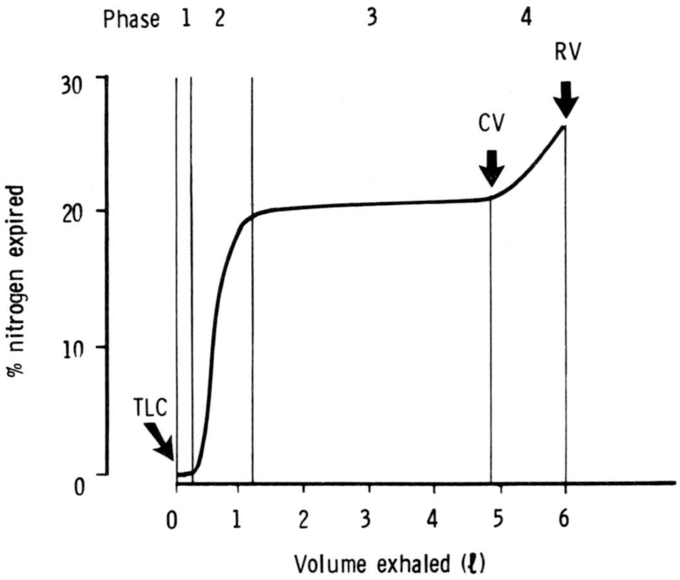

Figure 1.5 Single breath nitrogen concentration after a vital capacity breath of 100 per cent O_2 plotted against expired lung volume to indicate 'closing volume' (CV)

function are undoubtedly more discriminating than the FEV_1, for example in showing abnormalities in smokers in whom they may precede abnormalities in the FEV_1 by several years (Buist and Nagy, 1980). Even so, a 25 per cent change in a single measurement of R_{AW} or $\dot{V}_{max}$ 25 per cent could well be due to 'noise', while this would be most unlikely with even a 10 per cent change in FEV_1 which is used in most bronchodilator trials in asthma for example.

Ventilation, aerosol deposition and uptake

In assessing ventilation, tidal volume (V_T) and minute volume must be considered or controlled. V_T is distributed to the conducting airways (where the anatomical dead space V_D amounts to about 150 ml of the resting V_T) and to the alveoli (where the physiological dead space indicates areas of ventilation without perfusion $-\dot{V}/\dot{Q}$ imbalance, West, 1977). In health the combined dead spaces add up to 20–30 per cent of tidal volume $-V_D/V_T \leqslant 30$ per cent, indicating a minor degree of $\dot{V}/\dot{Q}$ imbalance largely dependent on gravity (West, 1963). Upright at rest pulmonary blood flow traverses only about the lower half of the lung, whereas the gradient of ventilation determined by pleural pressure has been shown to decrease from apex to base (Milic-Emili *et al.*, 1966). Recent work (Chamberlain *et al.*, 1983) has confirmed that aerosol particle deposition and ventilation are closely related in healthy smokers and non-smokers, the greater the ventilation the greater the deposition of particles irrespective of position and breathing rate. At higher respiratory rates they found that central deposition increased, especially in smokers.

Uptake of soluble particles will depend upon their regional distribution and that of pulmonary (and less so bronchial) blood flow.

In lung disease, $\dot{V}/\dot{Q}$ abnormalities are common and constitute 90 per cent of the causes of hypoxaemia. Ventilation may be impaired by airways obstruction (e.g. asthma, chronic bronchitis and emphysema), airways compression (e.g. tumours, pleural effusion) and lung collapse for instance; perfusion will be affected by constriction, obliteration or blockage of sections of the pulmonary circulation, as seen in heart failure, shock, lung collapse, emboli, fibrosis and emphysema (Wagner, 1976). By contrast alveolar-capillary block as such, is an uncommon cause of hypoxaemia. Radioisotope ventilation-perfusion scans may confirm mismatch, particularly where the clinical consequences are important, such as in lung cysts or bullae and pulmonary emboli where surgery and anticoagulation respectively may be required. Further aspects of these scans are discussed in another chapter.

Airways obstruction and receptor location

Aerosol deposition is profoundly affected by airways obstruction (Pavia *et al.*, 1977). In many cases bronchial smooth muscle constriction is the major factor, particularly in asthma and less so in chronic bronchitis and emphysema. The control of bronchial smooth muscle by the adrenergic and cholinergic nervous systems are therefore important. Beta-adrenergic nerves bronchodilate whereas cholinergic (and the scant α-adrenergic nerves) bronchoconstrict. Further the smooth muscle contains mast cells, important in allergen mediated constriction. Also bronchial infection, smoke, NO_2, ozone and SO_2 cause inflammation and bronchial hyper-reactivity with increased mucosal permeability giving ready access of mediators and irritants to both irritant and other receptors. Barnes *et al.* (1983) using autoradiographic methods have recently described the precise localization of β- and α-adrenergic and muscarinic receptors in the ferret. β-receptors were present in high density throughout the airways, the highest in bronchioles; α-receptors were sparse in large airways and numerous in small bronchioles, whereas cholinergic receptors were numerous in bronchial smooth muscle, sparse in proximal bronchioles and almost absent from distal bronchioles.

The localization of airways receptors *in vivo* in man has been attempted using radioaerosol techniques (Ruffin *et al.*, 1981). For example these authors used an inhaled β-agonist plus radioaerosol before and after an inhaled β-antagonist and radioaerosol to investigate the distribution of β_2-adrenoreceptors in asthmatics. Although no definite pattern of β_2-receptor distribution could be interpreted from the airway function responses, nevertheless, their work does suggest a means whereby aerosols may be utilized to elucidate receptor distribution in the future. Such techniques may be of considerable importance in locating target areas for aerosol therapy in a variety of lung disorders.

Conclusions

The aim of this chapter was to introduce and expand upon some of the factors determining aerosol inhalation, deposition and fate (either by mucociliary clearance or uptake by the bronchial or pulmonary circulation—the clearance of particles reaching the alveolar region is dealt with elsewhere). Anatomical and physiological facts have been dwelt upon, since a knowledge of these is important in assessing aerosol inhalation. Perforce some aspects are covered more fully than others. However, the hope is that subsequent chapters will prove complementary, and that the references will give additional background information.

References

BARNES, P.J., BASBAUM, C.B. and NADEL, J.A. (1983). Autoradiographic localisation of autonomic receptors in airway smooth muscle. *Am. Rev. Respir. Dis.*, **64,** 758–762

BUIST, A.S. (1981). Evaluation of lung function: tests of small airway function. *Curr. Pulmonology*, vol. 3, chapter 10. Edited by Simmons, D.H. New York; Wiley Medical

BUIST,A.S. and NAGY, J. (1980) A longitudinal study of smokers and non-smokers: 5–6 year follow-up using spirometry and the single-breath N_2 test. *Chest*, **77**, (2 Suppl.) 259

CHAMBERLAIN, M.J., MORGAN, W.K.C. and VINITSKI, S. (1983). Factors influencing the regional deposition of inhaled particles in man. *Clin. Sci.*, **64**, 69–78

CUMMING, G. and SEMPLE, S.J. (1980). Blood distribution by the pulmonary circulation. *Disorders of the Respiratory System*, 2nd edn, chapter 4. Oxford; Blackwell

DALY, I. de B. and HEBB, C.O. (1966). Pulmonary and Bronchial Vascular Systems: Their Reactions Under Controlled Conditions of Ventilation & Circulation. London; Arnold

DOUEK, E. (1979). Physiology of the nose and paranasal sinuses in Scott-Brown's Diseases of the Ear, Nose and Throat. 4th edn. Basic Sciences, Edited by Ballantyne, J. and Groves, J. London; Butterworths

DUBOIS, A.B., BOTELHO, S.Y., BEDELL, G.N., MARSHALL, R. and COMROE, J.H. (1956). A rapid plethysomographic method for measuring thoracic gas volume: a comparison with a nitrogen washout method for measuring functional residual capacity in normal subjects. *J. Clin. Invest.*, **35**, 322–326

ELLUL-MICALLEF, R. (1976). A look at the past. *Br. J. Dis. Chest*, **70**, 112–116

FOSTER-CARTER, A.F. (1963). Broncho-pulmonary anatomy. In *Chest Diseases*, edited by Perry, K.M.A. and Sellors, T.H. London; Butterworths

FREEDMAN, S. (1981). Lung volumes. In *Methods in Clinical Pharmacology. 2. Respiratory System*, pp. 3–11. Edited by Howell, J.B.L. and Tattersfield, A.E. London; MacMillan

GERRITY, T.R., GARRARD, C.S. and YEATES, D.B. (1981). Theoretical analysis of sites of aerosol deposition in the human lung. *Chest*, **80**, 898S–901S

HIGGENBOTTAM, T. and PAYNE, J. (1982). Glottis narrowing in lung disease. *Am. Rev. Respir. Dis.*, **125**, 746–750

HORSFIELD, K. (1974). The relation between structure and function in the airways of the lung. *Br. J. Dis. Chest*, **68**, 145–160

HORSFIELD, K. (1980). Gaseous diffusion in the lungs. *Br. J. Dis. Chest*, **74**, 99–120

HORSFIELD, K., DART, G., OLSON, D.E., FILLEY, S.F. and CUMMING, G. (1971). Models of the human bronchial tree. *J. Appl. Physiol.*, **31**, 207–217

HOWELL, J.B.L. and TATTERSFIELD, A.E. (1981) (Eds). Methods in Clinical Pharmacology. *Respiratory system*. London; MacMillan

IKEDA, S. (1974). *Atlas of flexible bronchofiberscopy*. Tokyo; Igeku Shoin Ltd. and London; University Park Press

LIPPMANN, M. (1977). Regional deposition of particles in the human respiratory tract: reactions to environmental agents. *Handbook of Physiology*, chapter 14, 213–232

LOURENÇO, R.V. and COTROMANES, E. (1982a). Clinical aerosols. I. Characterization of aerosols and their diagnostic uses. *Arch. Intern. Med.*, **142**, 2163–2172

LOURENÇO, R.V. and COTROMANES, E. (1982b). Clinical aerosols. II. Therapeutic aerosols. *Arch. Intern. Med.*, **142**, 2299–2308

MILIC-EMILI, J., HENDERSON, J.A.M., DOLOVICH, M.B., TROP, D. and KANEKO, K. (1966). Regional distribution of inspired gas in the lung. *J. Appl. Physiol.*, **21**, 749–759

MUIR, D.C.F. (1972) (Ed.). Clinical Aspects of Inhaled Particles. London; Heinemann

PAVIA, D., THOMSON, M.L., CLARKE, S.W. and SHANNON, H.S. (1977). Effect of lung function and mode of inhalation on penetration of aerosol into the human lung. *Thorax*, **32**, 194–197

PAVIA, D., BATEMAN, J.R.M. and CLARKE, S.W. (1980). Deposition and clearance of inhaled particles. *Bull. Europ. Physiopath. Resp.*, **16**, 335–366

POLGAR, G. and WENG, T.R. (1979). The functional development of the respiratory system. *Am. Rev. Respir. Dis.*, **120**, 625–695

PRIDE, N.B. (1981). Assessment of changes in airway calibre—tests of forced expiration in Methods in Clinical Pharmacology 2, Respiratory System, pp 13–23. Edited by Howell, J.B.L. and Tattersfield, A.E. London; MacMillan

PROCTOR, D.F. (1977a). The upper airways. I. Nasal physiology and defense of the lungs. *Am. Rev. Respir. Dis.*, **115**, 97–129

PROCTOR, D.F. (1977b). The upper airways. II. The larynx and trachea. *Am. Rev. Respir. Dis.*, **115**, 315–342

RUFFIN, R.E., DOLOVICH, M.B., OLDENBURG, F.A. and NEWHOUSE, M.T. (1981). The preferential deposition of inhaled isoproterenol and propranolol in asthmatic patients. *Chest*, suppl., **80**, 904–906

WAGNER, H.N. (1976). The use of radio-isotope techniques for the evaluation of patients with pulmonary disease. *Am. Rev. Respir. Dis.*, **113**, 203–218

WEIBEL, E.R. (1963). *Morphometry of the human lung.* Berlin; Springer

WEIBEL, E.R. (1979). Morphometry of the human lung: the state of the art after two decades. *Bull. Europ. Physiopath. Resp.*, **15**, 999–1013

WEST, J.B. (1963). Regional differences in gas exchange in the lung of erect man. *J. Appl. Physiol.*, **17**, 893–898

WEST, J.B. (1977). Ventilation-perfusion relationships. *Am. Rev. Respir. Dis.*, **116**, 919–943

YEATES, D.B. and ASPIN, N. (1978). A mathematical description of the airways of the human lungs. *Resp. Physiol.*, **32**, 91–101

YEH, H.C. and SCHUM, G.M. (1980). Models of human lung airways and their application to particle deposition. *Bull. Math. Biol.*, **42**, 461–480

YU, C.P., NICOLAIDES, P. and SOONG, T.T. (1979). Effect of random airway sizes on aerosol deposition. *Am. Ind. Hyg. Assoc. J.*, **40**, 999–1005

Chapter 2

Lung secretions

Maria Teresa Lopez-Vidriero

Introduction

Lung secretions include mucus secretion from the conducting airways and alveolar liquid. They have multiple functions which are divided into non-specific and specific. Some non-specific functions are dependent upon their chemical composition and physical properties, including viscoelasticity: trapping and clearance of particles, lowering surface-tension, lubrication, non-wettability, humidification of air, and dilution of toxic substances to mention only a few. Other non-specific functions rely on their cellular component; neutrophils and macrophages are the scavengers of the lung. Present in mucus are substances usually locally produced: lysozyme, bronchotransferrin and antiproteases which have antimicrobial and antiproteolytic actions.

The conducting airways are lined by a mucus-secreting ciliated epithelium with very distinctive structure at different levels of the airways. As a result of this the chemical composition, rheological properties and cellular components of mucus also have a regional variation. The regional variation in the nature of mucus may reflect the need for different defence mechanisms at various levels of the respiratory tract, i.e. more mucus and a higher viscosity is needed in the large airways to protect the peripheral airways and alveoli against inhaled particles.

This chapter will consider briefly the sources of lung secretions, their chemical composition and physical properties, and their control and functions.

Lung secretions have been divided into tracheobronchial, bronchiolar and alveolar in an attempt to understand better the diagnostic and therapeutic uses of aerosols in respiratory medicine and their application in research.

Tracheobronchial secretion

Origin

The airways are lined by a ciliated mucus-secreting epithelium. In the trachea and bronchi the epithelium is pseudostratified and columnar; as the airways become smaller the epithelium decreases in height consisting, in the terminal bronchioli, of a single layer of cuboidal cells. In the respiratory bronchioli the ciliated epithelium becomes even thinner and is continuous with that of the alveolar duct and alveolus.

By electron microscopy ten cell types have been identified in human airways, eight are of epithelial endodermal origin (basal, ciliated, mucous, serous, Clara, 'special type', intermediate and brush cells) one ectodermal Kultschitsky and one migratory (lymphocyte) (Jeffery, 1978).

The epithelial cells have been classified according to their position within the epithelium as basal or superficial, the presence of cilia—ciliated and non-ciliated—and to the presence of secretory granules as secretory or non-secretory. In human trachea the mean secretory cell density is approximately 6800 mm^{-2} of epithelium. Four secretory cell types have been identified in human airways: mucous cells, Clara cells, serous cells, and the 'special type' cells.

Mucous cell

This cell is also known as goblet cell because of its chalice-like shape. In recent years light and electron microscopy studies have shown that the number of secretory granules influences the shape of the cell, and the term mucous cell is preferred since it includes not only the goblet cell but also those with a smaller number of granules.

The cytoplasm of the mucous cell is electron-dense, the rough endoplasmic reticulum is located mainly at the base of the cell and the nucleus is irregular in outline. The secretory granules are electron-lucent, sometimes have an electron-dense core, and are confluent.

Serous cell

The serous cell has been identified in the human lung, but only in the fetal stage, and very little is known of its fate after birth although it is likely that it transforms into a mucous cell. This transformation has been described in rat epithelium exposed to irritants and drugs (Jeffery *et al.*, 1976). The serous cell cytoplasm is electron-dense with abundant rough endoplasmic reticulum and an irregular nucleus near the base of the cell. The secretory granules are electron-dense, discrete, spherical and enclosed by a membrane. The granules are about 600 nm in diameter and their number ranges between 1 and 34.

Brush cell

The brush cell has finger-like projections—microvilli—at its free surface, and morphologically it resembles that found in the gut brush border. The microvilli are 1–2 μm high, while the cytoplasm is darker than that of the ciliated and intermediate cell and contains vesicles, fibrils and often glycogen. These cells are rare in human airways and their function(s) remain unknown, but their similarities with those found in the gut suggest that they are responsible for liquid absorption.

Intermediate cell

This cell type is called intermediate because it lacks both secretory granules and cilia and its apical processes are few and shorter than those found in the brush cell. The electron-density of the cytoplasm can be dense or lucent. They are capable of transformation into any of the epithelial cell types.

Basal cell

The basal cell touches the basement membrane but does not reach the lumen. It has a small amount of cytoplasm and an electron-dense nucleus. The basal cell is the stem cell from which other superficial cells develop by maturation.

Kultschitsky cell

This is also known as an argyrophil or the Feyrter cell, and it has been identified in human airways (Bensch *et al.*, 1965). Kultschitzky cells are frequently found in the fetus and newborn and are less common in the adult. Neuroepithelial bodies, which are clumps of 10–30 serotonin containing argyrophilic cells have been described in human airways including bronchioles as well as in the alveolar epithelium.

These cells are part of the so-called diffuse neuroendocrine system.

Ciliated cells: Structure

The ciliated cells are characterized by their long cytoplasmic projections and numerous microvilli (*Figure 2.1*).

These cells are found in the entire respiratory tract except in the anterior part of

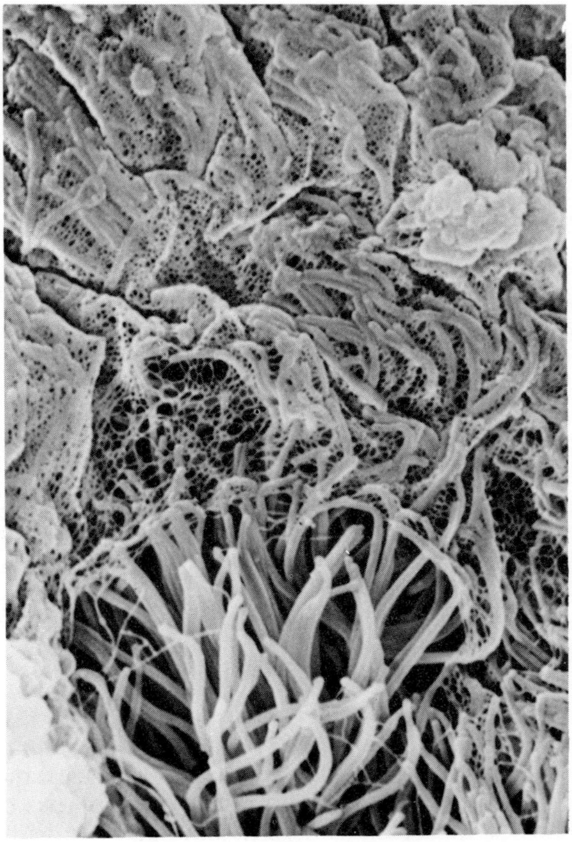

Figure 2.1 Scanning electron micrograph of human bronchial epithelium (×6666)

the nasal cavity and in the alveoli. Their number has been estimated to be around 3 $\times 10^{12}$ and they commonly occur as groups or clusters and are interspersed with mucus-secreting cells. The proportion of ciliated cells in the surface epithelium varies with the size of the airways, but whether the variation is towards an increase or decrease is not clear. Jeffery and Reid (1975) found that in the rat airway there is a gradual increase from 17 per cent in the upper trachea, to 35 per cent in the extrapulmonary bronchi, 53 per cent in the intrapulmonary and 65 per cent in the bronchioli. In contrast, the studies of Serafini and Michaelson (1977) in human and canine airways have shown that the percentage of ciliated cells decreased from 53 per cent in the trachea to 45 per cent in the first airway generation, 23 per cent in the third and 15 per cent in the fifth generation. The discrepancy between these findings could be due to a species difference and methodology.

Cilia are cellular projections, containing fibrils surrounded by cytoplasm and enclosed by the membrane of the cell (Sleigh, 1977)—they are densely packed at about 8 per μm^2 or 200 per cell, with a diameter of 0.25 μm. The length varies at different levels of the airways, for example they are longer in the trachea (5–7 μm) than in the seventh airway generation (3–4 μm) (Serafini and Michaelson, 1977).

A cilium consists of three main structural regions: the ciliary shaft, the basal body and ciliary roots. The ciliary shaft is composed of longitudinal fibrils—the axoneme—which has a highly characteristic structure of 9 outer and 2 central microtubules (*Figure 2.2b*). The outer microtubules consist of two microtubules, one complete (microtubule A) and one incomplete (microtubule B). These microtubules are attached laterally to each other to make a doublet. Microtubules A and B are in turn composed of 13 protofilaments, and 4 or 5 protofilaments are shared by both microtubules. The microtubules are composed of a contractile protein-tubulin. Two types of tubulin have been identified in both the A and B outer fibrils. The two central microtubules are also made up of protofilaments containing tubulin which differs in its amino acid composition from those of the outer fibrils.

Functional structures exist between outer microtubules and between outer and central tubules. Dynein arms connect the A microtubule to the B microtubule of the adjacent doublet, pairs of arms are borne at intervals of 17 nm along the A microtubule. The outer dynein arm is longer than the inner arm and has an extra segment.

The major protein component of the axoneme is an ATPase protein known as dynein. Biochemical and electron microscopic studies have shown that the dynein arms consist of ATPase or dynein protein.

When the outer dynein arms are biochemically removed the axonemes continue to move but at a low frequency. The actual bending of the cilium is due to an active sliding of the doublet microtubules. The dynein molecules attached to the A microtubule undergo cyclical changes in shape as they engage and disengage with the microtubule B of the adjacent doublet. Cations are required to activate dynein, but magnesium is the only cation essential for motility.

Peripheral radial links, also known as nexin arms, have been described joining the A microtubules of adjacent doublets or between the inner arm of an A microtubule and the adjacent B microtubule. In addition, from the A microtubule an accessory structure—radial link or radial spoke—projects centrally toward the central tubules. The radial spoke terminates in a dilated breach which appears to connect with the lateral projections of the central microtubules and contain an ATPase protein dynein 2+ which differs from that isolated from the dynein arms.

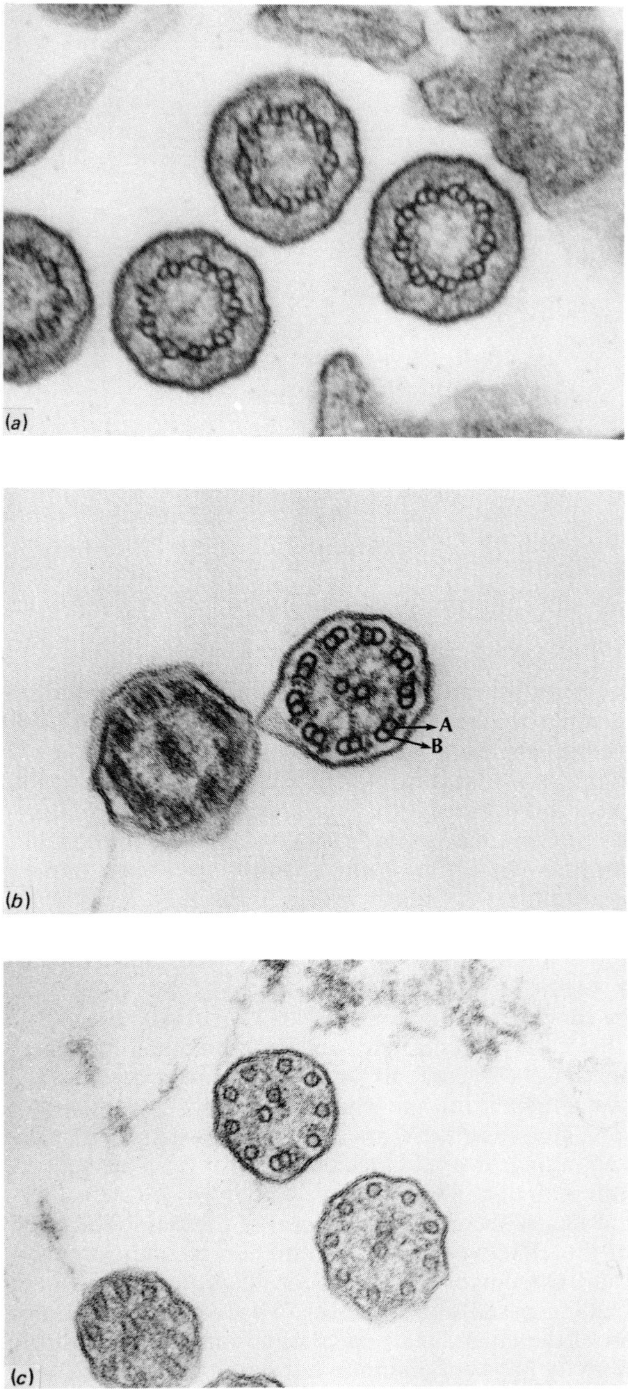

Figure 2.2 Transmission electron micrographs of cross sections of cilia showing the normal microtubular arrangement at the base (a) at the middle of the shaft (b) and at the tip of the cilium (c) (×100 000)

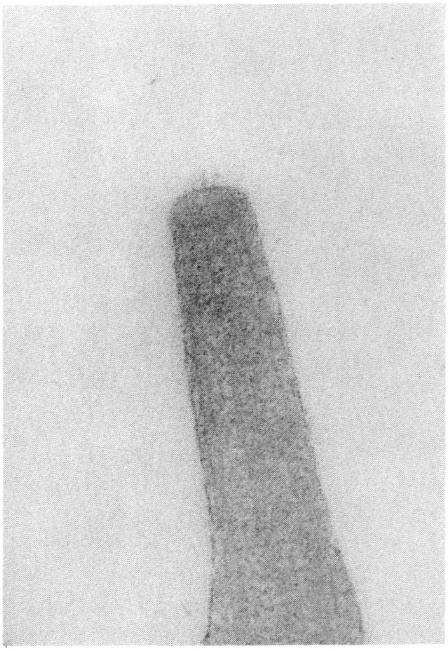

Figure 2.3 Transmission electron micrograph of the tip of a cilium showing the claws (×100000)

This characteristic axonemial structure exists all along the cilium except at the tip and base. At the tip of the cilium the microtubule B first terminates and the peripheral outer doublets become single microtubules then the microtubules A disappear and only the central microtubules remain (*Figure 2.2*). In contrast at the base only the outer tubules exist.

A crown of short projections or claws has been identified at the tips of the cilia, these projections penetrate into the mucus during the effective stroke and propel the mucus (*Figure 2.3*).

At the *ciliary base*, below the cell surface the outer doublets become triplets by the addition of another incomplete microtubule—microtubule C. The microtubules rotate in such a way that microtubule A is nearest to the centre of the cilium. The microtubules are connected by functional structures of various configurations.

A specialized region of the ciliary membrane—ciliary necklace—has been identified in somatic cilia, including rat trachea, in the transition region where the ciliary membrane joins the plasma membrane and where extensions from the outer doublets to the ciliary membrane are present. Comparative studies suggest that the ciliary necklace may be involved in the control of localized membrane permeability and may play a role in the timing of ciliary beat (Gilula and Satir, 1972).

A basal foot projects at right angles from the mid-region of the basal body and points toward the direction of the effective stroke. Several contractile proteins—alpha actinin, actin, myosin and tropomyosin—have been identified in different regions of the basal body including basal foot processes. These proteins are also found in the contracted region of the ciliary shaft and extend into the core of the microvilli. Because ATPase activity has been identified in basal bodies it is likely that these structures are involved in the cilia movement.

Attached to the basal bodies are the *ciliary roots* which help to maintain the position of the cilium and are the main anchorage of the axonema.

Cilia: Function

The beat cycle of mucus-propelling cilia consists of an effective stroke and a recovery stroke during which the cilium moves clockwise. At the beginning of the cycle the cilia are in the rest position, that is at the end of an effective stroke, thus each beat starts with a recovery stroke. During the effective stroke the cilium is fully extended and penetrates the mucus by 0.5 μm, while in the recovery phase it is bent and moves to one side of the cell keeping near to the surface. The duration of the recovery stroke is twice as long as the effective stroke, 29 and 15 milliseconds respectively (Sleigh, 1981).

Ciliated cells are usually found in groups and the cilia within a group beat in a coordinated fashion which is probably due to viscochemical coupling. The direction of beat and wave propagation varies between groups of cells but the overall direction of beat—oropharyngeal—is similar between regions.

Human respiratory ciliary beat frequency (CBF) at different levels of the airways is controversial. *In vitro* studies have shown either a gradual decrease or no change in CBF from trachea to subsegmental bronchus (Rutland and Cole, 1981; Dulfano *et al.*, 1981).

Variations in ciliary beat frequency of 6 to 16 Hz, have been observed in normal human bronchial tissue (Lopez-Vidriero and Clarke, (1982). The mechanisms responsible for this variation are unknown but it is likely that changes in levels of intracellular cAMP and electrolytes—magnesium and calcium—could be involved.

Control of ciliary activity

In human respiratory epithelium, ciliary activity is independent of nervous control and mechanical stimulation and appears to be a spontaneous activity which arises from a small group of active cilia that initiate the metachronal waves within a small region.

Ciliary activity is influenced by physical and chemical factors: temperature, radiation, pH, and viscoelastic properties.

The control of ciliary activity has been studied in great detail both *in vivo* and *in vitro* in Protozoa and the frog palate, and in various mammals including the rat, the rabbit and the cat (Sleigh, 1977). It is surprising how little work has been done in human respiratory epithelium, particularly in bronchial epithelium. Furthermore, most of the investigations have used mucociliary transport as an indirect method for assessing the effect of drugs on ciliary activity, and it is impossible to separate the effect on mucus secretion from the effect on ciliary activity or both.

The results published in the literature are confusing and controversial and are most likely due to differences in the techniques, animal species and organs investigated.

The more consistent findings are the cilioexcitatory effect of cholinergic and beta-adrenergic agonists. The effect of α adrenoreceptors is not clear. Terbutaline, a selective β_2 agonist increases ciliary activity of human bronchial epithelium *in vitro* (Clarke and Lopez-Vidriero, 1983). More studies are needed for a better understanding of control of ciliary activity in man.

Intercellular junctions

Functional and ultrastructural studies on secretory epithelium suggest that the specificity of water and ion transport is a consequence of the physical characteristics of the intercellular junctions (Oschman and Berridge, 1971). Different types of intercellular junctions have been described in the tracheobronchial epithelium of guinea pigs and rats: tight junctions, gap junctions and rectilinear arrays (Inoue and Hogg, 1977; Schneeberger, 1980). Tight junctions seal the space between cells and thereby provide a barrier which protects the milieu interna from the external environment.

Three types of tight junctions—1, 2 and 3—have been identified in the surface epithelium of rats. They differ in the degree of interconnection of the luminal fibrils (Schneeberger, 1980). In type 1 the luminal fibrils are sparsely interconnected, in type 2 richly interconnected and in type 3 characterized by a narrow interconnected network of fibrils.

The morphology of the tight junctions varies not only depending on the cell type—ciliated or mucus-secreting—but also on its level in the airways—extrapulmonary or intrapulmonary. Type 1 tight junction is found almost exclusively between ciliated cells in the extrapulmonary airways, while in the bronchioles the junctional pattern changes to type 2. Mucous cells have type 3 junctions, and Clara cells type 2. The factors governing the morphology of tight junctions are still unclear. Changes in the tightness of the intercellular junctions have been described in relation to the secretory cycle, the junction becoming 'leaky' when the mucous cell is actively secreting (Inoue and Hogg, 1977). These structural changes associated with mucus discharge suggest that water, ions and small soluble macromolecules are probably released with the secretion from the granules.

Gap junctions are rare. They are found only between secretory cells of the extrapulmonary airways. The location of gap junctions near the base of the cells seems to indicate that they may serve to connect secretory to basal cells.

Submucosal glands

Submucosal glands are found in airways with cartilage in the wall, they lie between the epithelium and plates of cartilage and between and occasionally external to the plates of cartilage (Jeffery and Reid, 1977). Their density has been estimated to be 1 gland per square millimetre of epithelium. Submucosal glands represent 40 times the volume of the surface epithelial mucous cells and are probably the more important source of mucus.

Four regions can be identified in the submucosal gland: the ciliated duct, the collecting duct, the mucous tubule and the serous tubule.

The ciliated duct forms the first part of the main duct system and opens into the surface epithelium. It is lined by ciliated mucus-secreting epithelium, but contains less mucous cells than surface epithelium. The ciliated duct gives way to the collecting duct, and the ciliated epithelium is replaced by non-ciliated cells. The duct cell cytoplasm is strangely eosinophilic and contains numerous mitochondria. At the proximal end of the duct they are 30 μm high, and within a short distance they increase to 70 μm. These cells have been found to possess a high metabolic activity, and it has been postulated that their function in the glands is to control the ionic and water concentration of the gland secretion.

The duct is about 1 mm in length and runs obliquely to the surface; it is usually single but branching has been observed.

An important feature is that the blood capillaries are more numerous around the collecting duct than around the secretory tubules. The mucous tubules arise directly from the collecting duct. The serous tubules are situated at the end of mucous tubules either singly or in groups. Occasionally serous tubules arise directly from the collecting duct like buds. The mucous tubules are larger (500 μm) than the serous (50–180 μm). The mucous and serous cells comprise their own separate and discrete regions within a gland, the ratio between mucous and serous cells being 1:1. The anatomical arrangement of the secretory tubules ensures that the secretion of the serous granules passes over that of the mucous. Both secretions pass into the collecting duct; it is here that ionic and water adjustments of mucus probably take place before it is discharged into the lumen.

The morphological features of the serous and mucous cells of the gland are similar to their counterpart in the surface epithelium.

Myoepithelial cells are found beneath the serous, mucous and collecting duct cells and resemble smooth muscle cells. Contraction of these cells doubtless contributes to discharging secretion from the gland.

The 'clear cell', which has the features of an immunoblast, is found between the cells of the secreting tubules and collecting duct and the basement membrane.

Mast cells and Kultschitsky cells are occasionally found to penetrate the acinar basement membrane; chemical mediators and regulatory peptides have been shown to influence submucosal gland secretion.

Innervation

Our knowledge of the distribution and concentration of nerve ganglia, fibres and endings in the human lung is still fragmentary. Studies using light microscopy established the nerve supply to the large airways especially to the smooth muscle and submucosal layer (Richardson, 1979).

The parasympathetic (cholinergic) innervation consists of afferent and efferent pathways. The afferent or sensory fibres originate in the surface epithelium, submucosal layer, smooth muscle and interalveolar surfaces and terminate in the vagal nuclei. The efferent pathway starts in the ganglia which are mainly located external to the smooth muscle and cartilage as well as in the submucosa, and ends in the smooth muscle and submucosal glands. Ultrastructural studies have confirmed the presence of sensory nerve endings in the human tracheal epithelium, which are located in the basal portion of the ciliated and mucous cells (Rhodin, 1966). The role of intraepithelial nerves is unclear. It is apparent from human organ culture studies that acetylcholine causes discharge of submucosal glands but has no effect on the secretory cells of the surface epithelium (Sturgess and Reid, 1972). It is possible that intraepithelial nerves are concerned with the function of tight junctions, since administration of acetylcholine increases the leakiness of tight junctions between epithelial cells.

The existence of sympathetic innervation has been less clearly established in the human lung. Preganglionic fibres leave the spinal cord to form a synapsis with the prevertebral ganglia; postganglionic fibres originate in the ganglia and supply the smooth muscle of the bronchi and blood vessels. Whether the submucosal glands receive sympathetic innervation or not is still under debate.

Non-adrenergic inhibitory nerves were first described in the guinea pig trachealis muscle (Coburn and Tomita, 1973). Richardson and Beland (1976) demonstrated the presence of non-adrenergic inhibitory nerves in the smooth muscle of the human trachea and bronchi. The large opaque vesicles found in the axons are similar to those found in the gastrointestinal tract. In recent years a wide range of biologically active peptides have been identified in nerve endings e.g. substance P, vasoactive intestinal peptide (VIP), and bombesin. In human airways some nerve endings adjacent to the submucosal glands have been shown to contain VIP (Dey and Said, 1980). This complex system is called the diffuse neuroendocrine system and although biological activity can be demonstrated for most of this new group of compounds, their role in normal function has not yet emerged.

Intracellular glycoproteins

The use of histochemical stains at different pH and autoradiographic techniques have demonstrated the presence of several types of glycoprotein in the secretory cells of the surface epithelium and submucosal gland (Jones and Reid, 1978).

In man, the mucous cells of the surface epithelium contain acid glycoprotein both sialylated and sulphated and lack neutral glycoprotein. Submucosal glands have been studied in more detail in man than the surface epithelium. A great variety of types of glycoprotein has been described. Four types of acid glycoprotein have been identified in the mucous cell: (1) sialylated susceptible to neuroaminidase; (2) sialyated resistant to neuroaminidase; (3) sulphated identified by alcian blue stain after hydrolysis and autoradiographic studies of uptake of radioactive sulphate but not staining with specific sulphate stains; and (4) as above but staining with specific sulphate stains. A mucous cell may contain one or more of these four types of glycoprotein, either present in one granule or from a mixture of granules, but it is of interest to note that they only occur in certain combinations. The intracellular secretion of the serous cell consists of a PAS positive material associated with two acidic groups, sialic acid and sulphate. The serous cell is characterized by a high degree of sulphation. In addition to the acid glycoprotein a serous cell granule may contain the protein lysozyme.

Normal human airways show a marked range in the proportion of various types of intracellular glycoproteins but in any single individual the distribution throughout the airways is similar and there is less variation between the glands in one individual than between individuals.

Tracheobronchial secretion *in situ*

Half a century ago Lucas and Douglas (1934) put forward the hypothesis that for the satisfactory functioning of the mucociliary system, the tracheobronchial secretions *in situ* were composed of two layers of different physical properties. A liquid layer in which the cilia beat which is known as the periciliary or sol layer and a viscous layer lying on the tips of the cilia called the gel or mucus layer. Since a two layer system, epiphase and hypophase, has also been described for surfactant in the alveolus the same terminology could be used for the tracheobronchial tree.

Using electron microscopy the hypophase has been identified as an electron-lucent zone, indicating that it contains a small amount of macromolecular material (Sanderson and Sleigh, 1981). Its origin, configuration and control are still hypothetical. Alveolar surfactant, Clara cell secretion and ciliated cells have been proposed as the possible origin of the hypophase. Since ciliated cells are found at all levels of the airways, except in alveoli, it is more likely that the ciliated cells secrete the hypophase.

Using radioactively labelled precursors of mucus glycoprotein, (^{3}H) glucose and sodium (^{35}S) sulphate, Gallagher *et al.* (1978) found that ciliated cells of the cat's trachea incorporated (^{3}H) glucose and most of it was located in the luminal border of the cell. Whether this material represents the glycocalix or the liquid hypophase is not clear. The numerous microvilli present in the ciliated cells may be responsible for ion and water absorption from the hypophase.

The epiphase or mucus layer has been identified not only in rat and rabbit but also in human airways (Sturgess, 1977). The airway mucus forms a three-dimensional fibrous network, the thickness being greatest at the trachea and gradually becoming thinner with subsequent airway generations. The thickness of the epiphase varies from 8–12 μm in the trachea to 2–5 μm in lobar bronchi.

In the trachea the fibrous network is smooth and cohesive, but often series of overlapping plaques are observed which give a characteristic layering appearance to the epiphase. In the main bronchus a more complex three-dimensional arrangement occurs, although plaques are also present at this level. By contrast in the intrapulmonary airways the fibrous network becomes more expanded with a random arrangement of fibrils and loss of smooth sheets of mucus. This difference in appearance may reflect either changes in chemical composition or reabsorption of water and ions.

Within the mucus layer, the mucus close to the cell surface forms more open networks while the luminal side forms more cohesive plaques. This finding may reflect changes in entanglement or cross-linking of macromolecules; similar changes have been described in expectorated mucus from patients with bronchorrhoea (Lopez-Vidriero *et al.*, 1977a).

Control of tracheobronchial mucus secretion

The neurohumoral control of airway secretion has been studied both *in vivo* and *in vitro* in a wide range of animal species including goose, rat, cat, dog, monkey and ferret. Unfortunately relatively little is known about the control of secretion in humans and it is restricted to *in vitro* studies. Extrapolation of results from animal studies to man should be done with extreme caution, since the type of innervation and its distribution, presence or absence of glands and the type and distribution of mucus-secreting cells differ between animals and man (Jeffery and Reid, 1977).

While there is no direct evidence that parasympathetic stimulation increases mucus secretion in man, *in vitro* studies have shown that parasympathomimetic drugs increase both mucus glycoprotein secretion and ion transport (Sturgess and Reid, 1972; Shelhamer *et al.*, 1980; Knowles *et al.*, 1982). Atropine reduces mucus glycoprotein secretion but there is a resting secretion which is not under parasympathetic control (Sturgess and Reid, 1972).

The role of the sympathetic nervous system is still controversial, some *in vitro* studies have shown that β_2 agonists increase mucus glycoprotein secretion (Phipps *et al.*, 1982) while others found no effect on either mucus glycoprotein secretion or ion transport (Sturgess and Reid, 1972; Boat and Kleinerman, 1975; Shelhamer *et al.*, 1980; Knowles *et al.*, 1982).

Similar controversial findings have been reported in relation to α agonists, which seem to increase mucus glycoprotein secretion (Phipps *et al.*, 1982; Shelhamer, 1980) but have no effect on ion transport.

The role played by regulatory peptides of the non-adrenergic/neuroendocrine diffuse system in the control of mucous secretion is beginning to be explored.

Vasoactive intestinal peptide (VIP) decreases mucus glycoprotein in normal tissue but has no effect on hypertrophied glands (Coles *et al.*, 1981).

A better understanding of the effect of chemical mediators of inflammation and allergy on mucus secretion is needed. Limited information is available on the effect of chemical mediators on mucus glycoprotein secretion but is lacking on their role in water and ion transport. Histamine, which is the main chemical mediator of allergy, increases mucus glycoprotein secretion but at relatively high dose (Shelhamer *et al.*, 1980). Early studies by Sturgess and Reid (1972) showed that histamine at similar concentration had no effect.

Prostaglandins A_2, D_2 and $F_{2\alpha}$ but not E_2, and arachidonic acid increase mucus glycoprotein secretion and there is evidence that lipoxygenase products generated by the airways also stimulate secretion (Shelhamer *et al.*, 1982).

Leukotrienes, LTD_4 and LTC_4, are constituents of the slow-reacting substance of anaphylaxis (SRS-A) and are 1000 times more potent secretagogues than acetylcholine (Shelhamer *et al.*, 1982).

Hydrocortisone but no other corticosteroids, e.g. β-methasone, dexamethasone and triamcinolone, increases mucous glycoprotein secretion but only in some specimens of bronchus.

Several nucleotides, cyclic AMP and cyclic GMP have been investigated *in vitro* and here again the findings are controversial. Shelhamer *et al.* (1980) found that cyclic GMP increased mucus glycoprotein secretion while cyclic AMP had no effect. In contrast Whimster and Reid (1973) showed that cyclic AMP and theophylline, a phosphodiesterase inhibitor, stimulate mucus secretion.

When interpreting this information it should be remembered that the secretory cycle consists of different stages: incorporation of precursor, synthesis, transport and discharge and that these stages can be independent, that is a drug may influence synthesis without changing discharge (Coles, 1977).

In addition, stimulation of the myoepithelial cells surrounding the glands can result in discharge of secretion without having an effect on the secretory cycle itself.

Further studies are needed to elucidate the mechanisms involved in the control of both mucus glycoprotein secretion and water and ion transport in man.

Tracheobronchial secretion: chemical composition

Tracheobronchial mucus is a mixture of secretions from the surface epithelium, submucosal glands and tissue fluid transudate.

Tracheobronchial mucus, whether aspirated, expectorated or collected from a tracheostomy tube also contains secretion from the bronchioles—Clara cell—and alveoli—surfactant. Histochemical studies have shown that there are regional differences in the distribution of intracellular glycoprotein, that is the mucus glycoprotein component is not uniform along the tracheobronchial tree.

In addition regional differences exist in water and ion transport across the epithelium. Airway mucus becomes increasingly complex from peripheral airways to the trachea. Therefore our knowledge of the chemical composition and viscoelastic properties of tracheobronchial mucus is based not only on a mixture of secretions from different tissue and cell sources, but also on a mixture of substances from any given source. This is important when studying the correlations between lung mucociliary clearance and chemical composition or rheological properties of mucus.

The volume of mucus produced daily by a normal human tracheobronchial tree is not known with certainty. Based on studies in subjects with tracheostomy, the daily volume was found to be 7 and 21 ml (Toremalm, 1960). It is possible that this volume is an overestimation since the airways of these subjects are not entirely normal and the tracheostomy tube could be inducing reflex mucus hypersecretion.

Several methods are being used for collecting mucus from normal airways but they involve either invasive techniques (bronchial lavage) or pharmacological manipulation: prostaglandin $F_{2\alpha}$, acetylcholine administration (Lopez-Vidriero *et al.*, 1977b).

Material obtained from bronchial lavage is suitable for chemical analysis but unsuitable for rheological studies. Most of our knowledge of the chemical composition and viscoelastic properties of airway mucus is derived from expectorated secretion obtained from abnormal airways.

Airway mucus consists of water, dialyzable material and macromolecular constituents. Water is the main constituent by weight and in normal secretion it accounts for 95 per cent of the total weight. Dialyzable material—salts and small molecules—represent only 1 per cent. Mucus glycoprotein (2–3 per cent), proteins (0.1–0.5 per cent) and lipids (0.3–0.5 per cent) are the major macromolecular constituents. Recently a new macromolecular component of airway mucus—glycosaminoglycan—has been identified in secretion from normal canine airways *in vivo* and human airways *in vitro* (Bhaskar *et al.*, 1982a; Coles *et al.*, 1982). The origin and function of this constituent is not clear and further studies are needed.

Mucus glycoprotein is the main macromolecular constituent and is responsible for the viscoelastic behaviour of airway secretion. Mucus glycoprotein is a homogeneous, polydisperse macromolecule with an average molecular weight of 3 to 7×10^6 but smaller and larger molecules are also present (Creeth *et al.*, 1977). This macromolecule is made up of a polypeptide core with sugar chains attached along its length through *O*-glycosidic linkages between threonine or serine and *N*-acetyl galactosamine. Serine and threonine account for more than 40 per cent of the total amino acid content, cysteine molecules are also present but in very small amounts. Carbohydrates contribute up to 50–80 per cent of the total weight, the oligosaccharide side chains are branched and have an average length of 8 to 10 sugars although as few as 2 and as many as 20 have been identified. The oligosaccharides most commonly found in bronchial mucus are fucose, galactose, galactosamine, *N*-acetyl galactosamine and *N*-acetyl neuraminic acid. Sulphate radicals are attached to the oligosaccharide side chains and usually those chains appear to be longer than those containing *N*-acetyl neuraminic acid.

The sugar chains protect the polypeptide core against proteolytic degradation but these are regions devoid of sugars—the so-called naked peptide regions—which are susceptible to enzymatic degradation.

The native mucus glycoprotein, that is the macromolecule isolated from the mucus without using degradative methods, is made up of small glycopeptide sub-units (3×10^5 to 1×10^6 MW). The glycopeptide sub-units are cross-linked through disulphate bonds and there is evidence that a small peptide belonging to the glycopeptide may be involved. Intramolecular and intermolecular disulphide bonds are not the only linkages responsible for gel formation. Negatively charged radicals such as *N*-acetyl-neuraminic acid and sulphate influence the tertiary structure. Chaotropic agents like urea and guanidium solubilize mucus, indicating that hydrogen bonds can also contribute to gel formation. Very little is known about mucus glycoprotein–lipid interaction but recent studies have shown that they play an important role in gel formation (Bhaskar and Reid, 1982; Bhaskar *et al.*, 1982b).

Plasma type glycoproteins and proteins have been identified in normal airway mucus. Lysozyme, bronchotransferrin and secretory piece are locally produced by the mucous cells of the surface epithelium and submucosal glands and by the serous cell of the glands.

Immunoglobulins, in particulage IgA dimer (10S), IgM and IgE are locally produced by plasma cells and mast cells located in the mucosa, while IgA (7S) and IgG derive mainly from tissue fluid transudate.

Proteins play several roles in the airways, some influence viscoelastic properties by interacting with other macromolecules, others protect the airways against infection or damage by proteases.

Lipids contribute to almost a third of the total macromolecular material and have been identified not only in bronchoalveolar lavage, but also in sputum and in secretion from bronchial explants (Bhaskar *et al.*, 1982a and b; Coles *et al.*, 1982; Bhaskar and Reid, 1982).

Neutral lipids, phospholipids and glycolipids have been identified but very little is known about their origin and functions. Surfactant membrane of mucous granules and tissue fluid transudate are known sources of lipids but further studies are needed.

Airway mucus consists of soluble phase known as sol and an insoluble phase called gel. Sol and gel phases are obtained by using high speed centrifugation. The soluble phase contains mainly proteins and a small amount of mucus glycoprotein which is always of low molecular weight. In contrast the gel contains mainly mucus glycoprotein of high molecular weight, proteins and lipids (Lopez-Vidriero and Reid, 1980; Bhaskar *et al.*, 1982b).

Tracheobronchial mucus: physical properties

The rheological properties of airway mucus—viscosity and elasticity—have been increasingly accepted as the key physical properties required for its main function, that is mechanical coupling with cilia (King *et al.*, 1974; Litt, 1981). Rheology is defined as the study of deformation and flow properties of matter. Airway mucus behaves as a special liquid/solid material. As a liquid it exhibits viscous behaviour, that is when a force is applied it shows continuous deformation (flow) and expends energy. The deformation persists as long as the force is applied and when the force is removed the deformation ceases and there is no recovery. For a Newtonian or ideal liquid viscosity is independent of the shear stress, airway mucus like most biological materials is a non-Newtonian liquid and its viscosity varies according to the force supplied. Different patterns of non-Newtonian behaviour can be identified: pseudoplastic, dilatant and plastic. Airway mucus is a pseudoplastic liquid: its viscosity decreases with increasing shear rate (shear thinning). At intermediate shear rates ($<10s^{-1}$) it may show thyxotropic behaviour—the decrease in viscosity is partly recovered after removal of the stress. The apparent viscosity is the ratio of the total shear stress to total shear rate at a given value of shear rate.

An ideal solid can be deformed when a force is applied and stores energy returning to its original shape when the force is removed. This is known as ideal or linear elasticity. When after removal of the applied force the material shows permanent deformation it is known as elastic hysteresis and is a feature of semisolid materials.

Mucus is a viscoelastic semisolid material—when a stress is applied four phases can be identified. First it behaves as a solid and shows an initial deformation which is followed by a second phase of viscoelastic behaviour characterized by retarded deformation. The third phase is denoted by a period of steady flow in which the rate of deformation is constant. When the force is removed there is only partial recovery of the strain indicating permanent deformation (phase four).

Elasticity, like viscosity, is also frequency dependent, but in contrast it increases with increasing frequency. When subjected to weak forces mucus reacts more like a solid, while with strong forces it behaves more like a liquid. This different pattern of behaviour has important implications for mucus transport via the ciliary escalator or during cough.

Several mechanical models of viscoelastic behaviour have been prepared, in which the viscous component has been represented by a dashpot or shock absorbing element and the elastic component by a spring. The complexity of airway mucus is such that it is impossible to represent it with discrete models, Maxwell and Voigt elements or even with more elements, dashpots and springs, both in series and parallel combination.

A wide variety of instruments is available to study the rheological properties of mucus (Lopez-Vidriero *et al.*, 1977a). Some measure only viscosity (Ferranti Shirley viscometer) while others measure both viscosity and elasticity (modified rotational viscometer, Weissenberg rheogoniometer and magnetic rheometer). Two basic methods are used for testing viscoelastic properties, the creep test and the dynamic or oscillatory test. The creep test involves application of an instantaneous, small stress and the measurement of displacement or strain induced in the sample is measured. The ratio between stress and strain represents elasticity. In the dynamic test the stress is applied sinusoidally and the strain transmitted by the sample is measured. The ratio between stress and strain is the mechanical impedance G* which represents viscoelasticity. The mechanical impedance is the vector sum of the storage modulus G' and G''. The storage modulus—elasticity—is the component in phase with the stress. The loss modulus (G'') is the component out of phase; dynamic viscosity is obtained by dividing loss modulus by frequency. The elegant studies of King *et al.* (1974) have established without doubt that the gel-like properties of mucus are essential for coupling with cilia and hence transport. Mucus from different sources can act as mechanical couplers and even more important synthetic polymers with an optimal degree of cross-linking can also act as mechanical couplers. The ideal viscoelastic properties for mucus transport have been studied in the frog palate preparation and although they may not be entirely representative of the requirements for mucus transport in human airways, at least they have shown that elasticity is more important than viscosity for mucus transport (King *et al.*, 1974; Puchelle *et al.*, 1981).

There is strong evidence that the gel-like (viscoelastic) properties of mucus are mainly due to disulphide cross-links between glycopeptide sub-units, but other types of cross-linkages may also contribute. Recent studies indicate that optimal mucus transport *in vitro* is not only dependent upon the number of cross-links but also upon the manner in which they are introduced and arranged.

Mucus exhibits many physical properties such as adhesiveness, tackiness, pourability, wettability, consistency and spinnability but relatively little is known about their role in mucus transport as mechanical couplers and also in cough.

Tracheobronchial mucus: functions

The tracheobronchial tree is anatomically and physiologically designed to protect the peripheral airways—bronchioles—and the functional region of the lung—the alveoli—against inhaled particles. The host defence mechanisms of the tracheobronchial tree are divided into non-specific and specific. The non-specific mechanisms include a large variety of resources: anatomical, physical, chemical and cellular. The anatomy of the tracheobronchial tree with its characteristic pattern of branching and the presence of a mucus layer can affect the airflow and pattern of deposition of particles. The presence of irritant receptors in the trachea and large airways, particularly in the bifurcations where particle impaction is more likely to occur, provide the airways with at least three essential defence mechanisms: cough and mucus hypersecretion and bronchoconstriction. Mucus hypersecretion can be stimulated via a nervous reflex and probably by local release of chemical mediators. Mucus hypersecretion has various functions, it increases impaction of inhaled particles, makes cough more efficient, i.e. for expectoration of noxious substances, and protects the surface epithelium against physical and chemical injury. Mucus hypersecretion in the trachea and large airways can be induced by stimulating irritant receptors in the nasopharyngeal epithelium and as a result the lower respiratory tract is prepared in advance to cope with an abnormal environment (Phipps and Richardson, 1976).

Airway mucus plays a key role in the mucociliary defence mechanism, an active ciliated epithelium depleted of mucus does not transport particles (King *et al.*, 1974). Airway mucus is a gel with special viscoelastic properties suited to be propelled by respiratory cilia. This is one reason why in the frog palate preparation the transport rate of bronchial mucus is slower than that of frog palate mucus. There seems to be a close relationship between rheological properties of mucus, pattern of ciliary movement and function. The presence, depth and viscoelastic properties of the hypophase (periciliary layer) are also important for mucus transport.

Chemical constituents of mucus like lysozyme, bronchotransferrin and interferon are bactericidal, others have antiprotease activity—α_1 antitrypsin and antichymotrypsin and protect the airways against enzymatic degradation. Also present in mucus are substances—complement and opsonins—that enhance bacterial adherence to phagocytic cells.

The cellular component of the tracheobronchial tree, i.e. surface epithelium and phagocytic cells, contribute to the defence mechanism of the lung. The surface epithelium with its tight intercellular junctions forms a protective barrier. When this barrier is breached, as happens with viral infection and chemical damage by aspiration or inhalation, respiratory tract infections are frequent. The phagocytic cells found in the tracheobronchial mucus are neutrophils and to a lesser extent macrophages. These cells ingest and digest (detoxification) organisms and foreign particles and are removed via the mucociliary escalator.

The specific defence mechanisms of the tracheobronchial tree are the humoral and cell-mediated immune responses, which are highly complex mechanisms and still incompletely understood. The specific defences are not present at birth but acquired and they involve highly specific stimuli that cause equally specific responses.

Immunoglobulins are antibodies produced by the antigenic challenge of B lymphoid cells. Serum-derived immunoglobulins IgA (7S), IgG, IgM and IgE are found in normal mucus in relatively small amounts but increase during an inflammatory process. Precipitation, agglutination, opsonization cytolisis through complement activation and neutralization are their main functions for protecting the mucous membranes against foreign proteins and bacteria.

The locally produced immunoglobulin S-IgA(11S) is highly resistant to proteolytic digestion. This is due to the presence of the secretory piece. The exact biological role of S-IgA is not completely documented. It has a neutralizing activity against viruses whether they are inhaled or ingested, but it seems to lack activity against bacteria. There is evidence that S-IgA protects the mucosa against allergic reactions.

The existence of local T cell-mediated immunity in airways is still uncertain.

Bronchiolar secretion

Small airways are the target site of initial damage and dysfunction in chronic airways obstruction (Hogg *et al.*, 1968). In the normal human lung two types of cells line the distal airways: a secretory cell—the Clara cell first described by Clara (1934)—and a ciliated cell. Unfortunately little is known about the nature of the secretory granules, the chemical composition, physical properties or the neurohormonal regulation of secretion in these cells.

Bronchiolar secretion: origin

Bronchioles are the airways distal to the last plate of cartilage and proximal to the alveolar region. The bronchioles are no longer lined by a pseudostratified epithelium, nor have they cartilage, glands or a continuous muscularis. They are characterized by the presence of a columnar epithelium, in which a unique type of secretory cell replaces the mucous cell and by an increase in the thickness of the muscularis and separation of smooth muscle fascicles by connective tissue.

Two major cell types are present in the bronchioles: the ciliated and the Clara cell. The ciliated cells are similar to those in the bronchi except that they are shorter. These cells are more numerous at first, but in small bronchioles Clara cells dominate the epithelium. Striking interspecies differences have been reported in their number, distribution and presence of cytoplasmic organelles. Clara cells are found in a greater part of the bronchial tree of small compared to large animals (Cutz and Conen, 1971).

The Clara cells are identified by the characteristic apical bulge into the lumen and the presence of electron-dense granules which in the human appeared mottled. They have prominent microvilli on their free surfaces similar to those found in Type II cells. Lateral plasma membranes form complex interdigitations, desmosomes, with adjacent cells. Their cytoplasm contains a prominent Golgi zone, rough endoplasmic reticulum and numerous mitochondria, features of a secretory cell. The electron-dense granules, usually in the apical part of cell, are round or oval and measure 0.4–0.6 μm in diameter (Cutz and Conen, 1971).

The Clara cells are among the more metabolically active cells in the lungs. They contain a large number of enzymes which are frequently located at the apex, i.e. lysosomal enzymes, esterases, peroxidases, lipases and protease inhibitors. It has been suggested that lipases may be responsible for the breakdown of surfactant. Since these cells lie distally to the mucus-secreting areas of the tracheobronchial tree, just as the serous tubules generally are distal to the mucous tubules in the glands, it is possible that their secretions serve to alter the physical properties of the secretions released higher up in the bronchial tree.

Intracellular: Clara cell secretion

The exact nature of the secretion produced by the Clara cells is not known but there is increasing evidence that these cells are not the source of alveolar surfactant.

Cytochemical studies have shown that the secretory granules contain lipids which are bound to a non-lipid component (Azzopardi and Thurlbeck, 1969), phospholipids, protein and carbohydrate (Cutz and Conen, 1971).

The presence of lipids has been confirmed by using radiolabelled precursors ^{3}H-palmitate and ^{3}H-acetate (Petrik and Collet, 1974). The presence of protein is supported by autoradiographic studies with ^{3}H-leucine (Ebert *et al.*, 1976).

The presence of neutral glycoproteins in the secretory granules is still controversial. Histochemical studies indicate that the PAS positive material is a neutral glycoprotein (Azzopardi and Thurlbeck, 1969; Cutz and Conen, 1971), but recently Widdicombe and Pack (1982) concluded that glucose and glucosamine are not taken up by the Clara cells which is against glycoprotein synthesis.

Bronchiolar secretion *in situ*

The extracellular lining of bronchioles has been studied in great detail in rats (Gil and Weibel, 1971; Ebert and Terracio, 1975). The bronchiolar lining is continuous with that of the alveoli and consists, like the latter, of two layers: hypophase and epiphase. The hypophase, where the cilia beat, contains a small amount of macromolecular material and has a similar electron-density to the hypophase of the tracheobronchial tree.

The epiphase appears considerably thicker than that seen over the alveolar surface. In Gil and Weibel's study, osmiophilic material, alveolar surfactant, was seen in the epiphase at the air/liquid interface.

These studies indicate that both alveolar surfactant and Clara cell secretion contribute to the bronchiolar lining.

Bronchiolar secretion: control

Relatively few studies have been made of the neurohumoral regulation of Clara cell secretion.

Beta adrenergic agonists increase secretion both *in vivo* and *in vitro* at high ($10\,mg\,kg^{-1}$) and low doses ($5\,\mu g$) and the effect is blocked by propranolol. Analogues of cAMP (dibutyryl and 8 bromo) increase secretion *in vitro*, these findings indicate that the β-adrenergic effect is mediated by cAMP (Massaro *et al.*, 1981).

Conflicting results have been reported on the effect of pilocarpine, when this cholinergic agonist is administered *in vivo* it increases secretion while *in vitro* it has an inhibitory effect (Massaro *et al.*, 1981). It is likely that the *in vivo* effect is mediated by extrapulmonary mechanisms.

An interesting observation is that Clara cell secretion is stimulated by increased ventilatory volume and this effect seems to be mediated by cGMP.

Chemical composition/physical properties/function

Study of the chemical composition and physical properties of bronchiolar secretion has been beset by technical obstacles in particular in the collection of secretion both from *in vivo* and *in vitro* preparations.

Our knowledge of its composition is derived from cytochemical and ultrastructural studies: protein, lipid and carbohydrate are present intracellularly but whether they are secreted as lipoprotein, glycoprotein or glycolipid is not known.

There is more speculation than knowledge regarding its physical properties. Functional studies carried out in excised lungs suggest that the bronchiolar secretion acts as a surfactant-like material stabilizing the small airways (Macklem *et al.*, 1970). Mucociliary clearance in distal airways is slower than in large airways, the reduction in ciliary activity and decrease in height of the cilia in this region doubtless influencing mucus transport. The histochemical features of the secretory granules indicate that the secretion is different from that of the mucous cells and thus will have different viscoelastic properties, probably being less viscous.

Alveolar secretion

Alveolar surfactant: origin

The alveolar epithelium is composed of a continuous layer of squamous pneumonocytes—type I cells—and agranular pneumonocytes—type II cells. Type I cells cover 95 per cent of the alveolar surface; they are flattened cells with broad and thin extensions 0.1 to 0.3 μm thick. Cytoplasmic organelles are sparse and pynocytic vesicles are often observed. Type II cells are cuboidal which explains why, although more numerous than type I cells, they only occupy 5 per cent of the alveolar surface. They have blunt microvilli and contain multivesicular bodies, osmiophilic lamellated indurian bodies, mitochondria, peroxisomes, rough endoplasmic reticulum and a prominent Golgi apparatus (Sorokin, 1961; Petrik, 1971).

A third cell type—brush alveolar or type III cell—was first described by Meyrick and Reid (1968) in rat lung and is also present in human alveoli although very rarely (Weibel, 1973). Their function is unknown but like their counterpart in the large airways they may play a role in water absorption.

Both type I and II cells are covered by a glycocalyx which is thicker in type II cells (400 Å) than in type I cells (100 Å). Enzymes in particular alkaline phosphatase sterases and catalases containing peroxisomes are present in type II cells (Petrik, 1971). The function of peroxisomes has been linked to gluconeogenesis, carbohydrate oxidation, lipid metabolism and respiration and it has been suggested that they may play a role in protecting the cell against oxygen toxicity (deCuve, 1969).

Intracellular pulmonary surfactant

Macklin (1954) was probably the first to suggest that alveolar surfactant was produced by type II cells. Indirect evidence that these cells are responsible for the synthesis, storage and secretion of surfactant was provided by cytochemical studies (Sorokin, 1961) and investigations in fetal lungs (Wang *et al.*, 1971). Cell culture studies provided definite evidence that the type II cells synthesise and secrete surface-active material (Mason and Dobbs, 1980).

Alveolar liquid *in situ*

An extracellular duplex lining consisting of an epiphase and a hypophase has been identified in mammalian lung alveoli using vascular perfusion fixation (Weibel and

Gil, 1968) and freeze-fracture techniques (Kuhn, 1972). The film facing the alveolar space—the epiphase—is rich in highly surface active phospholipids while the hypophase contains mainly proteins, carbohydrate and phospholipids but in a different physicochemical configuration (Scarpelli *et al.*, 1973).

Synthesis and control

Our knowledge of the metabolic pathways associated with the synthesis of the different components of surfactant—phospholipids, protein, carbohydrate—is still fragmentary (King, 1982). Most of the work has centred on the metabolic pathways of diphosphotidyl choline. The combination of cytidine diphosphate (CDP)—choline and diaglycerol forms phosphotidyl choline. Most of the phosphatidic acid which is the precursor of diaglycerol goes through the Kennedy pathway (King, 1982), but it can also be formed by the reduction of acyldihydroactenone.

The pathway followed for the synthesis of phosphatidyl glycerol is not completely known and additional information is required.

The regulation of the secretion of surfactant is affected by β-adrenergic agonists (Brown and Longmore, 1981; Oyarzun and Clements, 1978) probably acting through cAMP. Cholinergic drugs modulate the secretion of surfactant but it has been suggested that they are acting via the β-adrenergic system (Massaro *et al.*, 1982). Prostaglandins can also affect surfactant secretion but more work is needed in this area (Massaro *et al.*, 1982; Oyarzun and Clements, 1978).

The effect of glucocorticoids on surfactant secretion in fetal lungs is well established (Strang, 1977) and they are being used in the treatment of the respiratory distress syndrome (RDS). Thyroid hormones—L-thyroxine—also increase surfactant secretion (Wu *et al.*, 1973).

Different modes of ventilation, even sighs, and ventilatory rate influence surfactant secretion (Oyarzun and Clements, 1978; Thet *et al.*, 1979; Massaro, 1981).

Chemical composition

Pulmonary surfactant is a complex lipoprotein material consisting of lipid (90 per cent), protein (8 per cent) and carbohydrate (2 per cent). The lipid composition is given in *Table 2.1*.

Dipalmitoyl phosphatidylcholine (DPPC) is the major phospholipid component and it is the only phospholipid present in sufficient amount to form a monomolecular film over the entire alveolar surface at functional residual capacity (FRC).

Although several phospholipids have surface active properties, DPPC lowers the surface tension of surfactant below 10 μdyn cm^{-1}. Other phospholipids also have an effect on the physical properties of surfactant; unsaturated phosphatidylcholine and

TABLE 2.1. Lipid composition of pulmonary surfactant

Saturated phosphatidylcholine	45%
Unsaturated phosphatidylcholine	25%
Phosphatidyl glycerols	5%
Phosphatidyl ethanolamines	3%
Neutral lipids	10%
Other phospholipids	2%

phosphoglycerol accelerate the surface adsorption and spreading of surfactant (King and Macbeth, 1981).

Several proteins have been identified in alveolar lavage fluid, the major protein component, apolipoprotein A, is a large molecule 3.5–4.0 × 10^4 MW and is probably synthesized only by type II cells. Apolipoprotein A may be involved in the formation of tubular myelin and facilitates the interfacial adsorption of surfactant. A smaller protein molecule, apolipoprotein B (MW $\simeq 10^4$), is also present in alveolar fluid and investigations suggest that it may be a breakdown product of the apolipoprotein A.

Recent findings indicate that apolipoprotein B facilitates the uptake of phospholipid by type II cells (Chander *et al.*, 1981).

The ultimate fate of surfactant is not completely known. Surfactant is cleared by: ingestion by alveolar macrophages (King and Martin, 1980); uptake and metabolism by type II cells (Desai *et al.*, 1978); and transport to large airways by the mucociliary escalator.

Osmiophilic lamellated bodies have been identified in the mucus layer (epiphase) of large airways (Yoneda, 1976).

Lipids with surface activity have been identified in sputum from patients with chronic bronchitis (Havez, 1969).

Saturated phosphatidylcholines have been described in sputum from patients with cystic fibrosis, bronchiectasis and chronic bronchitis (Galabert *et al.*, 1981).

On the other hand, animal studies suggest that tracheal clearance does not play a major role in the clearance of alveolar surfactant (Fisher *et al.*, 1979).

Physical properties/functions

Pulmonary surfactant lowers surface tension at the air-alveolar interface and by doing so reduces the work of expanding the lung. In recent years interest has been focused on the surface active properties of various biological and synthetic surfactants and their clinical use in the management of respiratory distress syndrome not only in infants but also in adults.

The cationic nature of some phospholipids, in particular DPL, enables them to be attached quite firmly to any negatively charged surface. As a result of this their long carbohydrate chains provide a hydrophobic surface which acts as a water-repellent and helps to keep the alveolar surface dry.

Cationic phospholipids are widely used in industry as fabric softeners and this property may contribute to maintain the integrity of the alveolar architecture (Hill, 1981).

Alveolar macrophages

Alveolar macrophages play a key role in the non-specific defence mechanism of the lung. They are large pleomorphic cells 20–40 μm in diameter; they are characterized by a ruffled surface membrane with numerous foot processes and a large number of intracytoplasmic granules—lysosomes and phagosomes. Most alveolar macrophages derive from the haematopoietic system and although some studies indicate that they can also originate from epithelial type II cells, interstitial histiocytes and mesenchymal cells, these findings need to be investigated further (Brain *et al.*, 1977).

The main function of the alveolar macrophage is to phagocytose almost any foreign material as well as endogenous cells and materials reaching the alveoli. Phagocytosis is a complex process which involves adhesion, ingestion and digestion. Adhesion is influenced by the physicochemical properties of both the particle and the surface membrane of the macrophage. Adhesion can be due to electrostatic attraction or attachment to specific receptors. Certain proteins—opsonins—render the extracellular particle more adherent to the surface membrane and coating of the particles by surfactant enhances phagocytosis. Ingestion can take place either by interiorization of vacuoles, surface cavitation or pseudopodic formation. Lysosomal hydrolases, proteases and elastases digest a variety of organic materials including antigens. The oxygen dependent enzymatic system—peroxidases—is of great importance in the bactericidal activity of alveolar macrophages.

Macrophages leave the alveoli via three different pathways. The more important clearance pathway is directly via the airways, the particle-laden macrophages reach the mucociliary escalator by passing along the bronchiolar ciliated epithelium or from alveolus to alveolus through the pores of Kohn. Between 1×10^6 and $5 \times 10^6\,h^{-1}$ macrophages are cleared by the airways and the clearance time is approximately 24 hours.

The mechanisms involved in the movement of particles and macrophages from the alveolus to the bronchiolar ciliated epithelium are still at the hypothetical rather than factual phase. A chemotactic gradient has been suggested by some authors but this will apply only to macrophages and has not been confirmed. The other proposed mechanisms involve physical properties and mechanical forces. Gross (1953) proposed the existence of a viscosity gradient within the alveolar fluid layer owing to evaporation of water from the fluid film, respiratory movements helping particles to drift along the broncho-alveolar junction. Kilburn (1968) favoured the hypothesis that particles and macrophages were removed from the alveoli by the influence of surface forces. For Hilding (1965) it was the cohesion forces of the bronchiolar 'mucus' together with the propulsive power of cilia. More recently Sorokin and Brain (1975) proposed that there is a flow of fluid from the alveoli to the bronchioles, which is fed by transudation from the pulmonary blood flow capillaries as well as by cell secretions and is helped by respiratory movements of the lungs.

In the second pathway the macrophages also reach the bronchiolar lumen via the lymphoid tissue located at the broncho-alveolar junction. The macrophages migrate into the septal interstitium and are then carried by the interstitial fluid to the lymphoid tissue. The time course of this clearance pathway is 1 to 14 days.

Macrophages can also be transported from the interstitial tissue centrifugally in the lymphatic fluid to subpleural or paraseptal positions or to the hilar lymph nodes and thoracic duct and finally to the systemic circulation. This pathway contributes very little to alveolar clearance and the half-life for this transport is of the order of 100 days.

Lung secretions in disease

Mucus hypersecretion is a protective mechanism of the tracheobronchial tree against inhaled irritants, infection and acute antigen challenge. When the stimulus persists for a long period of time the mucus secreting structures—mucous cells and glands—respond with hyperplasia and hypertrophy and the protective mechanism becomes disease. The basic difference between health and disease is that a normal individual does not produce sputum spontaneously, while in disease cough and expectoration—hypersecretion—are always present whether in a chronic form as seen in chronic bronchitis, bronchiectasis and late stages of cystic fibrosis or intermittently as in asthma and the early stages of cystic fibrosis. Mucous gland hypertrophy and an increase in number and size of secretory cells within the surface epithelium are the major pathological features of mucus hypersecretion and are found in chronic bronchitis as well as in cystic fibrosis and occasionally in asthma. Thickening of the basement membrane, mucosal oedema and shedding of the epithelium are characteristic findings in asthma and they contribute to the narrowing of the airway lumen (Lopez-Vidriero and Reid, 1983).

Abnormalities of the ciliated cells have been described in patients with chronic bronchitis, cystic fibrosis, bronchiectasis and asthma. The most common abnormalities are blebbing of the surface membrane, compound cilia and increase or decrease in number of doublets, singlets or accessory singlets (*Figures 2.4*, *2.5* and *2.6*). Similar abnormalities have been found in normal bronchial tissue (Fox *et al.*, 1981).

There is no direct evidence that ciliary activity is affected *in vivo* in chronic bronchitis, asthma, cystic fibrosis and bronchiectasis. In all these diseases mucociliary transport has been found to be impaired *in vivo* but whether it is due to abnormalities of mucus or cilia or both is not clear. *In vitro* studies of ciliary activity in nasal epithelium from patients with chronic bronchitis, cystic fibrosis and bronchiectasis suggest that ciliary activity is within normal limits (Rutland and Cole, 1981). These results are based on measurements taken only from vigorously beating cilia; when studying differences between normal and disease and between diseases objective rather than subjective criteria for measuring ciliary activity should be applied (Lopez-Vidriero and Clarke, 1982).

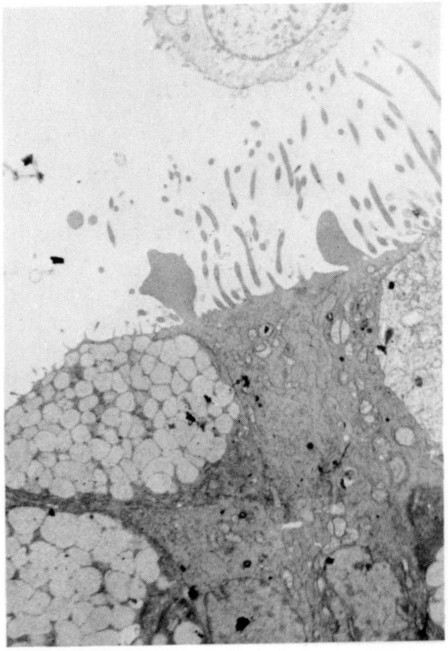

Figure 2.4 Transmission electron micrograph showing cytoplasmic blebs on the apical portion of a ciliated cell (×2850)

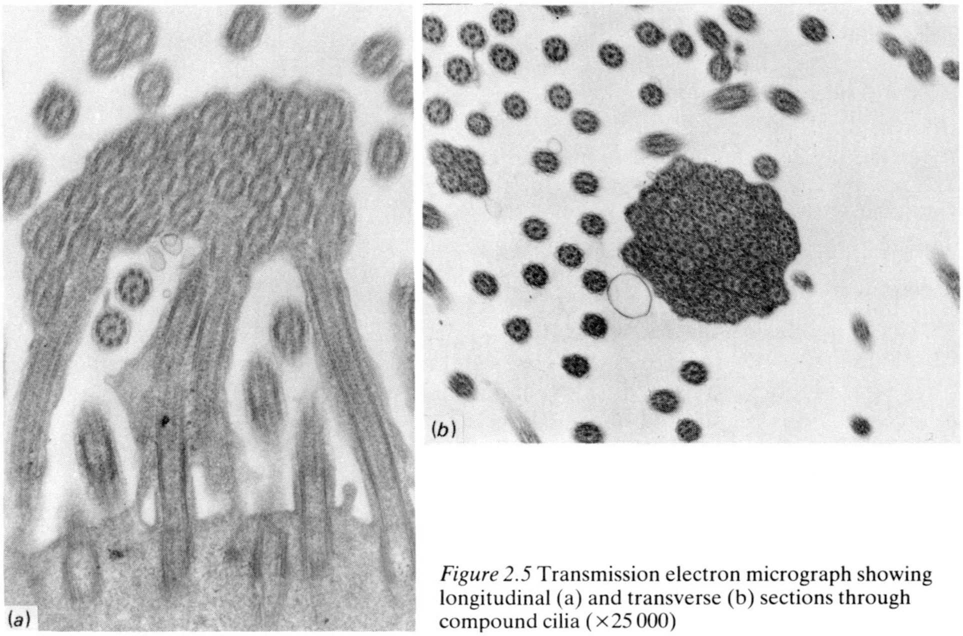

Figure 2.5 Transmission electron micrograph showing longitudinal (a) and transverse (b) sections through compound cilia (×25 000)

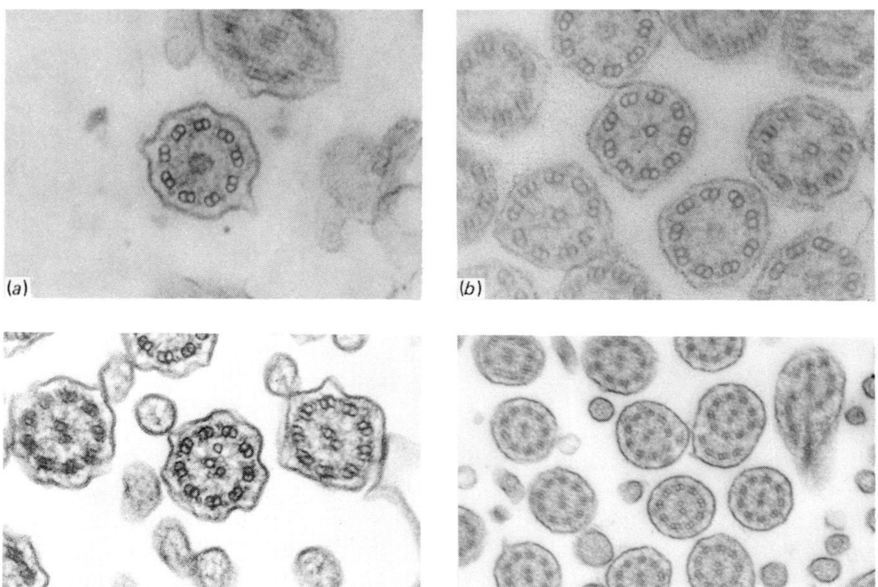

Figure 2.6 Transmission electron micrographs of abnormal axonemes of cilia in transverse section: (a) missing central microtubules (×66 666), (b) missing one central microtubule (×66 666) and (c and d) supernumerary outer microtubules (×33 333, 66 666)

Changes in the type of intracellular glycoprotein are common to all diseases characterized by mucus hypersecretion (Jones and Reid, 1978). There is an increase in the cell population producing acid glycoproteins and in particular those containing neuraminidase resistant and sulphated glycoproteins. These changes have been described in chronic bronchitis, cystic fibrosis and in some cases of asthma (Jones and Reid, 1978; Lopez-Vidriero and Reid, 1983).

A great deal is known about the chemical constituents, viscoelastic properties and transportability of airway mucus in various diseases particularly chronic bronchitis, cystic fibrosis, asthma and bronchiectasis (Lopez-Vidriero *et al.*, 1977; Puchelle *et al.*, 1981). In contrast information regarding the nature of normal mucus is sparse, making it almost impossible to ascertain if differences between normal and disease are quantitative, qualitative or both.

Airway mucus from patients with hypersecretion contains more macromolecular material than normal mucus and this is due to an increase in the mucus glycoprotein component, tissue fluid transudate (proteins), lipids and, when infection is present, DNA (Lopez-Vidriero *et al.*, 1977).

Although there is an overlap between various diseases in the concentration and proportion of glycoprotein, proteins, lipids and DNA, certain relevant differences exist (Lopez-Vidriero *et al.*, 1977a). The total amount of macromolecular material and proportion of its constituents vary more between macroscopic types of sputum—non-infected and infected—within a disease than between diseases for a given macroscopic type. Infected sputum, in particular from cystic fibrosis, contains large amounts of DNA and the protein component tends to be higher than in non-infected and infected sputum from other diseases. Asthmatic sputum shows a wide variation in chemical constituents, while tissue fluid transudate component and lipids tend to be higher than in chronic bronchitic sputum. Recent studies have shown that asthmatic sputum possesses a feature which is not found in other diseases—no mucus glycoprotein is found in the sol phase; the clinical implications of this finding are not known (Bhaskar and Reid, 1982).

Information is lacking on the effect of disease on mucosal transport of water and ion transport, which may affect the periciliary layer and mucus hydration.

The viscoelastic properties of normal secretion are still almost unknown. The apparent viscosity of sputum produced by normal individuals after inhaling prostaglandin $F_{2\alpha}$ falls within the low range of chronic bronchitis sputum. Unfortunately no information is available on the elastic properties of normal secretion. The viscoelastic properties of sputum from various diseases follow the same pattern of variation as that described for its chemical constituents. All diseases show a wide variation in levels of viscosity and elasticity and they seem to be trends rather than differences between diseases and macroscopic types of sputum (Lopez-Vidriero *et al.*, 1977a; Mitchell-Heggs, 1977). Infected sputum tends to be more viscous than non-infected and within infected sputum no differences have been found between sputum from chronic bronchitis, cystic fibrosis and bronchiectasis. Asthmatic sputum tends to be more viscous than chronic bronchitic sputum.

Mitchell-Heggs (1977) measured the elasticity of non-infected and infected sputa from patients with chronic bronchitis, cystic fibrosis, bronchiectasis and asthma over a range of frequencies (0.01–0.791 Hz). He found that sputum elasticity increased with shear rate but at any one shear rate there was a wide variation between sputum samples, and no differences emerged either between macroscopic types or between diseases. At low frequencies viscosity and elasticity are strongly correlated in all diseases, samples with high viscosity being more elastic and vice versa. In contrast at high frequencies sputum from chronic bronchitics and cystic fibrotics showed no correlation. It is probable that these findings may have an important effect on mechanical coupling and cough. During cough high shear rates are applied to the mucus and the dissociation between viscosity and elasticity could facilitate the propulsion of mucus by cough.

The optimal viscoelastic properties of mucus for clearance of secretion by cough are not as well defined as those required for ciliary transport. If the mucus is either too thin or too thick it will be cleared inefficiently by cough (Clarke *et al.*, 1970).

Experimental animal studies have shown that in SO_2 induced mucus hypersecretion the viscoelastic properties of mucus change, but they do so in such a way that they increase *in vitro* transportability, which suggests some compensatory mechanism to overcome the increased load and loss of ciliated epithelium (King, 1978).

Transportability of airway mucus from different diseases, in particular chronic bronchitis, has been studied *in vitro* using the frog palate preparation (Puchelle *et al.*, 1981; Chen and Dulfano, 1978). In chronic bronchitis the transportability of mucus varies with the stage of the disease, and shows a gradual decrease with the duration and severity of the disease.

It is of interest to note that some samples with viscoelastic properties outside the predicted optimal range showed normal transport rates, suggesting that other factors influence the control of mucociliary transport.

Serum, urine and saliva from patients with cystic fibrosis contain a substance(s) that affects the pattern of beating of cilia *in vitro* (Spock *et al.*, 1967; Conover *et al.*, 1973; Wilson and Fudenberg, 1977). This substance, known as ciliary dyskinesia factor, is a small molecular weight protein ($5–9 \times 10^3$) possibly related to the complement, kinin or fibrinolytic systems. Ciliary dyskinesia factors have also been identified in serum from patients with chronic obstructive airways disease, particularly asthmatics (Wilson and Fudenberg, 1977). Serum from asthmatic patients also contains a ciliostatic factor which differs biochemically from that found in cystic fibrosis.

Recent studies have shown that the sol phase of some sputum samples from patients with extrinsic and intrinsic asthma cause ciliostasis of respiratory cilia *in vitro* (Dulfano *et al.*, 1982; Dulfano and Luk, 1982). The ciliary inhibitory effect seems to be related to the type of sputum—slurry type—and clinical stage of the disease rather than to the type of asthma. The reversibility of the inhibitory effect indicates that the mechanism is functional rather than secondary to structural damage of the ciliated epithelium. The sol phase of sputum from normal subjects and from patients with chronic obstructive lung disease, except in few individuals, has no ciliostatic effect *in vitro* (Dulfano *et al.*, 1982).

Bronchiolar secretion in disease

The major obstruction to airflow in chronic bronchitis occurs in the small airways (<2 mm in diameter) and it is mainly due to intrinsic changes in these airways.

Experimental animal models of human chronic bronchitis have shown that the bronchioles respond to chronic irritation by transforming their cell population. The number of Clara cells decreases and they are replaced by mucous cells (Jeffery and Reid, 1977). Similar findings have been reported by several authors in human airways (Cosio *et al.*, 1980; Ebert and Terracio, 1975; Bignon *et al.*, 1976) and there is evidence that the bronchioles secrete mucus glycoprotein (Ebert and Hanks, 1981).

The difficulty of obtaining mucus secretion from the peripheral airways without contamination with alveolar liquid impairs our knowledge of the nature of this secretion both in health and disease.

Alveolar secretion

Alveolar surfactant and its role in disease has been thoroughly investigated in the infant respiratory distress syndrome (IRDS) (Strang, 1977). Recent interest has focused on its role in adult respiratory diseases including respiratory distress syndrome (ARDS), chronic bronchitis, emphysema and cystic fibrosis. The results are sparse and it is too early to reach any meaningful conclusions.

References

AZZOPARDI, A. and THURLBECK, W.M. (1969). The histochemistry of the non-ciliated bronchiolar epithelial cell. *Am. Rev. Resp. Dis.*, **99**, 516–525

BENSCH, K.G., GORDON, A.B. and MILLER, L.R. (1965). Studies on the bronchial counterpart of the Kultschitsky (argentaffin) cell and innervation of bronchial glands. *J. Ultrastruct. Res.*, **12**, 668–686

BHASKAR, K.R. and REID, L. (1982). Application of density gradient methods for the study of mucus glycoprotein and other macromolecular components of the sol and gel phases of asthmatic sputa. *J. Biol. Chem.*, **256**, 7583–7589

BHASKAR, K.R. O'SULLIVAN, D.D., LOPEZ-VIDRIERO, M.T., REID, L., DRAZEN, J.M. and INGRAM, R.H. (1982a). Characterization of canine bronchial mucus before and after exposure to SO_2. *Chest*, **81**, 39S–41S

BHASKAR, K.R., O'SULLIVAN, D.D., LOPEZ-VIDRIERO, M.T. and REID, L. (1982b). Characterisation of sol and gel phases of infected and mucoid sputum samples from a chronic bronchitis patient. In *Mucus in Health and Disease*, edited by Chantler, E.N., Elder, J.B. and Elstein, M. pp. 361–364. New York and London; Plenum Press

BIGNON, J., DEPIERRE, A., ANDRE-BOUGARAN, J. and HEM, B. (1976). Contribution of morphometry, bronchial casts and electron microscopy to the study of airway obstruction in chronic obstructive lung disease. *Proc. R. Soc. Med.*, **69**, 128–129

BOAT, T.F. and KLEINERMAN, J.I. (1975). Human respiratory tract secretions. 2. Effect of cholinergic and adrenergic agents on *in vitro* release of protein and mucus glycoprotein. *Chest*, **67**, 325–345

BRAIN, J.D., SOROKIN, S.P. and GODLESKI, J.J. (1977). Quantification, origin and fate of pulmonary macrophages. In *Respiratory Defense Mechanisms*, Part II. Edited by Brain, J.D. and Proctor, D.F. pp. 849–892. New York, Basle; Marcel Dekker

BROWN, L.A.S. and LONGMORE, W.J. (1981). Adrenergic and cholinergic regulation of lung surfactant secretion in isolated perfused rat lung and in the alveolar type II cell in culture. *J. Biol. Chem.*, **256**, 66–72

CHANDER, A., CLAYPOOL, W.D. Jr. and FISHER, A.B. (1981). Mechanism of liposomal phosphatidyl choline uptake by granular pneumonocytes. *Physiologist*, **24**, 104

CHEN, T.M. and DULFANO, M.J. (1978). Mucus viscoelasticity and mucociliary transport rate. *J. Lab. Clin. Med.*, **91**, 423–431

CLARA, M. (1937). Zur histobiologie des bronchalepithels. *Z. Mikr. Anat. Forsch.*, **41**, 321–347

CLARKE, S.W. and LOPEZ-VIDRIERO, M.T. (1983). The effect of a beta 2 agonist on the activity of human bronchial cilia *in vitro*. *J. Physiol.*, **332**, 56P

CLARKE, S.W., JONES, J.G. and OLIVER, D.R. (1970). Resistance to two-phase gas-liquid flow in airways. *J. Appl. Physiol.*, **29**, 464–471

COBURN, R.F. and TOMITA, T. (1973). Evidence for non-adrenergic inhibitory nerves in guinea pig trachealis muscle. *Am. J. Physiol.*, **224**, 1072–1080

COLES, S. (1977). Regulation of the secretory cycles of mucous and serous cells in the human bronchial gland. In *Mucus in Health and Disease*. Edited by Elstein, M. and Parke, D.V., pp. 155–168. New York, Basel; Plenum Press

COLES, S.J., BHASKAR, K.R., O'SULLIVAN, D.D. and REID, L. (1982). Macromolecular composition of secretion produced by human bronchial explants. In *Mucus in Health and Disease*. Edited by Chantler, E.N., Elder, J.B. and Elstein, M., pp. 357–360. New York, London; Plenum Press

COLES, S.J., SAID, S.I. and REID, L. (1981). Inhibition by vasoactive intestinal peptide of glycoconjugate and lysozome secretion by human airways *in vitro*. *Am. Rev. Respir. Dis.*, **124**, 531–536

CONOVER, J.H., BONFORTE, R.J., HATHAWAY, P., PACIUC, S., CONOD, E.J., HIRSCHHORN, K. and KOPEL, F.B. (1973). Studies on ciliary dyskinesia factor in cystic fibrosis. Bioassay and heterozygote detection in serum. *Pediatr. Res.*, **7**, 220–223

COSIO, M.G., HALE, K.A. and NIEWOEHNER, D.E. (1980). Morphologic and morphometric effects of prolonged cigarette smoking on the small airways. *Am. Rev. Resp. Dis.*, **122**, 265–271

CREETH, J.M., BHASKAR, K.R., HORTON, J.R., DAS, I., LOPEZ-VIDRIERO, M.T. and REID, L. (1977). The separation and characterization of bronchial glycoprotein by density-gradient methods. *Biochem. J.*, **167**, 557–569

CUTZ, E. and CONEN, P.E. (1971). Ultrastructure and cytochemistry of Clara cells. *Am. J. Path.*, **62**, 127–142

de CUVE, C. (1969). The peroxisome. A new cytoplasm organelle. *Proc. R. Soc. Lond. (Biol.)*, **173**, 71–83

DESAI, R., TETLEY, T.D., CURTIS, C.G., POWELL, G.M. and RICHARDS, R. (1978). Studies on the fate of pulmonary surfactant in the lung. *Biochem. J.*, **176**, 455–462

DEY, R. and SAID, S. (1980). Immunocytochemical localization of VIP-immunoreactive nerves in bronchial walls and pulmonary vessels. *Fed. Proc.*, **39**, 1062

DULFANO, M.J. and LUK, C.K. (1982). Sputum and ciliary inhibition in asthma. *Thorax*, **37**, 646–651

DULFANO, M.J., LUK, C.K., BECKAGE, M. and WOOTEM, O. (1981). Ciliary beat frequency in human explants. *Am. Rev. Respir. Dis.*, **123**, 139–140

DULFANO, M.J., LUK, C.K., BECKAGE, M. and WOOTEM, O. (1982). Ciliary inhibitory effects of asthma patients' sputum. *Clin. Sci.*, **63**, 393–396

EBERT, R.V. and HANKS, P. (1981). Mucus secretion by the epithelium of the bronchioles of cigarette smokers. *Br. J. Dis. Chest*, **75**, 277–282

EBERT, R.V. and TERRACIO, M.J. (1975). The bronchiolar epithelium in cigarette smokers. Observations with the scanning microscope. *Am. Rev. Respir. Dis.*, **111**, 4

EBERT, R.V., KRONENBERG, R.S. and TERRACIO, M.J. (1976). Study of the surface secretion of the bronchiole using radioautography. *Am. Rev. Respir. Dis.*, **114**, 567–573

FISHER, H.K., HYMAN, M.H. and ASHCRAFT, S.J. Alveolar surfactant phospholipids are not cleared via trachea. *Fed. Proc.*, **38**, 1373

FOX, B., BULL, T.B., BAKEY, A.R. and RAWBONE, R. (1981). The significance of ultrastructural abnormalities of human cilia. *Chest*, **80**, 796–799

GALABERT, C., FILLIAT, M. and LAMBLIN, G. (1981). Lipid analysis of sputum from patients with chronic bronchial diseases. *Bull. Eur. Physiopath. Respir.*, **17**, 197–208

GALLAGHER, J.T., HALL, R.L., JEFFERY, P.K., PHIPPS, R.J. and RICHARDSON, P.S. (1978). The nature and origin of tracheal secretions released in response to pilocarpine and ammonia. *J. Physiol.*, **275**, 36P–37P

GIL, J. and WEIBEL, E.R. (1971). Extracellular lining of bronchioles after perfusion-fixation of rat lungs for electron microscopy. *Anat. Rec.*, **169**, 185–200

GILULA, N.B. and SATIR, P. (1972). The ciliary necklace. A ciliary membrane specialization. *J. Cell Biol.*, **53**, 494–509

GROSS, P. (1953). The mechanisms of dust clearance from the lung: A theory. *Am. J. Clin. Pathol.*, **23**, 116–120

HAVEZ, R. (1969). Freie und gebundone Formen des Surfactant in Expektorat. *Dtsch. Med. J.*, **21**, 1–13

HILDING, A.C. (1965). Mucociliary insufficiency and its possible relation to chronic bronchitis and emphysema. *Med. Thorac.*, **22**, 329–345

HILL, S. (1981). What is the true role of surfactant in the lung? *Thorax*, **36**, 1–4

HOGG, J.C., MACKLEM, P.T. and THURLBECK, W.M. (1968). Size and nature of airway obstruction in chronic obstructive lung disease. *New Engl. J. Med.*, **278**, 1355–1360

INOUE, S. and HOGG, J.C. (1977). Freeze-etching study of the tracheal epithelium of normal guinea pigs with particular reference to intercellular junctions. *J. Ultrastruct. Res.*, **61**, 89–99

JEFFERY, P.K. (1978). Structure and function of mucus-secreting cells of cat and goose airway epithelium. In *Respiratory Tract Mucus*. Ciba Foundation Symposium 54, pp. 5–23. North-Holland; Elsevier Excerpta Medica

JEFFERY, P.K. and REID, L. (1975). New features of rat airway epithelium—a quantitative and electron-microscopic study. *J. Anat.*, **120**, 295–320

JEFFERY, P.K. and REID, L. (1977). The respiratory mucous membrane. In *Respiratory Defence Mechanisms*. Edited by Brain, J.D. *et al.* pp. 193–238. New York; Marcel Dekker

JEFFERY, P.K., REID, L. and WIDDICOMBE, J.G. (1976). Anatomical and physiological features of irritation of the bronchial tree. In *Air Pollution and the Lung*. Edited by Aharonson, E.F. *et al*. pp. 253–267. Chichester; Wiley

JONES, R. and REID, L. (1978). Secretory cells and their glycoproteins in health and disease. *Br. Med. Bull.*, **34**, 9–16

KILBURN, K.H. (1968). A hypothesis for pulmonary clearance and its implications. *Am. Rev. Resp. Dis.*, **98**, 449–463

KING, M. (1979). Rheological requirements for optimal clearance of secretions: ciliary transport versus cough. *Eur. J. Respir. Dis.*, **110** (Suppl.), 39–46

KING, M., GILBOA, A., MEYER, F.A. and SILBERBERG, A. (1974). On the transport of mucus and its rheologic stimulants in ciliated systems. *Am. Rev. Resp. Dis.*, **110**, 740–745

KING, R.J. (1982). Pulmonary surfactant. *J. Appl. Physiol.*, **53**, 1–8

KING, R.J. and MACBETH, M.C. (1981). Interaction of the lipid and protein components of pulmonary surfactant. Role of phosphatidyl glycerol and calcium. *Biochem. Biophys. Acta*, **647**, 159–168

KING, R.J. and MARTIN, H. (1980). Intracellular metabolism of the apoproteins of pulmonary surfactant in rat lung. *J. Appl. Physiol.*, **48**, 812–820

KNOWLES, M.R., MURRAY, G.F., SHALLAL, J.A., GATZY, J.T. and BOUCHER, R.C. (1982). Ion transport in excised human bronchi and its neurohumoral control. *Chest*, **81**, 115–135

KUHN, C.III. (1972). A comparison of freeze-substitution with other methods for preservation of the pulmonary alveolar lining layer. *Am. J. Anat.*, **133**, 495–508

LITT, M.L. (1981). Physicochemical determinants of mucociliary flow. *Chest*, **80**, 846–849

LOPEZ-VIDRIERO, M.T. and CLARKE, S.W. (1982). Objective criteria for measuring ciliary beat frequency in vitro. *Am. Rev. Respir. Dis.*, **125**, 244

LOPEZ-VIDRIERO, M.T. and REID, L. (1980). Respiratory tract fluid—chemical and physical properties of airway mucus. *Eur. J. Respir. Dis.*, **110**, 21–26

LOPEZ-VIDRIERO, M.T. and REID, L. (1983). Pathological changes in asthma. In *Asthma*. Edited by Clark, T.J.H. and Godfrey, S., pp. 79–98, 2nd edn, London; Chapman and Hall

LOPEZ-VIDRIERO, M.T., DAS, I. and REID, L. (1977a). Airway secretion: Source, biochemical and rheological properties. In *Respiratory Defense Mechanisms*. Edited by Brain, J.D., Proctor, D.F. and Reid, L., pp. 247–288. New York, Basel; Marcel Dekker

LOPEZ-VIDRIERO, M.T., DAS, I., SMITH, P. and REID, L. (1977b). Bronchial secretion from normal human airways after inhalation of prostaglandin $F_{2\alpha}$, acetylcholine histamine and citric acid. *Thorax*, **32**, 734–739

LUCAS, A.M. and DOUGLAS, L.C. (1934). Principles underlying ciliary activity in the respiratory tract. II. A comparison of nasal clearance in man, monkey and other mammals. *Arch. Otolaryng.*, **20**, 518–541

MACKLEM, P.T., PROCTOR, D.F. and HOGG, J.C. (1970). The stability of peripheral airways. *Respir. Physiol.*, **8**, 191–203

MACKLIN, C.C. (1954). The pulmonary alveolar mucoid film and the pneumocytes. *Lancet*, **1**, 1099–1104

MASON, R.J. and DOBBS, L. (1980). Synthesis of phosphotidylcholine and phosphatidylglycerol by alveolar type II cells in primary culture. *J. Biol. Chem.*, **255**, 5101–5107

MASSARO, D. (1981). The cellular and molecular basis of pulmonary alveolar stability. *Lab. Clin. Invest.*, **98**, 155–165

MASSARO, D., CLERCH, D.L. and MASSARO, G.D. (1982). Surfactant secretion: evidence that cholinergic stimulation of secretion is indirect. *Am. J. Physiol.*, **243**, C39–C45

MASSARO, G.D., FISCHMAN, C.M., CHIANG, M.J., AMADO, C. and MASSARO, D. (1981). Regulation of secretion in Clara cells. Studies using the isolated perfused rat lung. *J. Clin. Invest.*, **67**, 345–351

MEYRICK, B. and REID, L. (1968). The alveolar brush cell in rat lung—a third pneumocyte. *J. Ultrastruct. Res.*, **23**, 71–80

MITCHELL-HEGGS, P. (1977). Physical properties of bronchial secretion. In *Mucus in Health and Disease*. Edited by Elstein, M. and Parke, D.V., pp. 203–215. New York, Basel; Plenum Press

OSCHMAN, J.L., and BERRIDGE, M.J. (1971). The structural basis of fluid secretion. *Fed. Proc.*, **30**, 49–56

OYARZUN, M.J. and CLEMENTS, J.A. (1978). Control of lung surfactant by ventilation, adrenergic mediators and prostaglandins in the rabbit. *Am. Rev. Respir. Dis.*, **117**, 879–891

PETRIK, P. (1971). Fine structural identification of peroxisomes in mouse and rat bronchiolar and alveolar epithelium. *J. Histochem. Cytochem.*, **19**, 339–348

PETRIK, P. and COLLET, A.J. (1974). Quantitative electron microscopic autoradiography of in vivo incorporation of ^{3}H choline, ^{3}H leucine, ^{3}H acetate and ^{3}H galactose in non-ciliated bronchiolar (Clara) cells of mice. *Am. J. Anat.*, **139**, 519–534

PHIPPS, R.J. and RICHARDSON, P. (1976). The effects of irritation at various levels of the airway upon tracheal mucus secretion in the cat. *J. Physiol. (Lond.)*, **261**, 563–581

PHIPPS, R.J., WILLIAMS, I., PACK, R.J. and RICHARDSON, P. (1982). Adrenergic stimulation of mucus secretion in human bronchi. *Chest*, **81**, 19S–20S

PUCHELLE, E., ZAHM, J-M. and AUG, F. (1981). Viscoelasticity, protein content and ciliary transport rate of sputum in patients with recurrent and chronic bronchitis. *Biorheology*, **18**, 659–666

RHODIN, J. (1966). Ultrastructure and function of the human tracheal mucosa. *Am. Rev. Respir. Dis.*, **93**, 1–15

RICHARDSON, J.B. (1979). Nerve supply to the lungs—State of the Art. *Am. Rev. Resp. Dis.*, **119**, 785–802

RICHARDSON, J.B. and BELAND, J. (1976). Non-adrenergic inhibitory nerves in human airways. *J. Appl. Physiol.*, **41**, 764–771

RUTLAND, J. and COLE, P. (1981). Non-invasive sampling of nasal cilia for measurement of beat frequency and study of ultrastructure. *Lancet*, **2**, 564–565

RUTLAND, J., GRIFFIN, W. and COLE, P. (1981). Nasal brushing and measurement of ciliary frequency. *Chest*, **80**, 865–867

SANDERSON, M.J. and SLEIGH, M.A. (1981). Ciliary activity of cultured rabbit tracheal epithelium: beat pattern and metachrony. *J. Cell Sci.*, **47**, 331–347

SCARPELLI, E.M., WOLFSON, D.R. and COLACICCO, G. (1973). Protein and lipid-protein fractions of lung washings: Immunological characterization. *J. Appl. Physiol.*, **34**, 750–753

SCHNEEBERGER, E.E. (1980). Heterogeneity of tight junction morphology in extrapulmonary and intrapulmonary airways of the rat. *Anat. Rec.*, **198**, 193–208

SERAFINI, S.M. and MICHAELSON, E.D. (1977). Length and distribution of cilia in human and canine airways. *Bull. Europ. Physiopath. Respir.*, **13**, 551–559

SHELHAMER, J.H., MAROM, Z. and KALINER, M. (1980). Immunologic and neuropharmacologic stimulation of mucous glycoprotein release from human airways *in vitro*. *J. Clin. Invest.*, **66**, 1400–1408

SHELHAMER, J.H., MAROM, Z., SUN, F., BACH, M.K. and KALINER, M. (1982). The effects of arachinoids and leukotrienes on the release of mucus from human airways. *Chest*, **81**, 36S–37S

SLEIGH, M.A. (1977). The nature and action of respiratory tract cilia. In *Respiratory Defense Mechanisms*. Part I. Edited by Brain, J.D., Proctor, D.F. and Reid, L., pp. 247–288. New York, Basel; Marcel Dekker

SLEIGH, M.A. (1981). Ciliary function in mucus transport. *Chest*, **80**, 791–795

SOROKIN, S.P. (1961). A morphological and cytochemical study of the great alveolar cell. *J. Histochem. Cytochm.*, **14**, 884–897

SOROKIN, S.P. and BRAIN, J.D. (1975). Pathways of clearance in mouse lungs exposed to iron dioxide aerosols. *Anat. Rec.*, **181**, 581–625

SPOCK, A., HEICK, H.M., CRESS, H. and LOGAN, W.S. (1967). Abnormal serum factor in patients with cystic fibrosis of the pancreas. *Pediatr. Res.*, **1**, 173–177

STRANG, L.B. (1977). *Neonatal Respiration Physiological and Clinical Studies*. Oxford; Blackwell Scientific Publications

STURGESS, J. (1977). Bronchial mucous secretion in cystic fibrosis. *Modern Probl. Pediatr.*, **19**, 129–140

STURGESS, J. and REID, L. (1972). An organ culture study of the effects of drugs on the secretory activity of the human bronchial submucosal glands. *Clin. Sci.*, **43**, 533–543

THET, L.A., CLERCH, L., MASSARO, G.D. and MASSARO, D. (1979). Changes in sedimentation of surfactant in ventilated excised rat lungs. Physical alterations in surfactant associated with the development and reversal of atelectasis. *J. Clin. Invest.*, **64**, 600–608

TOREMALM, N.G. (1960). The daily amount of tracheo-bronchial secretions in man. *Acta Orolaryngol. (Suppl.)*, **158**, 43–53

WANG, N.S., KOTAS, R.V., AVERY, M.E. and THURLBECK, W.M. (1971). Accelerated appearance of osmiophilic bodies in fetal lungs following steroid injection. *J. Appl. Physiol.*, **30**, 362–365

WEIBEL, E.R. (1973). Morphological basis of alveolar-capillary gas exchange. *Physiol. Rev.*, **53**, 419–495

WEIBEL, E.R. and GIL, J. (1968). Electron microscopic demonstration of an extracellular duplex lining layer of alveoli. *Respir. Physiol*, **4**, 42–57

WHIMSTER, W.F. and REID, L. (1973). The influence of dibutyryl cyclic adenosine monophosphate on human bronchial mucous gland discharge. *Exp. Mol. Pathol.*, **18**, 234–240

WIDDICOMBE, J.G. and PACK, R.J. (1982). The Clara cell. *Eur. J. Respir. Dis.*, **63**, 202–220

WILSON, G.B. and FUDENBERG, H.H. (1977). Ciliary dyskinesia factors in cystic fibrosis and asthma. *Nature*, **266**, 463–464

WU, B., KIKKAWA, Y., ORZALESI, M.M., MOTOYAMA, E.K., KAIBARA, M., ZIGAS, C.J. and COOK, C.D. (1973). The effect of thyroxine on the maturation of fetal rabbit lung. *Biologia Neonat.*, **22**, 161–168

YONEDA, K. (1976). Mucous blanket of rat bronchus. An ultrastructural study. *Am. Rev. Respir. Dis.*, **114**, 837–842

Chapter 3

Physical properties and mechanisms of deposition of aerosols

John E. Agnew

Aerosols

An aerosol comprises air plus fine liquid or solid particles suspended in the air. The properties of an aerosol are largely determined by interaction between the air and the particles. The particles must be sufficiently large not to diffuse like gas molecules and sufficiently small to remain airborne for some length of time. This implies a size range of about 0.01 to 100 μm (Fuchs, 1964; Morrow, 1981). An aerosol with liquid particles may be termed a 'mist'; the names 'dust' and 'smoke' are applied to solid particle aerosols produced respectively by dispersion and condensation (Fuchs, 1964). Liquid aerosol particles are essentially spherical although deformable but solid particles may vary greatly in shape.

A crucial factor to interaction between the air and the particles is the frequency with which gas molecules collide with any individual particle. The mean free path, λ, travelled by a molecule in air between successive collisions with other gas molecules is about 0.1 μm (under ordinary atmospheric conditions). For an aerosol particle of diameter, d, smaller than λ, collisions with gas molecules may be regarded as separate discrete events. The force exerted by the air on a moving particle is effectively determined by the cross-sectional target area the particle presents to moving gas molecules and by the velocity of the particle relative to the air. Resistance to relative motion of the particle is therefore proportional to the product of velocity and d^2.

With increasing particle size a transition occurs to sizes for which the air can be regarded as a continuous medium. The resistance offered by the air to a moving particle is then approximately given by Stokes' Law—and depends on the product of velocity, particle diameter and air viscosity. The derivation of Stokes' Law assumes there is no velocity discontinuity at the particle/air interface; in effect that the particle is surrounded by a very thin layer of air stationary with respect to the particle. Less force is exerted by the air on the particle when this condition is not met. The resulting reduction in resistance constitutes the phenomenon of 'slip' and can be important for particles of less than about 1 μm diameter (Fuchs, 1964; Vincent, 1980). Resistance greater than predicted by Stokes' Law tends to occur with increasing particle size or velocity; the force exerted on a 2–5 μm particle at airway bifurcations where an abrupt change occurs in airflow direction may, even under tidal breathing conditions, be some 5 per cent higher than that calculated from Stokes' Law. If necessary, correction factors—based on the product of particle diameter and velocity—may be applied (Vincent, 1980) but, in general, Stokes' Law does provide an adequate guide to particle/air interaction under most conditions of practical relevance.

It follows that where particles of different size have initially the same velocity the ratio of retarding force (proportional to d) to mass (proportional to d^3) is much higher for small particles than for large. Small particles accordingly travel a much shorter 'stop' distance before becoming stationary with respect to the air. This is made use of in the spinning disc generator (Chapter 4) for separating unwanted small satellite particles from the primary particles generated.

Gravitational sedimentation

In addition to air/particle interactions, particles in an aerosol are subject to external force fields (gravitational or electrostatic) and to particle/particle interactions. In practice however, interaction between particles may almost always be dismissed as negligible compared with the other forces (Fuchs, 1964).

Under Stokes' Law conditions, the velocity (v) at which a particle falls under gravity is given by

$$v = \tau g(1 - \exp(-t/\tau)) \tag{3.1}$$

with

$$\tau = \frac{\rho d^2}{18\eta}$$

where ρ is particle density, η is air viscosity and g is the gravitational constant. In fact, the exponential term rapidly approaches zero, simplifying the equation to

$$v_g = \tau.g \tag{3.2}$$

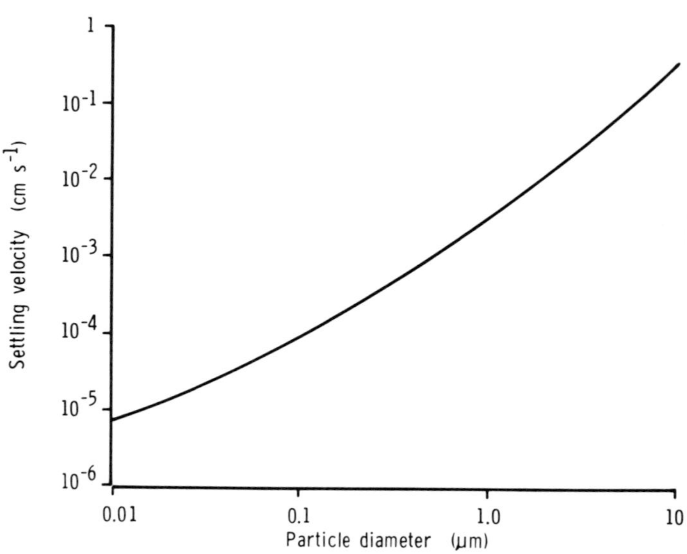

Figure 3.1 Terminal settling velocities for unit density particles, based on data for spherical oil drops falling in air at 23°C and standard atmospheric pressure (Fuchs, 1964). For particles not of unit density the velocities shown should be multiplied by particle density (in g cm^{-3})

The physical counterpart of this is that particles falling under gravity rapidly acquire a steady settling velocity (v_g) at which gravitational force is exactly balanced by air resistance. From Equation (3.1) it may be calculated that a unit density 4 μm particle reaches 90 per cent of its terminal settling velocity in less than 10^{-2} s; this represents less than 1 per cent of the typical transit time for airflow through any single generation of the bronchial tree for aerosols inhaled at 30 ℓ min^{-1} (a calculation based on the Weibel (1963) airways model). For all practical considerations of aerosol deposition in the lungs, particles may thus be considered to reach their terminal settling velocities instantaneously in stationary air. The dependence of settling velocity on particle size is illustrated in *Figure 3.1*—the values for small particles being corrected for slip (Fuchs, 1964).

Effect of inertia

When airflow containing aerosol particles is deflected, the force exerted by the air on the particles has to overcome the particles' inertia if they are to follow the change in airflow direction. For airflow of velocity U incident on a spherical obstacle of diameter D, the proportion of particles initially travelling towards the obstacle which will actually strike it is (Vincent, 1980) a function of a dimensionless number, the Stokes' number,

$$\mathrm{Stk} = \frac{\rho d^2 U}{18\eta D} \tag{3.3}$$

The higher the value of Stk the more readily particles will diverge from the airflow streamlines and the more likely they are therefore to deposit by impaction on the obstacle.

Particle size

Comparing Equations (3.1) and (3.3) it can be seen that both gravitational settling velocities and the inertial tendency not to follow changes in the direction of airflow streamlines depend on the product ρd^2. The square root of this product is known as the aerodynamic diameter of the particle. This is frequently used to describe the effective size of a particle under conditions where inertial impaction and gravitational sedimentation are the principal causes of deposition (roughly from d = 0.5 μm upwards). The concept of aerodynamic diameter may be applied to a particle of any shape, however irregular, and may be defined properly as the diameter of a unit density sphere which would undergo sedimentation at the same rate as the particle in question.

Sizes of solid aerosol particles may be measured by optical or electron microscopy after deposition on a suitable surface. For airborne particles geometrical diameters may be determined by various light scattering techniques. These include methods based on diffraction of laser beams as small particles diffract light through greater angles than large particles. Knowledge of particle density—not necessarily identical to that of the bulk material used in preparing the particles (Lippmann and Albert, 1969)—is required to translate geometrical diameters into aerodynamic diameters. Alternatively deposition properties may be used to assess aerodynamic diameters directly. Sedimentation is used in the horizontal elutriator based on the fact that deposition from an aerosol flowing between two horizontal plates depends on plate separation and length, settling velocity and mean air flow but not on the velocity profile of the airflow (Vincent, 1980). Impaction is used in the cascade impactor which consists of a series of air-jets impinging onto glass discs (or other inserts). Relatively large particles are deposited at the first impactor stage where low velocity at a coarse jet means that the smaller particles can easily follow the change in airflow direction. Progressively higher velocities at progressively finer jets lower stage-by-stage the size of particles able to follow the changes occurring in airflow direction.

Many aerosol preparations contain a very wide range of particle sizes and are classified as 'heterodisperse'. Often a plot of the particle size distribution resembles a Gaussian curve when particle number or mass is plotted against the logarithm of particle diameter (*Figure 3.2b*). For radioaerosol particles homogeneously prepared from radioactive solution, distribution of radioactivity is identical to that of mass. When pre-formed particles are surface-labelled with a radioactive agent radioactivity distribution will be the same as that of particle surface area. Re-plotting the log-normal distributions of *Figure 3.2b* on a linear scale (*Figure 3.2c*) emphasizes the important practical point that an extended 'tail' of large particle sizes may be present. The distribution pattern of deposited particle mass in the lungs may significantly depend on the fate of relatively few particles carrying a relatively high proportion of the total mass available. This is obviously important to the deposition pattern both of inhaled radioactive tracers and of inhaled drugs.

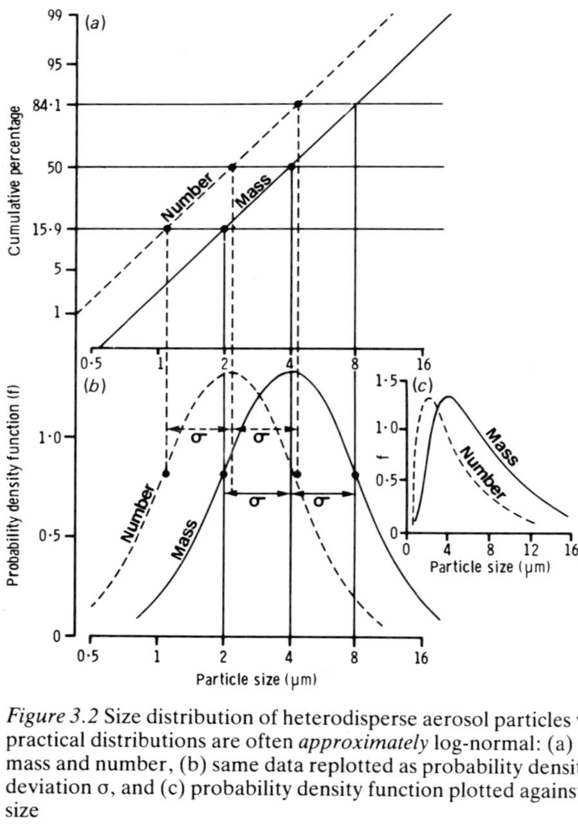

Figure 3.2 Size distribution of heterodisperse aerosol particles with a log-normal size distribution; practical distributions are often *approximately* log-normal: (a) cumulative probability plots for particle mass and number, (b) same data replotted as probability density, showing Gaussian curves of standard deviation σ, and (c) probability density function plotted against particle size but with a linear scale for size

Techniques for measuring particle size often yield estimates of particle number or mass in wide particle size bands. It is then convenient and accurate to plot the data in cumulative form on probability paper (*Figure 3.2a*); mean size and range can be directly obtained from the cumulative plot. Mean size (for particle number or for mass) can be expressed as the geometric mean diameter (GMD)—which is the diameter corresponding to 50 per cent probability on the cumulative plot. Size range can be read from the cumulative plot as the ratio of the diameter for 84.1 per cent cumulative probability to that for 50 per cent probability. This is the same as the ratio of the 50 per cent diameter to the 15.9 per cent diameter and is termed the geometric standard deviation (GSD). The values of 84.1 per cent and 15.9 per cent correspond to mean ±SD (σ) of the Gaussian curve (*Figure 3.2b*); ratios must be calculated because the horizontal scale is logarithmic.

A valuable property of the log-normal particle size distribution is that number, particle surface and mass all have the same GSD (and hence parallel cumulative probability plots). A measurement of MMAD (i.e. GMD for mass) plus GSD can therefore be translated into a measurement of mean and range for the distribution of particle number or surface area (Marple and Rubow, 1980).

Aerosols with a GSD of greater than 1.22 are generally termed 'heterodisperse'. The term 'monodisperse' is applied to those of lower GSD (Morrow, 1981) and usually carries the implication that the particles behave as though they are all of the same one size. The name 'multimodal' (Hiller *et al.*, 1982) has been applied to aerosols consisting of mixed monodisperse aerosols of different (and readily distinguishable) sizes.

Particle deposition in the upper airways

Far fewer large airborne particles are likely to reach the lungs when air is inhaled via the nose rather than via the mouth. Over a wide range of inhalation conditions, the nasal route functions as a much more effective particle filter than the oral route—and thus tends to protect the lungs against particulate pollutants in the atmosphere. In consequence the nose itself constitutes an important deposition site for some industrial pollutants—as in the furniture and shoe manufacturing industries and in chrome handling; ulceration and malignant changes in the septum and middle turbinates of exposed workers are attributed to localized dust deposition at these sites (Hounam and Morgan, 1977).

Experimental studies on head deposition during nose breathing have been reviewed by Lippmann (1977) who showed that the majority of results lay close to values predicted by a Task Group of the International Commission on Radiological Protection (*Figure 3.3*), indicating that deposition is proportional to $\log(d^2F)$ (where d = particle diameter and F = inhalation flow rate). The nasal passages are however distensible and there is some evidence that resistance rather than flow rate is the important determinant of deposition (Hounam and Morgan, 1977; Lippmann, 1977). Nasal resistance varies greatly between different people and this may account for marked inter-subject variability in nasal deposition.

The relationship of head deposition to $\log(d^2F)$ for mouth breathing also shown in *Figure 3.3* was obtained by direct measurement of radioaerosol deposition immediately after inhalation via a mouthpiece. During exercise most people tend to shift from nasal to mouth breathing—thereby lessening protection of the lung against particulate pollutants. Protection during natural mouth breathing may

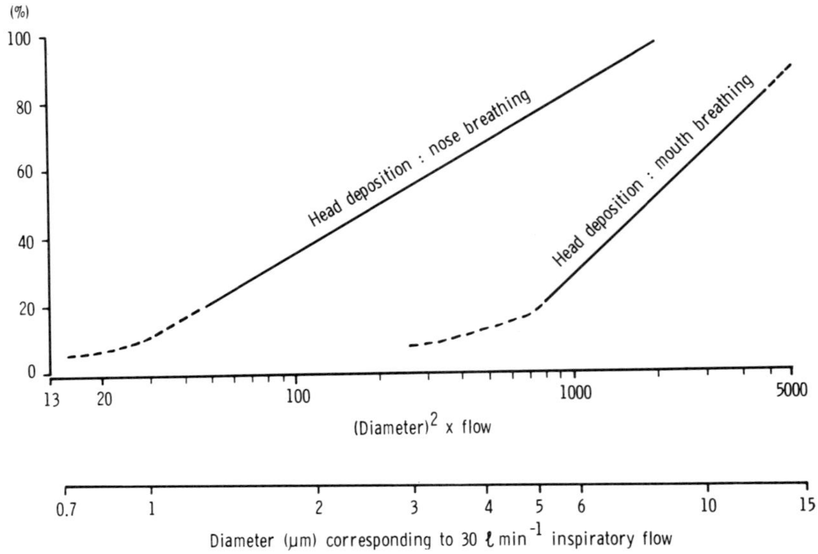

Figure 3.3 Deposition of inhaled particles in the head. The line for nose breathing is that of the International Commission on Radiological Protection which has been shown by Lippmann (1977) to correspond well to experimental results from a number of authors. The line for mouth breathing is based on experimental data of Lippmann (1977) using inhalation via a mouthpiece

however be higher than for inhalation through a mouthpiece (Hounam and Morgan, 1977; Swift and Proctor, 1982). Calculations based on the premise that this is so suggest that a negligible proportion of particles greater than 10 μm aerodynamic diameter can reach the lungs during natural oronasal breathing (Swift and Proctor, 1982). With inhalation via a mouthpiece, a significant proportion of such particles can, as shown in *Figure 3.3*, escape filtration in the head and therefore reach the lungs.

Nasal deposition of very small particles (<0.01 μm) may be produced by diffusion (Hounam and Morgan, 1977) but the dependence of head deposition on log (d^2F) from 1 μm upwards (nasal breathing) and from 4–5 μm upwards (mouthpiece breathing) indicates deposition predominantly by impaction, and transit times via either route are too short for significant sedimentation to occur.

Particle deposition in the lungs

Experimental studies have shown that some 90 per cent of inhaled 0.5 μm diameter particles normally reappear in the exhaled air under quiet tidal breathing conditions; even more can be recovered if tidal inhalation is followed by deep exhalation (Davies *et al.*, 1972; Taulbee *et al.*, 1978). These results show that no very effective mechanisms exist in the human lung for depositing particles of this size. Smaller particles tend to undergo greater deposition because of their increased diffusional mobility whereas large sizes are associated with a marked increase in total deposition which approaches 100 per cent for particles in the 5–10 μm range (Chan and Lippmann, 1980; Stahlhofen *et al.*, 1980). Deposition of large particles is generally attributable to the combined effects of inertial impaction and gravitational sedimentation. The former becomes predominantly important as particle size or velocity increase. The way both processes function in the lung may, roughly, be considered in terms of simple geometry (*Figure 3.4*). A change in airflow direction at an airway bifurcation may be represented by airflow through a curved tube (Landahl, 1950; Martonen, 1982). Particles of mass m in an aerosol entering the tube at velocity U are subjected to a centrifugal force of magnitude mU^2/r, where r is the radius of curvature of the airflow streamlines. Air/particle interaction provides an opposing force trying to keep the particle travelling along the streamline.

Particles initially at a distance less than Δ from the outer wall will be sufficiently displaced from their initial streamlines to come into contact with the airway wall. The value of Δ—which defines a 'limiting trajectory'—depends on the relative magnitude of the centrifugal and air/particle interaction forces. Fractional deposition is equal to the shaded area (*Figure 3.4*; top right) as a fraction of the total

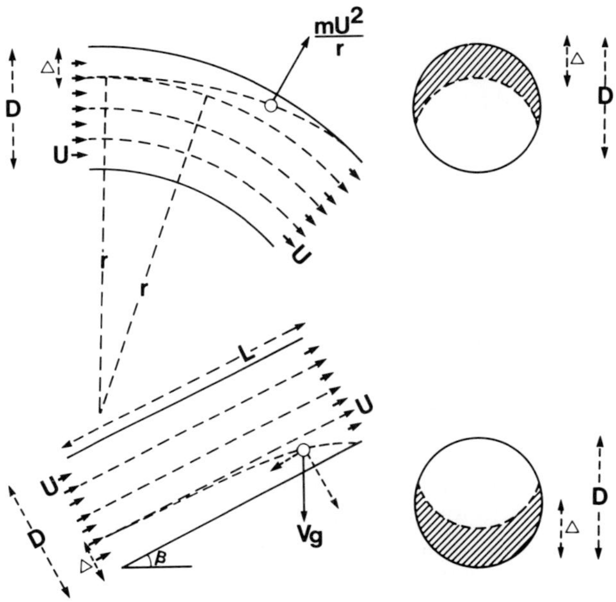

Figure 3.4 Deposition mechanisms for 1–10 μm particles in the conducting airways; geometrical illustration of the basis for semi-quantitative predictions of particle deposition per airway generation

cross-sectional area. A similar limiting trajectory may be defined for gravitational sedimentation. A particle entering an inclined tube and initially travelling at an angle β to the horizontal has a component of its gravitational settling velocity ($v_g \cos \beta$) directed towards the lower airway wall and a component ($v_g \sin \beta$) parallel to the airway walls. This latter component will tend to slow down the particle relative to the air for upwards flow (as illustrated) but speed it up for downwards flow. But the important component of v_g is that directed towards the airway wall. The limiting trajectory is defined by an initial distance Δ from the lower wall which depends on the value of $v_g \cos \beta$ relative to the transit time of the aerosol through the airway (L/U providing $v_g \sin \beta << L/U$). Deposition is again represented by the shaded area as a fraction of the total cross-sectional area (*Figure 3.4*; bottom right).

Both inertial and gravitational deposition may be enhanced by growth of hygroscopic aerosols in the lung. Martonen *et al.* (1982) have drawn attention to discrepancies between theoretical and experimental assessment of hygroscopic growth. Their experimental evidence suggests that dry NaCl particles entering the trachea at a flow rate of 30 ℓ min^{-1} with 5 μm diameter should have grown to 5.9 μm diameter on reaching the terminal bronchioles. This would have little effect on deposited particle distribution. A very different situation arises with small hygroscopic particles which can grow in diameter by a factor of two in the first few airway generations (Martonen *et al.*, 1982). Equations for predicting hygroscopic growth rates and particle equilibrium sizes for salts of varying molecular weights and solubilities are given by Ferron (1977).

Two different mechanisms can sometimes enhance particle deposition. Elongated fibres in particular can be deposited by 'interception' if part of the particle surface comes into contact with an airway wall even though the particle's centre of gravity may lie in an air streamline relatively distant from the wall. Perhaps, however, electrostatic attraction is the deposition mechanism least measured or appreciated in some practical situations. Several forms of aerosol generator can give rise to highly charged particles. Although the mechanisms by which this occurs are, in detail, poorly understood (John, 1980), any aerosol produced by high

TABLE 3.1. Lung deposition of neutral and of charged carnauba wax particles (results of Melandri *et al.* (1977))

Particle diameter (μm)	0.33	0.65	1.10
Charges per particle	29	45	95
% deposition for charged particles	32.9	30.6	35.4
%deposition for uncharged particles	26.9	24.3	29.8

Inhalation flow rate 24 ℓ min^{-1}

velocity dispersion of liquid or solid material is liable to give charged particles (unless a charge neutralizing system is used). Quite large charges may be produced—measured in hundreds or even thousands of elementary charge units per particle (John, 1980). These tend to be fairly rapidly neutralized in the atmosphere but will effect deposition if inhalation—either in the industrial setting or in the laboratory—occurs immediately after particle generation. Some experimental data on the deposition of charged particles are summarised in *Table 3.1*.

The effect of electric charge on deposition is believed to result chiefly from formation of image charge in the airway walls rather than from electrostatic interaction between particles. Essentially an airway constitutes an electrically conducting cylinder such that a charged particle within it gives rise to image charges in the walls—charge carriers (ions) of like sign being repelled towards the outer surface of the wall; charge carriers of the opposite sign being attracted to the inner surface *and* exerting an attractive force on the aerosol particle. On the whole, the present evidence is that quite high charges are needed on particles of 1–10 μm diameter to give comparable deposition to that arising from inertial and gravitational forces (Chan and Yu, 1982). Calculated estimates of particle deposition in the lungs are therefore often based on the presumption that inertial impaction and gravitational sedimentation—together with diffusion for submicronic particles—are the only significant mechanisms of deposition.

Patterns of aerosol deposition in the lung

While overall lung deposition of inhaled particles is relatively amenable to experimental measurement, information about distribution within the lung may be more important but far less easy to measure. If receptor sites for an inhaled drug (Chapter 9) or bronchoprovocation agent (Chapter 10) are either known or hypothesized, how may the inhaled agent be 'targeted' onto the appropriate sites? If the receptor sites are unknown how may data about changes in effectiveness resulting from changes in the mode of inhalation be translated into estimates of where the receptor sites may be situated? Imaging of radioactive aerosols (including those formed by intermixing radioactive tracers with aerosolised drugs) can illustrate whether deposition is predominantly in the more central airways or predominantly in the lung periphery. Imaging techniques however cannot distinguish deposition in the alveoli from that in the small airways and can only give a very approximate indication of distribution within the large airways.

Detailed assessments of particle distribution at large airway bifurcation regions—based on experiments with model bifurcations or tracheobronchial casts—have shown very irregular patterns of deposition with much of the deposited material occurring in localized hot spots both at the carina and further downstream (Lee and Wang, 1977; Bell, 1978; Schlesinger *et al.*, 1982). The detailed irregularities of deposition result from localized variations in airflow patterns. Localized concentrations may vary by more than one hundredfold in the immediate vicinity of a bifurcation. Thus very high local concentrations of inhaled irritants may occur at hot spot sites and may play a crucial role in the pathogenesis of disease related to deposited pollutants. Comparison of deposition patterns with cyclic and steady inhalation flows suggests that localized carinal deposition may be enhanced by turbulence or by high peak flow rates (Schlesinger *et al.*, 1982).

A different approach to the assessment of overall distribution patterns is to make use of mathematical modelling—applying formulae for particle impaction, sedimentation and diffusion to models of the airways.

Such calculations can be used to estimate the magnitude of deposition at successive airway generations but are ill-suited to calculating very detailed aspects of deposition. Modelling studies must obviously suffer from all the limitations of the deposition formulae and anatomical models on which they are based; they therefore cannot claim to offer exact deposition calculations.

Almost all published studies are based on symmetric lung models (a notable exception being that of Gerrity *et al.*, 1981) and thus make no allowance for lung asymmetry; they also often ignore the effect of secondary flow patterns on deposition and treat the entry of gas into the airways as though all velocity profiles were square. The ways in which secondary flow patterns may affect impaction and interception are discussed by Bell (1978), who concludes that they are likely to influence the detailed pattern, but not the overall magnitude of deposition at an airway bifurcation. Bulk transfer of aerosol from tidal to reserve air is also often neglected in model calculations although recovery of tidally inhaled 0.5 μm particles after maximal expiration suggests that some 10 per cent of non-deposited particles can transfer from tidal to reserve air under quiet breathing conditions (Davies *et al.*, 1972; Taulbee *et al.*, 1978).

Yet despite their drawbacks, modelling calculations offer an effective route to semi-quantitative estimates of how much deposition is attributable to different mechanisms. They can also estimate the effect on deposition of changes in inhalation conditions or lung dimensions.

Perhaps the first factor which should be considered in applying deposition modelling to the lungs (even though ignored in many published studies) is the effect on deposition of differences in lung size—either differences in total lung capacity or in the degree of lung inflation at the time of inhalation. The importance of lung volume (V_L) is indicated in *Figure 3.5* which demonstrates markedly increased deposition of 4 μm particles at low lung volume (2400 ml) than at high lung volume (4800 ml). This figure is derived by applying the impaction and sedimentation formulae of Landahl (1950) to the regular dichotomy airways model of Weibel (1963). This combination of formulae and anatomical model has been quite widely used in published studies—for instance those of Lippmann and Albert (1969) and Gerrity *et al.* (1979). The data of Weibel (1963) apply to a lung volume of V_L = 4800 ml. The results in *Figure 3.5* for V_L = 2400 ml are based on scaling the tabulated model dimensions on the assumptions that volumes of individual airway units are proportional to V_L, cross-sectional areas to $V_L^{2/3}$ and diameters and lengths to $V_L^{1/3}$.

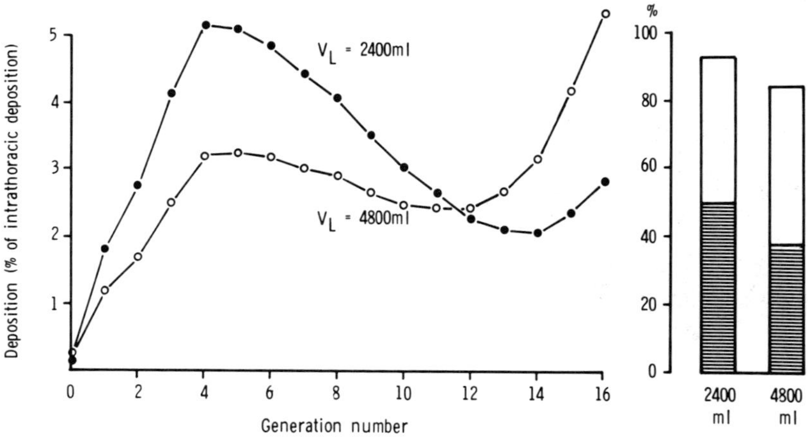

Figure 3.5 Effect of lung volume on the distribution of tracheobronchial deposition, calculations based on applying the impaction and sedimentation formulae of Landahl (1950) to the regular dichotomy airways model of Weibel (1963) with scaling for lung volume as described in the text. Inhalation conditions: particle size = 4 μm (unit density), V_T = 900 ml, breath-hold pause = 0.4 s, inspiratory (and expiratory) flow rate = 30 ℓ min^{-1}. Right-hand columns show total deposition (percentage of particles entering the trachea) plus (shaded) total tracheobronchial deposition

A two-fold justification exists for these scaling factors. First, diameters and lengths of bronchi and bronchioles in excised lung preparations tend to change in proportion to the cube root of lung volume as lung inflation increases or decreases (Klingele and Staub, 1971; Hughes *et al.*, 1972). Secondly autopsy studies suggested that a bronchial cross-sectional area measurement (summed over right and left main, upper and lower bronchi) was proportional to $V_L^{0.69}$ and a bronchial perimeter measurement (summed over the same bronchi) to $V_L^{0.33}$ (Thurlbeck and Haines, 1975).

Although Weibel model calculations are usually based on V_L = 4800 ml, the lower value of 2400 ml (*Figure 3.5*) may well be a better guide to inhalation conditions for a person of normal size inhaling tidally from functional residual capacity. While the smaller lung volume predicts greater impaction in the more proximal conducting airways it also predicts less sedimentation in the most distal conducting airways (generation 14 to 16) where sedimentation is believed to be the predominant deposition mechanism. At V_L = 2400 ml, airflow entering generation 14 contains fewer particles than at V_L = 4800 ml (because of greater proximal deposition). In addition the effect of increased airflow velocity (due to diminished cross-sectional area) plus diminished airway lengths more than counterbalances the effect of reduced airway diameters on the distances required for gravitational settling. Overall lung deposition accordingly changes very little (*Figure 3.5*). Similarly there is little change in total calculated tracheobronchial deposition over generations 0–16 inclusive (shown shaded in the right hand section of *Figure 3.5*).

Decreasing particle size—say from 4 μm to 2 μm as illustrated in *Figure 3.6*—reduces both impaction and sedimentation and therefore reduces deposition over all the tracheobronchial generations. If little or no breath-hold pause follows

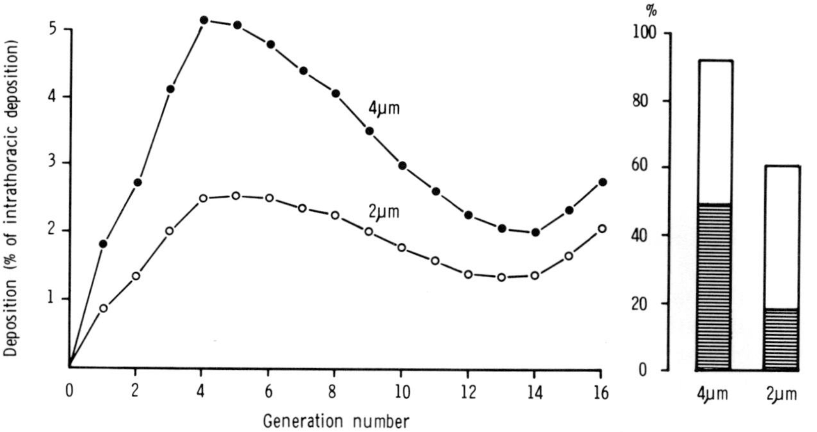

Figure 3.6 Effect of particle size on distribution of tracheobronchial deposition. Inhalation conditions: V_L = 2400 ml, V_T = 900 ml, breath-hold pause = 0.4 s, inspiratory (and expiratory) flow rate = 30 ℓ min^{-1}. Method of calculation and meaning of right-hand columns are as for *Figure 3.5*

inspiration then total deposition must also be reduced for 2 μm as compared to 4 μm particles. A significant proportion of 2 μm particles inhaled at moderate flow rates can escape deposition by either impaction or sedimentation during inspiration and expiration. It is under such conditions that a post-inspiration breath-hold pause can significantly increase total deposition. During a breath-hold pause airborne particles of any size larger than about 0.5 μm are deposited predominantly by sedimentation and the fraction remaining airborne decreases exponentially with time, the rate of decrease being determined by the dimensions of the airspaces where the aerosol is situated (Gebhart *et al.*, 1981). This forms the basis of the 'aerosol probe' or 'aerosol persistence' method for estimating mean airspace dimensions (Chapter 5). The effect of a varying length of breath-hold pause is illustrated for 2 μm particles in *Figure 3.7*. Total deposition increases substantially over the first few seconds of the pause. So too does deposition in the alveolar region (generations distal to the terminal bronchioles which are numbered as generation 16 in the Weibel system). There is however no major change in tracheobronchial deposition (generations 0–16) or in the distribution of deposited activity within the tracheobronchial region. The enhanced therapeutic effect achieved with bronchodilator

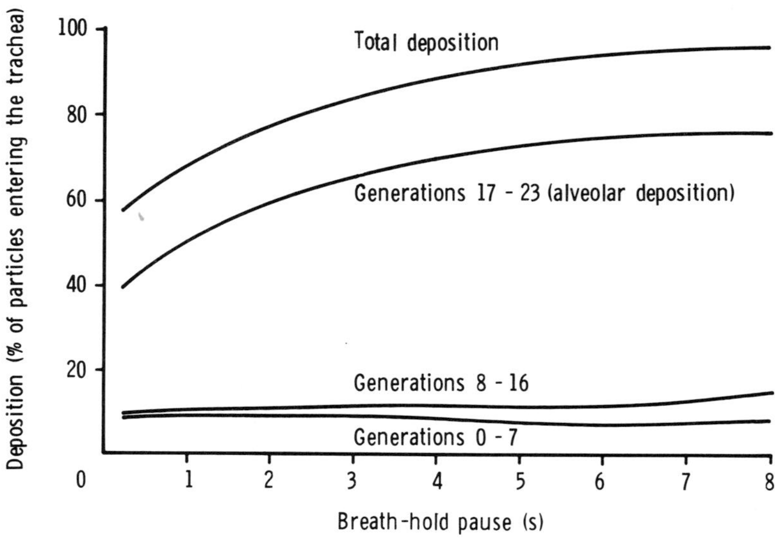

Figure 3.7 Effect of breath-hold pause on distribution of tracheobronchial deposition, calculated for 2 μm unit density particles inhaled at 30 ℓ min^{-1} (V_L = 2400 ml, V_T = 900 ml)

drugs by means of a breath-hold pause (Chapter 9) therefore presumably either arises from an increase in total deposition *per se* or is inadequately modelled by these simple calculations.

The relatively undramatic effect of particle size illustrated in *Figure 3.6* derives partly from the fact that deposition per generation is plotted as a percentage of total deposition in the lungs in order to concentrate on the *distribution* of deposition and partly from the extent to which deposition in distal generations is determined by the proportion of particles surviving passage through the preceding generations. The values for impaction and sedimentation probabilities tabulated in *Table 3.2* emphasize that these basic probabilities as calculated by the Landahl formulae depend on the square of particle diameter in accord with Equations (3.1) and (3.3). Impaction is approximately proportional to particle velocity ($\propto V_L^{-2/3}$) divided by airway diameter ($\propto V_L^{1/3}$) and therefore changes in inverse proportion to lung

TABLE 3.2. Calculated impaction and sedimentation probabilities at two different airway sites (percentage of airborne particles reaching the airway in question which would be deposited by either mechanism acting on its own)

	Subsegmental bronchi (generation 4)		*Terminal bronchioles (generation 16)*	
	4 μm	2 μm	4 μm	2 μm
V_L = 4800 ml				
Impaction	2.60	0.66	0.35	0.09
Sedimentation	0.08	0.02	5.43	1.44
V_L = 2400 ml				
Impaction	5.06	1.32	0.70	0.18
Sedimentation	0.05	0.01	3.46	0.91

These probabilities are calculated by applying the formulae of Landahl (1950) to the symmetric airways model of Weibel (1963); scaling for lung volume as described in the text

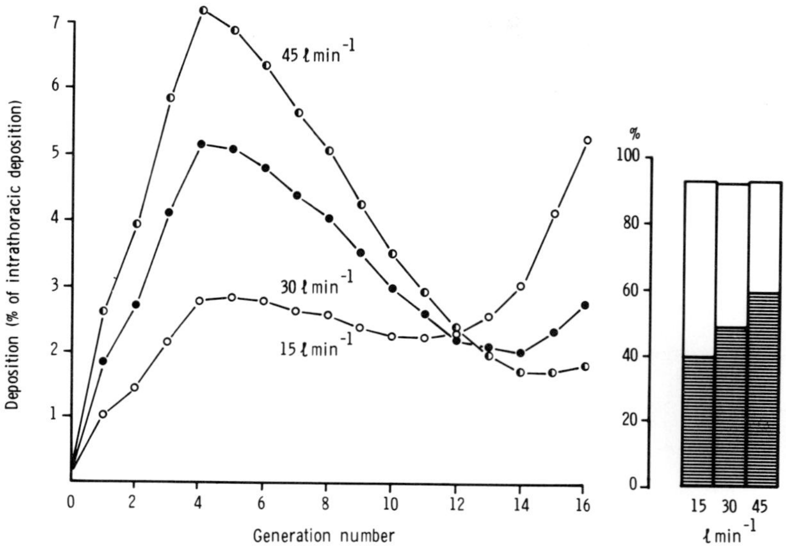

Figure 3.8 Effect of flow rate on distribution of tracheobronchial distribution. Flow rates shown are for inspiratory and expiratory flow. Inhalation conditions: $V_L = 2400$ ml, $V_T = 900$ ml, breath-hold pause = 0.4 s. Method of calculation and meaning of right-hand columns are as for *Figure 3.5*

volume. Sedimentation can, considered in an over-simplified way, be taken as inversely proportional to velocity ($\propto V_L^{-2/3}$) and airway diameter ($\propto V_L^{1/3}$) but proportional to airway length ($\propto V_L^{1/3}$). It therefore tends to change in inverse proportion to $V_L^{2/3}$.

Increasing velocity in the airways enhances impaction but decreases sedimentation. Inhalation flow at the mouth can therefore (*Figure 3.8*) have a marked effect on the pattern of tracheobronchial deposition. High flow enhances impaction and therefore increases deposition in the large airways. Low flow enhances sedimentation and therefore increases deposition in the more distal small airways and in the alveoli. The effect of changing inhalation flow is therefore quite different from that of increasing particle diameter. Changes in particle size are likely to alter total tracheobronchial deposition but not necessarily the pattern of distribution within the conducting airway generations (as illustrated in *Figure 3.6*). An obvious exception is that very large particles will tend to deposit completely in the first few airway generations.

The fact that inhalation flow but not particle size can significantly influence the *pattern* of tracheobronchial deposition has important implications for attempting to target therapeutic or other agents onto specific airway generations. Control of inhalation flow (*Figure 3.8*) may determine whether deposition is maximal at about the level of the subsegmental bronchi or much more evenly spread over the airway generations with high deposition in the more distal small airways. Attempts to control deposition sites in this way will also be influenced by lung volume. The data of *Figure 3.5* suggest that a small volume inhaled early in a vital capacity inhalation will tend to give more pronounced large airways deposition than one inhaled later in the vital capacity inhalation when the airways are more expanded. Aerosol administered very near the end of an inhalation manoeuvre may not however be able to penetrate fully into the tracheobronchial tree.

TABLE 3.3. Deposition of nonhygroscopic and hygroscopic (NaCl) aerosol particles in the conducting airways: modelling calculations by Martonen (1982)

	Nonhygroscopic particles	*NaCl particles* (a) *Experimental growth rate*	*NaCl particles* (b) *Theoretical growth rate*
*Particle size on inhalation (μm)	3.0	3.0	3.0
*Particle size at terminal bronchioles (μm)	3.0	4.2	5.2
Total tracheobronchial deposition (% of particles entering trachea)	19	29	47
% of tracheobronchial deposition in generations			
0–6	38.4	37.1	40.0
7–10	24.6	24.4	24.5
11–16	37.0	38.5	35.5

Inspiratory flow rate = 40 ℓ min^{-1}
*Aerodynamic diameters

Mathematical modelling also offers a chance to estimate the influence of hygroscopic growth on the deposited particle distribution within the tracheobronchial tree. A rapidly growing hygroscopic particle may have quite different impaction and sedimentation probabilities in distal airways from those applicable in the absence of hygroscopic growth. The modelling calculations of Martonen (1982) based on the Weibel model suggest however that the chief effect of hygroscopic growth may be on total tracheobronchial deposition rather than on the distribution within the tracheobronchial generations—an example of this modelling work is summarized in *Table 3.3*. The experimental growth rate data include allowance for the influence of the laryngeal jet on aerosol-air mixing in the upper airways whereas the theoretical growth curve assumes that each particle is surrounded by an atmosphere of constant temperature and relative humidity. The model calculations based on the theoretical growth curve therefore probably overestimate total tracheobronchial deposition (Martonen, 1982).

The use of hygroscopic radioaerosol particles could possibly be of value in ventilation imaging if a sufficiently small initial size (plus slow inhalation) minimized large airways impaction while increased size by the end of inspiration (plus a post-inspiration breath-hold) maximized sedimentational deposition in the alveolar region. This argument only stands however if hygroscopic growth occurs fairly slowly. If in fact—as has been suggested both for NaCl and for medicinal aerosols (Martonen *et al.*, 1982)—hygroscopic growth occurs predominantly in the first one or two airway generations then its chief effect will be to enhance total tracheobronchial deposition.

Modelling calculations based on the Weibel model have also been used to predict the effect of electric charge on the distribution of tracheobronchial deposition (Chan and Yu, 1982): as low a charge as 50 units per particle was estimated to give a dramatic increase in deposition of 2 μm particles (inhaled at 15 and 20 ℓ min^{-1}) distal to generation 4. With 5 μm particles changes only in small airway deposition were predicted to occur.

The difficulty however with model calculations—both for hygroscopic and electrostatic effects—is generally that of knowing how fast a hygroscopic growth is likely to occur or how much charge is initially carried per particle. In practice these are usually unknown for aerosols used in the medical field, with the obvious exceptions of particles that are not hygroscopic and have been through a charge neutralizer.

Effect of bronchoconstriction

Many experimental studies have demonstrated reduced lung penetration of aerosol particles in patients with airways obstruction. Deposition may occur predominantly in the central airways or may be patchy and irregular with localized zones of hyperdeposition throughout the lung image. Modelling techniques can be used to illustrate the average tendency towards more central deposition but are not easily applied to characterizing more irregular patterns of deposition. Two different simple approaches have been applied to the Weibel model (with $V_L = 4800$ ml): (a) the airways were assumed to be coated with a thick uniform layer of mucus and (b) all airways from the subsegmental bronchi to the terminal bronchioles were assumed to be constricted by the same percentage diameter reduction (Agnew *et al.*, 1982). For 5 μm particles inhaled at 30 ℓ min^{-1} the same reduction in deposition distal to the terminal bronchioles (from 45 to 20 per cent) was achieved by (a) a 200 μm mucus blanket and (b) a 30 per cent bronchoconstriction. However the first modification increased deposition fairly uniformly over generations 5–12, whereas

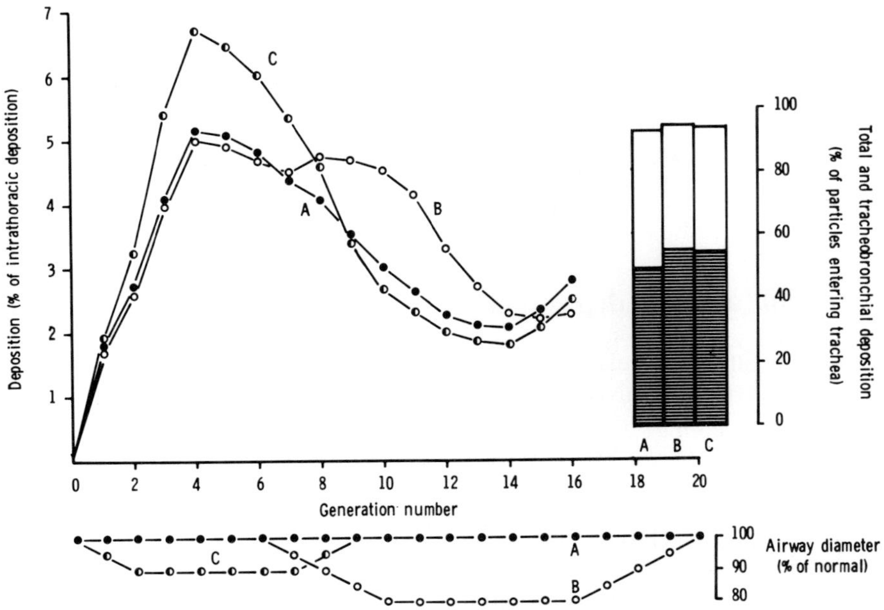

Figure 3.9 A modelling estimate of the effects of bronchoconstriction based on comparing zero bronchoconstriction (A) with predominantly small airways bronchoconstriction (B) and predominantly large airways bronchoconstriction (C). The patterns of bronchoconstriction (percentage reduction in airways diameter and generations affected) are illustrated at the bottom of the figure. Inhalation conditions: particle size = 4 μm (unit density), $V_L = 2400$ ml, $V_T = 900$ ml, breath-hold pause = 0.4 s, inspiratory (and expiratory) flow rate = 30 ℓ min^{-1}. Method of calculation and meaning of right-hand columns are as for *Figure 3.5*

the second modification predominantly increased deposition only over generations 5–8.

The influence on tracheobronchial deposition of more modest, but equally artificial, patterns of bronchoconstriction is depicted in *Figure 3.9*. Compared with normal deposition at V_L = 2400 ml (pattern A) neither pattern B, 20 per cent bronchoconstriction of the small airways, nor pattern C, 10 per cent bronchoconstriction of the large airways, have any significant effect on total deposition. The effect on the ratio of tracheobronchial to alveolar deposition is small but there is a shift in the pattern of deposition within the tracheobronchial region. Pattern B if applicable uniformly to the lung represents a 50 per cent increase in deposition over generations 10 to 12. In the context of measuring mucociliary clearance with deposited particles (Chapters 6 and 7) this implies an increased number of particles with a long clearance path from deposition site to the trachea. A non-uniform pattern of small airways constriction coupled with an uneven distribution of ventilation creates the conditions for localized zones of high impaction probability relatively close to the lung periphery. This mechanism may account for the 'spotty' deposition pattern sometimes seen in patients with chronic bronchitis or emphysema (Santolicandro and Giuntini, 1979). The large airways pattern of bronchoconstriction (pattern C) illustrates how a relatively small degree of airway narrowing can enhance deposition in the more central airways. Deposition at these sites is also sensitive to airflow velocity (*Figure 3.8*) so that changes in the distribution of ventilation leading to changes in peak velocities in the larger bronchi could also significantly enhance central deposition.

The role of aerosols in clinical ventilation imaging (Chapter 5) is dependent on sufficient particles surviving the journey through the central airways to give an image of peripheral ventilation. This clearly requires reasonably small particles and reasonably low inhalation flows. The clinical test is whether adequate images can be obtained in patients with severe airflow obstruction. The relationship of aerosol deposition patterns to lung function is therefore considered further in Chapter 5. The converse question is also considered there: can abnormalities in aerosol deposition be usefully interpreted as evidence of localized airways dysfunction?

The concept of 'alveolar deposition'

When looking at simple model calculations it is easy to interpret deposition distal to a particular generation as 'alveolar deposition', the generation in question being taken to represent the terminal bronchioles. The experimental counterpart is that insoluble particles deposited on the ciliated conducting airways (trachea to terminal bronchioles) are assumed to be completely cleared from the lungs within 24 hours (by mucociliary transport or by cough); while particles deposited in the alveolar region (respiratory bronchioles and alveoli) are assumed to undergo negligible clearance in that time, as discussed in Chapter 8. 'Alveolar deposition' is then simply the percentage of particles remaining within the lung at 24 hours post inhalation.

The assumption of a fast, 'tracheobronchial' clearance phase complete within 24 hours appears to be substantially valid in healthy non-smoking subjects. It is not correct for all patients with airflow obstruction. Mean retention of an insoluble ^{99m}Tc-labelled aerosol in 10 patients with chronic airways obstruction has been shown to fall by a further 6.5 per cent of initial deposition from 24 hours to 48 hours post inhalation, with one patient's retention falling by 24 per cent (Agnew *et al.*, 1981). This is likely to represent delayed tracheobronchial clearance rather than any abnormally fast mechanism of alveolar clearance.

As used experimentally, the term 'alveolar deposition' is to some extent a misnomer. A variety of experimental studies have shown persistence of tracheobronchially deposited particles well beyond 24 hours. Some 1 per cent of intratracheally administered ^{133}Ba-barium sulphate particles are retained in the rat trachea at 24 hours and most of them are still present after 30 days (Patrick and Stirling, 1977). More than two-thirds of similarly administered teflon particles deposited on the first bifurcation of the rabbit lung have been shown to clear with a half-time of 39 hours (Svartengren *et al.*, 1981), suggesting that the main carina or deeper bifurcations of the human lung may, because of inefficient local clearance, also represent zones of prolonged retention (as well as zones of high localized deposition) and in consequence be subject to particular risk from deposited pollutants. Autoradiography has demonstrated that when prolonged tracheobronchial retention occurs the particles deposited on the airways (intratracheal barium sulphate and inhaled uranium oxide) may remain on the airway surface for up to 24 hours but then tend to penetrate the epithelium to a depth of about 10 μm (Gore and Patrick, 1982).

Another difficulty over pretending that experimental 'alveolar deposition' corresponds to an anatomical division of the airways is that the more distal small airways are, as discussed in Chapter 2, very poorly supplied with mucus secreting glands and goblet cells in healthy people. Mucus is a pre-requisite for mucociliary transport (Sadé *et al.*, 1970) and studies of *in vitro* lung preparations have suggested that both mucus and mucociliary transport may be virtually absent in normal terminal bronchioles (Iravani and Van As, 1972).

A small proportion of particles can thus evade mucociliary clearance in the trachea and, very probably, a much larger proportion in the distal small airways.

However 24-hour particle retention (whether called 'alveolar deposition' or not) has a very important role when radioaerosols are used for mucociliary clearance testing. It constitutes the only practicable means of separating those particles which can be, and those which cannot be, cleared with mucus from the lungs within 24 hours. In the case of patients with chronic airways obstruction a 48-hour reading should ideally be substituted for the 24-hour one to allow for impaired mucociliary transport rates. This may however be difficult in practice with short-lived radionuclide labels. Even with careful control of inhalation conditions the proportion of particles which can be cleared within 24 hours varies markedly from one subject to another and within repeated tests on the same subject. If clearance at differing times after inhalation is expressed as a percentage of the total initial deposition those tests with the highest proportion of particles available for clearance (lowest 'alveolar deposition') may falsely appear to give the fastest clearance.

The two upper curves (labelled '1') in *Figure 3.10*, represent typical patterns of whole lung retention in a normal subject and in a patient with chronic airways obstruction. Retention in the patient at 6 hours is slightly lower than in the normal person. But if retention at 24 hours—much lower in the patient—is subtracted from all readings, the resulting 'tracheobronchial' retention curves (labelled '2') suggest a very different comparison. Retention over the whole 0–6 hour period, and beyond, is much greater in the patient than in the normal subject. Clinical mucociliary clearance data for inhaled radioaerosols should in principle always be converted in this way. The exceptions to this rule are when deposition is so central

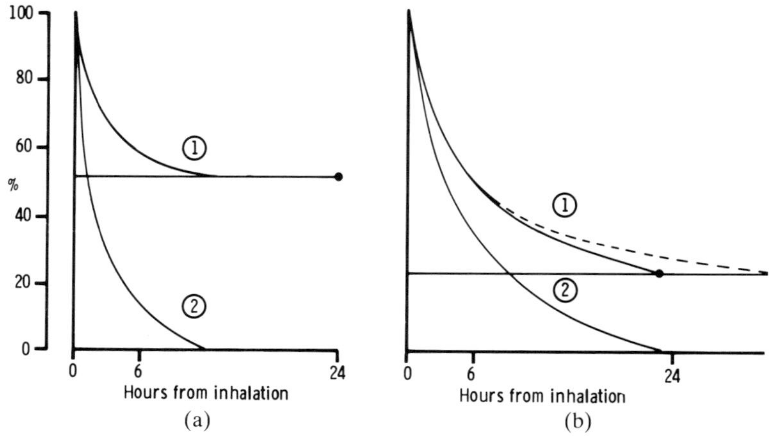

Figure 3.10 Schematic illustration of whole-lung (1) and tracheobronchial (2) retention curves in (a) a normal subject and in (b) a patient with chronic airways obstruction inhaling radioaerosol particles under the same conditions. Whole lung retention appears to fall more slowly in the normal subject than in the patient simply because of the far smaller amount of radioactivity deposited on the conducting airways. Subtracting whole-lung retention at 24 hours gives tracheobronchial retention which falls faster in the normal subject than in the patient. Tracheobronchial clearance may not however (dashed line) be complete by 24 hours in the patient in which case the calculated tracheobronchial retention values will be lower than they should be (and the margin between normal subject and patient will appear less than it should)

that retention at 24 hours can be dismissed as negligible or when tests with virtually identical deposition patterns are to be compared, in particular when the patient acts as his own control in studies of drug treatments (Chapter 6) or physiotherapy (Chapter 7) administered after radioaerosol inhalations so that they cannot affect the pattern of radioaerosol deposition.

The justification for expressing clearance results as 'tracheobronchial' retention curves by subtracting 24-hour retention from the whole lung data is *not* that 'tracheobronchial' retention derives from an anatomically correct specification of deposition sites but that it does in practice seem to relate only to particles deposited on airways mucus and not to particles deposited elsewhere. If however clearance of particles on mucus is not complete by 24 hours (as represented by the dashed line in *Figure 3.10*) a falsely high 'alveolar deposition' value will be subtracted from the whole lung data and 'tracheobronchial' clearance will seem faster (retention lower) than it really is.

Measurement of 'alveolar deposition'

Extensive experimental investigation of alveolar deposition in normal non-smoking subjects has revealed considerable inter-subject variability but also a very clear overall dependence on the product of (diameter)^2 and flow for unit density particles in the 1–12 μm range (Lippmann and Albert, 1969; Lippmann, 1977; Foord *et al.*, 1978; Stahlhofen *et al.*, 1980 and 1981). This implies that impaction in the conducting airways is the principal factor determining how many particles reach the alveolar zone or, to be more exact, are deposited in sites from which clearance does not occur within 24 hours. The results of Foord *et al.* (1978) are depicted in *Figure 3.11*, where each point represents the mean of 3–7 experimental observations on

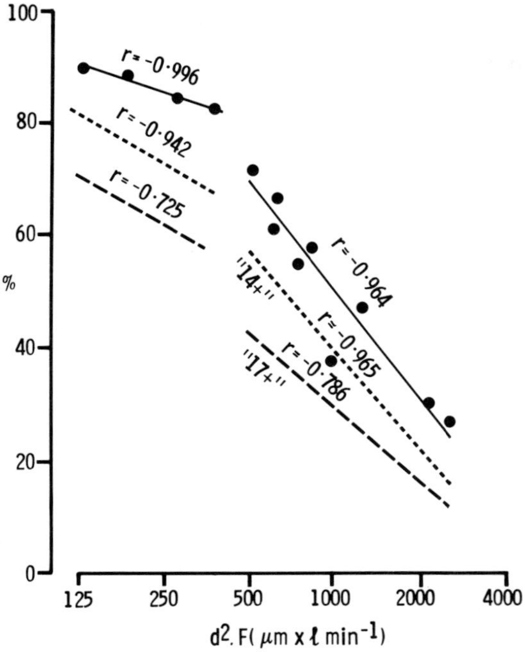

Figure 3.11 Dependence of experimentally measured 'alveolar deposition' on the product (diameter)^2 × flow. The points represent mean data for normal non-smoking subjects studied by Foord *et al.* (1978) with particle sizes from 2.5 to 7.5 μm (unit density) and inhalation flows from 15 to 60 ℓ min^{-1}. The continuous lines represent least-squares fits to their data. Deposition was also calculated for the experimental inhalation conditions corresponding to each data point using the same method of calculations as for *Figures 3.5–3.9*. The lower dashed lines represent deposition in and distal to generation 17; the upper dashed lines represent deposition in and distal to generation 14. The latter correlate better than the former with log (d^2F) and lie closer to the experimental data: the possible implications are discussed in the text

normal non-smokers at inhalation flow rates ranging from 15 to 60 ℓ min^{-1} and (unit density) particle sizes from 2.5 to 7.5 μm. The dashed lines comprise theoretical predictions derived from the modelling approach outlined earlier in this chapter, namely applying the impaction and sedimentation formulae of Landahl (1950) to the airways model of Weibel (1963); the calculations were performed for each of the inhalation conditions studied by Foord *et al.* (1978) but using a mean value of V_L estimated from data they tabulated about vital capacities and expiratory reserve volumes. If 'alveolar deposition' is defined—as anatomically it should be—to be deposition distal to generation 16 ('17+' in the figure), agreement with the experimental data is poor and correlation with log (d^2F) is considerably less than observed experimentally. If 'alveolar deposition' is calculated as that distal to generation 13 (i.e. '14+' in the figure) both agreement with experimental data and the correlation with log (d^2F) are improved. Two alternative reasons for this may be suggested:

(a) that the model calculations are wrong, or
(b) that a high proportion of particles deposited by sedimentation in the distal airways do not get cleared from the lung in the 'mucociliary' phase of clearance.

The first of these conclusions counsels caution in interpreting model predictions! The second is consistent with the possibility that the distal small airways contain very little mucus (Iravani and Van As, 1972); if they are thus relatively 'defenceless' against inhaled particles this is likely to contribute to their involvement in the early stages of smoking-relating damage (Niewoehner *et al.*, 1974).

Measured 'alveolar deposition' in smokers systematically tends to be lower than in non-smokers (Lippmann, 1977) but this could result either from better clearance of the tracheobronchial airways owing to the presence of more mucus or from higher tracheobronchial deposition owing to minor degrees of bronchoconstriction. Variations in the ratio of particles cleared rapidly from the lungs ('tracheobronchial deposition') to those cleared very slowly ('alveolar deposition') arising from smoking, non-disabling airways disease and normal inter-subject variations should ideally be taken into account when estimating the hazards arising from inhaled industrial dusts (Chapter 11).

Summary

Particle deposition in the tracheobronchial airways occurs by impaction and sedimentation for unit density particles of greater than 1 μm diameter and by diffusion for particles of less than 0.1 μm diameter. Large particles may fail to reach the lungs because of impaction in the upper airways; this particularly applies to atmospheric aerosols inhaled via the nose. Both hygroscopic and electric charge effects can enhance tracheobronchial deposition but the importance of these mechanisms for aerosols with medical applications is at present uncertain. In general, inspiratory flow rate, particle size and, in disease, bronchoconstriction are likely to effect the magnitude of tracheobronchial deposition. Flow rate, lung volume and bronchoconstriction are likely to affect the distribution of tracheobronchial deposition.

'Alveolar deposition', measured by 24-hour retention, is neither well defined anatomically nor (in patients with severe airways disease) always reliable. But it does provide the essential means of differentiating deposited particles able to move with the airways mucus from those unable to move with the mucus when deposited particles are used to assess mucus clearance rates.

References

AGNEW, J.E., LITTLE, F., PAVIA, D. and CLARKE, S.W. (1982). Mucus clearance from the airways in chronic bronchitis—smokers and ex-smokers. *Bull. Eur. Physiopath Resp.*, **18**, 473–484

AGNEW, J.E., BATEMAN, J.R.M., WATTS, M., PARAMANANDA, V., PAVIA, D. and CLARKE, S.W. (1981). The importance of aerosol penetration for lung mucociliary clearance studies. *Chest*, **80**, 843–846

BELL, K.A. (1978). Local particle deposition in respiratory airway models. In *Recent developments in aerosol science*. Edited by Shaw, D.T. New York; John Wiley, 97–134

CHAN, T.L. and LIPPMANN, M. (1980). Experimental measurements and empirical modelling of the regional deposition of inhaled particles in humans. *Am. Ind. Hyg. Assoc. J.*, **41**, 399–409

CHAN, T.L. and YU, C.P. (1982). Charge effects on particle deposition in the human tracheobronchial tree. In *Inhaled particles V*. Edited by Walton, W.H. Oxford; Pergamon, 65–75

DAVIES, C.N., HEYDER, J. and SUBBA RAMU, M.C. (1972). Breathing of half-micron aerosols. I. Experimental. *J. Appl. Physiol.*, **32**, 591–600

FERRON, G.A. (1977). The size of soluble aerosol particles as a function of the humidity of the air. Application to the human respiratory tract. *J. Aerosol Sci.*, **8**, 251–267

FOORD, N., BLACK, A. and WALSH, M. (1978). Regional deposition of 2.5–7.5 μm diameter inhaled particles in healthy male non-smokers. *J. Aerosol Sci.*, **9**, 343–357

FUCHS, N.A. (1964). *The Mechanics of Aerosols*. Oxford; Pergamon

GEBHART, J., HEYDER, J. and STAHLHOFEN, W. (1981). Use of aerosols to estimate pulmonary air-space dimensions. *J. Appl. Physiol.*, **51**, 465–476

GERRITY, T.R., GARRARD, C.S. and YEATES, D.B. (1981). Theoretic analysis of sites of aerosol deposition in the human lung. *Chest*, **80**, 898–901

GERRITY, T.R., LEE, P.S., HASS, F.J., MARINELLI, A., WERNER, P. and LOURENÇO, R.V. (1979). Calculated deposition of inhaled particles in the airway generations of normal subjects. *J. Appl. Physiol.*, **47**, 867–873

GORE, D.J. and PATRICK, G. (1982). A quantitative study of the penetration of insoluble particles into the tissue of the conducting airways. In *Inhaled particles V*. Edited by Walton, W.H. Oxford; Pergamon, 149–161

HILLER, F.C., MAZUMDER, M.K., WILSON, J.D., McLEOD, P.C. and BONE, R.C. (1982). Human respiratory tract deposition using multimodal aerosols. *J. Aerosol. Sci.*, **13**, 337–343

HOUNAM, R.F. and MORGAN, A. (1977). Particle deposition. In *Respiratory defence mechanisms*. Edited by Brain, J.D., Proctor, D.F. and Reid, L.M. New York; Marcel Dekker, 125–156

HUGHES, J.M.B., HOPPIN, F.G. and MEAD, J. (1972). Effect of lung inflation on bronchial length and diameter in excised lungs. *J. Appl. Physiol.*, **32**, 25–35

IRAVANI, J. and VAN AS, A. (1972). Mucus transport in the tracheobronchial tree of normal and bronchitic rats. *J. Pathol.*, **106**, 81–93

JOHN, W. (1980). Particle charge effects. In *Generation of aerosols and facilities for exposure experiments*. Edited by Willeke, K. Ann Arbor, Michigan; Ann Arbor Science Publishers Inc., 141–151

KLINGELE, T.G. and STAUB, N.C. (1971). Terminal bronchiole diameter changes with volume in isolated, air-filled lobes of cat lung. *J. Appl. Physiol.*, **30**, 224–227

LANDAHL, H.D. (1950). On the removal of air-borne droplets by the human respiratory tract: I. The lung. *Bull. Math. Biophys.*, **12**, 43–56

LEE, W-C and WANG, C-S. (1977). Particle deposition in systems of repeatedly bifurcating tubes. In *Inhaled particles IV*. Edited by Walton, W.H. Oxford; Pergamon, 49–60

LIPPMANN, M. (1977). Regional deposition of particles in the human respiratory tract. In *Handbook of physiology: reaction to environmental agents*. Edited by Lee, D.H.K. *et al.* Bethesda, Md.; The American Physiological Society, 213–232

LIPPMANN, M. and ALBERT, R.E. (1969). The effect of particle size on the regional deposition of inhaled aerosols in the human respiratory tract. *Am. Ind. Hyg. Assoc. J.*, **30**, 257–275

MARPLE, V.A. and RUBOW, K.L. (1980). Aerosol generation concepts and parameters. In *Generation of aerosols and facilities for exposure experiments*. Edited by Willeke, K. Ann Arbor, Michigan; Ann Arbor Science Publishers Inc., 3–29

MARTONEN, T.B. (1982). Analytical model of hygroscopic particle behavior in human airways. *Bull. Math. Biol.*, **44**, 425–442

MARTONEN, T.B., BELL, K.A., PHALEN, R.F., WILSON, A.F. and HO, A. (1982). Growth rate measurements and deposition modelling of hygroscopic aerosols in human tracheobronchial models. In *Inhaled particles V*. Edited by Walton, W.H. Oxford; Pergamon, 93–108

MELANDRI, C., PRODI, V., TARRONI, G., FORMIGNANI, M., DE ZAIACOMO, T., BOMPANE, G.F. and MAESTRI, G. (1977). On the deposition of unipolarly charged particles in the human respiratory tract. In *Inhaled particles IV*. Edited by Walton, W.H. Oxford; Pergamon, 193–201

MORROW, P.E. (1981). An evaluation of the physical properties of monodisperse and heterodisperse aerosols used in the assessment of bronchial function. *Chest*, **80**, 809–813

NIEWOEHNER, D.E., KLEINERMAN, J. and RICE, D.B. (1974). Pathologic changes in the peripheral airways of young cigarette smokers. *N. Eng. J. Med.*, **291**, 755–758

PATRICK, G. and STIRLING, C. (1977). The retention of particles in large airways of the respiratory tract. *Proc. Roy. Soc. Lond. B*, **198**, 455–462

SADÉ, J., ELIEZER, N., SILBERBERG, A. and NEVO, A.C. (1970). The role of mucus in transport by cilia. *Am. Rev. Resp. Dis.*, **102**, 48–52

SANTOLICANDRO, A. and GIUNTINI, C. (1979). Patterns of deposition of labelled monodispersed aerosols in obstructive lung disease. *J. Nucl. Med. Allied Sci.*, **23**, 115–127

SCHLESINGER, R.B., GURMAN, J.L. and LIPPMANN, M. (1982). Particle deposition within bronchial airways: comparisons using constant and cyclic inspiratory flows. In *Inhaled particles V*. Edited by Walton, W.H. Oxford; Pergamon, 47–64

STAHLHOFEN, W., GEBHART, J. and HEYDER, J. (1980). Experimental determination of the regional deposition of aerosol particles in the human respiratory tract. *Am. Ind. Hyg. Assoc. J.*, **41**, 385–398a

STAHLHOFEN, W., GEBHART, J. and HEYDER, J. (1981). Biological variability of regional deposition of aerosol particles in the human respiratory tract. *Am. Ind. Hyg. Assoc. J.*, **42**, 348–352

SVARTENGREN, M., WIDTSKIÖLD-OLSSON, K., PHILIPSON, K. and CAMNER, P. (1981). Retention of particles on the first bifurcation and the trachea of rabbits. *Bull. Eur. Physiopath. Resp.*, **17**, 87–91

SWIFT, D.L. and PROCTOR, D.F. (1982). Human respiratory deposition of particles during oronasal breathing. *Atmos. Environ.*, **16**, 2279–2282

TAULBEE, D.B., YU, C.P. and HEYDER, J. (1978). Aerosol transport in the human lung from analysis of single breaths. *J. Appl. Physiol.*, **44**, 803–812

THURLBECK, W.M. and HAINES, J.R. (1975). Bronchial dimensions and stature. *Am. Rev. Resp. Dis.*, **112**, 142–145

VINCENT, J.H. (1980). The physics of gases and aerosols. In *Occupational Hygiene*. Edited by Waldron, H.A. and Harrington, J.M. Oxford; Blackwell, 1–38

WEIBEL, E.R. (1963). *Morphometry of the human lung*. Berlin; Springer-Verlag

Chapter 4

Production of radioaerosols

Stephen P. Newman

Choice of particles and radiolabel

Studies with radiolabelled aerosols produce some of the most reliable data on the deposition, retention and clearance of inhaled particles, giving much information that would be difficult, if not impossible to obtain by other means. Such techniques are accurate, sensitive, usually rapid to perform and generally involve little discomfort for volunteer subjects or patients. Other approaches, such as the use of magnetic particles, may in due course provide an alternative to the use of ionizing radiations, but for the time being, radiolabels remain the most practical means of tracing aerosols. Subsequent chapters in this book will describe in detail a wide range of applications of radiolabelled aerosols.

The majority of methods for producing radioaerosols involve the fragmentation of liquids into a system of droplets. These methods may be used to produce either solid or liquid aerosols. Aerosols consisting of liquid droplets may be produced if a relatively non-volatile solution is atomized. Alternatively, a system of solid particles becomes available if the solvents readily evaporate, leaving a smaller solid residue. Solid particles may also be produced by atomizing a suspension of previously prepared particles, again allowing the solvent to evaporate.

The choice of particle and label for radioaerosol studies will depend partly upon the objectives of the particular investigation being undertaken. Solid particles which are insoluble in body fluids have some advantages over liquid droplets. Since the latter are absorbed via airway surfaces and are hence removed very rapidly from the lung, they can only be used either for assessment of airway permeability (Chapter 8) or for other short-term measurements such as ventilation scanning (Chapter 5). Insoluble particles may be used for the measurement of mucociliary clearance (Chapter 6), a process which takes about one day to complete, and the 24 hour whole lung retention of such particles may be used as an index of alveolar deposition (Chapter 3). Insoluble particles tagged with long-lived radionuclides can be used to measure the rate of clearance from alveolated zones (Chapter 8). Both liquid and solid aerosols must be non-toxic, and should generally be biologically inert, although occasionally it is required to deliver drugs either labelled or mixed with radioactive materials in order that patterns of drug deposition may be assessed. Polystyrene and Teflon have proved particularly useful as solid test aerosols, since they are safe when deposited in the lung and can be firmly labelled with a variety of radionuclides.

In considering the radiolabelling of aerosols, it is important to draw a distinction between those radionuclides which emit gamma rays, and those which emit only beta rays. The majority of radionuclides emit both beta and gamma rays, but should be considered for practical purposes as gamma-emitters. Gamma rays can, depending upon their energy, be monitored satisfactorily by a detector located outside the body, while beta rays do not pass through tissue to any extent and can rarely be detected by an external probe. Since beta rays are densely ionizing compared to gamma rays, they give rise to relatively high radiation doses. The radionuclides ^{3}H and ^{14}C emit beta rays only, and can readily be labelled to a wide variety of organic compounds. Unfortunately, the deposition of ^{3}H and ^{14}C-labelled aerosols can only be assessed indirectly from plasma or urine levels of radioactivity by liquid scintillation counting, or from the recovery of label in mouth-washings. Useful techniques employing radioaerosols are largely confined to those radionuclides which emit gamma rays.

The gamma ray energy should be high enough ($\gtrsim$100 keV) for penetration through tissue, but low enough ($\lesssim$300 keV) to minimize the amount of radiation shielding required. Ideally, no beta rays should be emitted by the radionuclide of choice, since these needlessly increase the radiation dose. The half-life of the radionuclide should be as short as possible, but must of course be long enough to enable the study to be performed. Leaching or dissociation of the label from the particles should be small, and high specific activities should be obtainable. Physical characteristics of some of the various radionuclides which have been used to tag aerosols are shown in *Table 4.1*. ^{99m}Tc is the pre-eminent radionuclide label, since

TABLE 4.1. Physical characteristics of some gamma-emitting radionuclides used for aerosol labelling

Nuclide	*Physical half-life*	*Principal gamma-ray energy*	*Beta-rays*	*Production method*
^{11}C	20 minutes	511 keV	Yes	Cyclotron
^{18}F	1.8 hours	511 keV	Yes	Cyclotron
^{24}Na	15 hours	1.37, 2.75 MeV	Yes	Reactor
^{51}Cr	27 days	323 keV	No	Reactor
^{77}Br	58 hours	239, 521 keV	Yes	Cyclotron
^{82}Br	36 hours	560, 780 keV	Yes	Reactor
^{99m}Tc	6 hours	140 keV	No	Reactor
^{111}In	2.8 days	171, 245 keV	No	Cyclotron
^{113m}In	1.7 hours	393 keV	No	Reactor
^{123}I	13 hours	160 keV	No	Cyclotron
^{131}I	8 days	360 keV	Yes	Reactor
^{198}Au	2.7 days	412 keV	Yes	Reactor

it meets closely the criteria discussed above, and in addition has a versatile chemistry which enables it to be labelled to a wide variety of materials (Kelly, 1981). The half-life of ^{99m}Tc is 6 hours, permitting radioactive counting up to and beyond 24 hours, and negligible quantities of beta rays are emitted. As will be discussed later in this chapter, radiation doses resulting from ^{99m}Tc labelled compounds are low. The energy of ^{99m}Tc gamma rays (140 keV) is particularly suitable for use with a gamma camera. Gamma rays with higher energies, emitted by many alternative radionuclides, penetrate more readily through the lead collimators of the gamma camera.

For inhalation into the lung, particle size should be less than 10 μm (and preferably below 5 μm), or else the majority of particles will be unable to pass beyond the oropharynx. Submicronic particles are either exhaled or delivered entirely to alveolated zones, and as such are particularly useful for ventilation scanning. In order to obtain a spread of particles over small and large conducting airways, for instance to assess mucociliary clearance rates, particles in the 1–5 μm range are ideal. It is preferable, but not always essential, that test particles should be monodisperse (that is, all particles approximately the same size, Chapter 3). Monodisperse aerosols are more difficult to produce than heterodisperse aerosols, but have a marked advantage for studying deposition and clearance in that their aerodynamic behaviour can be more readily predicted. Some devices used to generate aerosols, such as the jet or ultrasonic nebulizer, yield heterodisperse aerosols, although auxiliary devices for modifying aerosol size are available. Other types of device, such as the spinning disc generator, make aerosols which are monodisperse. This chapter will consider in turn a variety of methods for producing radioaerosols within the respirable range, discussing how they may be used to generate both solid and liquid systems, with both monodisperse and heterodisperse size distributions.

Nebulizers

Jet nebulizer

This type of nebulizer is very widely employed, particularly in hospitals for administration of therapeutic agents, and for the delivery of radioaerosols used in ventilation scanning. A stream of compressed gas, from a compressor, an air cylinder, or even a foot-pump, is used to atomize a liquid into tiny fragments (Mercer, 1981). These nebulizers generally operate by the Venturi effect. The compressed gas is forced past the end of a narrow tube, the other end of which is

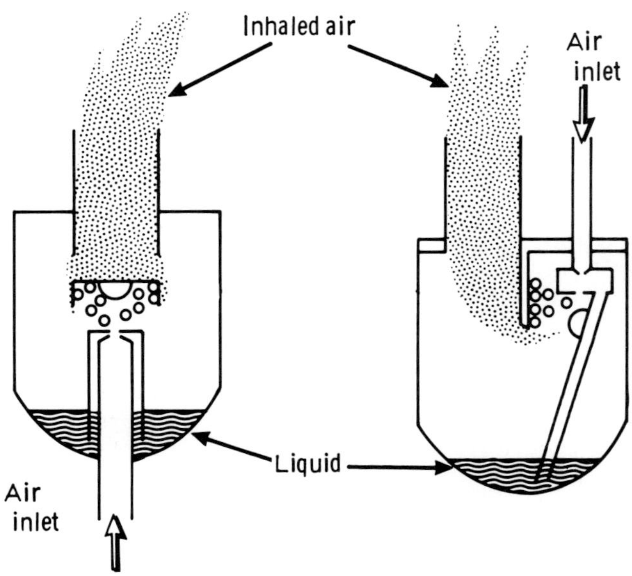

Figure 4.1 Two different designs of jet nebulizer. Liquid is drawn up a feed tube by a stream of compressed gas. The liquid fragments into droplets—larger droplets impinge on baffles and smaller droplets are carried away on the inhaled air stream

immersed in the liquid to be nebulized (*Figure 4.1*), and an area of negative pressure is created. The liquid is drawn up the tube, and is fragmented by the high velocity gas. More than 99 per cent of the total droplet mass consisting of large particles impinges on baffles which surround the nebulizer orifice, and is returned to the reservoir for re-nebulization. About 50 per cent of the liquid becomes permanently entrained upon the baffles, and constitutes a 'dead volume' unavailable for nebulization. Aerosol output rate is proportional to the flow rate of compressed gas through the device.

The Babington nebulizer is a variation on the jet nebulizer concept (Litt and Swift, 1972). In this device, the liquid to be nebulized flows as a thin film over the surface of a small hollow sphere, and air passing outwards through a circular or rectangular opening in the sphere is used to atomize the liquid.

The particle size obtained from a jet nebulizer depends upon the operating conditions, in particular upon the flow rate through the device, but generally droplets produced by the nebulizer may be characterized by a mass median diameter (MMD) in the range 1.2–6.9 μm and a geometric standard deviation (GSD) between 1.7–2.2 (Mercer, 1981), these sizes being measured as the aerosol leaves the device.

Ultrasonic nebulizers

Ultrasonic nebulizers are also widely used for therapy, diagnosis and research, especially in the United States. In this device (Mercer, 1981) the energy required to atomize a liquid is produced by a piezoelectric crystal, vibrating typically at a frequency in the 1–2 MHz range. Vibrations are transmitted through a coupling liquid to the nebulizer solution, and a fountain of droplets is formed in the reservoir (*Figure 4.2*). The smaller droplets are carried away in the inhaled airstream. The operating conditions of these nebulizers vary, and the mean particle size is inversely proportional to the operating frequency. MMD's of the liquid droplets at the

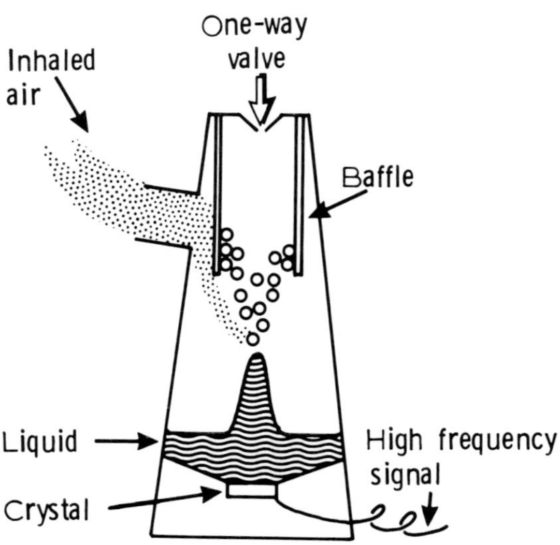

Figure 4.2 Ultrasonic nebulizer. Vibrations in a piezoelectric crystal cause the formation of both large and small droplets

nebulizer exit are typically in the 3.7–10.5 μm range, and GSD's between 1.4–2.0 (Mercer, 1981).

Modifications to particle size

Although the mean droplet size from nebulizers is generally 3 μm or greater, smaller solid particles (MMD typically 1 μm, depending upon the solute concentration) can be produced if the solvent evaporates, leaving a solid residue. This may be achieved if the solvent is highly volatile or if evaporation is brought about by passing the aerosol either through a jet of compressed air or through a heating chamber before inhalation.

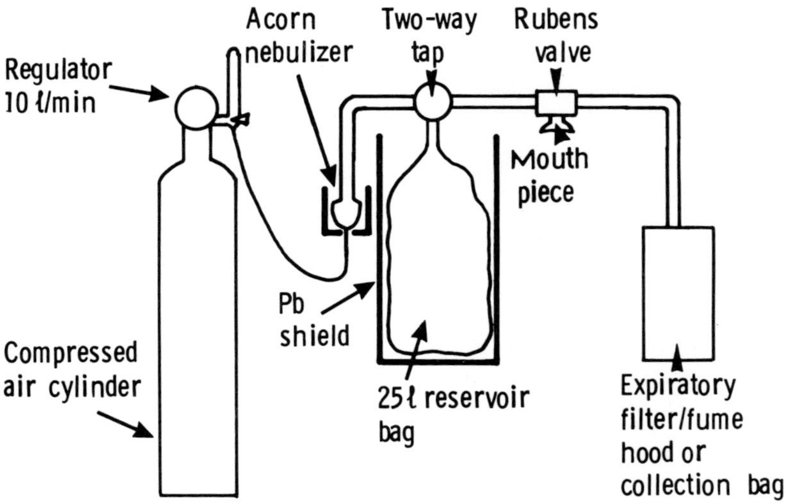

Figure 4.3 Schematic diagram of apparatus used to nebulize a solution of ^{99m}Tc-labelled compound and to administer this to patients for lung ventilation scanning (from Francis *et al.*, 1981). A plastic disposable jet nebulizer is shielded in a lead pot and the solution nebulized until the 25 ℓ reservoir is full. A two-way tap is then turned off and the patient subsequently inhales from the reservoir bag. An interval of 5 minutes between nebulization and inhalation is sufficient to ensure that large particles settle out within the reservoir bag and less than 5 per cent of the inhaled aerosol consists of particles >2 μm diameter. (The author would like to thank Chapman and Hall Ltd., publishers of *Nuclear Medicine Communications*, for permission to reproduce this figure)

The size distribution of nebulized aerosols is heterodisperse, but particles covering a much narrower size range can be selected from the spray. The simplest techniques for doing this involve the elimination of large particles either by allowing them to sediment under gravity, or by impacting them on baffles. Only the smaller particles in a distribution will remain suspended in air if the aerosol is temporarily stored in a settling bag (*Figure 4.3*) or is passed through a set of parallel plates. More complex forms of particle separator are available, which utilize the fact that very small particles may be conducted away by an airstream, while large particles are more readily filtered by impaction. For instance, starting with an aerosol which comprises particles from <1 μm to 10 μm diameter, it is possible to obtain an aerosol confined to the 1–2 μm range by conducting the submicronic particles to an exhaust, and then allowing particles >2 μm to impact on baffles so that they too are eliminated. The mean particle size is thus substantially reduced, enabling the particles to penetrate to more peripheral lung regions, and the spread of particle sizes is also small.

Nebulization of radioactive solutions

Jet and ultrasonic nebulizers have been used to produce aerosols of a variety of radiolabelled solutions, primarily for use in studies of aerosol deposition, and for ventilation scanning of the lung, as listed in *Table 4.2.* Aerosols containing the radionuclide ^{99m}Tc are widely used, often as sodium pertechnetate. Labelled compounds with a higher molecular weight, such as diethylenetriamine pentaacetic acid (D.T.P.A.) or gluconate are particularly useful, since their rates of absorption through airway surfaces (both bronchial mucosa and alveolar septa) are slower than those of small molecules.

TABLE 4.2. Nebulization of radiolabelled solutions

Material nebulized	*Label*	*Type of nebulizer*	*Object of study*	*Authors*
Pertechnetate	^{99m}Tc	Ultrasonic, jet	Deposition measurement	Asmundsson *et al.*, 1973
Pertechnetate	^{99m}Tc	Jet	Ventilation scanning	Kotrappa *et al.*, 1977
Phytate	^{99m}Tc	Ultrasonic	Development of prototype nebulizer	Wasnich, 1976
Albumin	^{113m}In	Jet	Ventilation scanning	Wollmer *et al.*, 1980
Pertechnetate	^{99m}Tc	Ultrasonic	Measurement of pulmonary clearance	Isitman *et al.*, 1974
Phytate	^{99m}Tc			
Chloride	^{111}In			
DTPA	^{111}In			
DTPA	^{99m}Tc	Jet	Measurement of alveolar epithelial permeability	Jones *et al.*, 1980
Antipyrene	^{123}I			
DTPA	^{99m}Tc	Jet	Ventilation scanning	Francis *et al.*, 1981
Gluconate	^{99m}Tc			

Bronchodilator drugs labelled with the beta-emitting isotope ^{3}H have been administered from both jet and ultrasonic nebulizers and the appearance of the label in body fluids used to assess both drug pharmacokinetics and deposition (Shenfield *et al.*, 1973). However, there have been no studies with gamma-labelled bronchodilators, owing to the difficulty of finding a suitable radionuclide. Beta-adrenergic bronchodilators comprise the elements hydrogen, carbon, nitrogen and oxygen, and while the radionuclides ^{11}C, ^{13}N and ^{15}O all emit gamma rays, their half lives are 20, 10 and 2 minutes, respectively. It is therefore difficult to synthesize the labelled drug before the label has decayed to negligible levels. There are no gamma-emitting isotopes of hydrogen. An alternative approach would be to attempt a covalent labelling of a bronchodilator with ^{18}F or ^{123}I, or to label the drug with a metal-ion nuclide such as ^{67}Ga, ^{99m}Tc, ^{111}In or ^{113m}In. However, this exercise would alter the chemical structure of the drugs, so that they may presumably no longer be pharmacologically active.

Drug deposition from nebulizers may be assessed without labelling the drug itself. If a mixture of drug and radioactive solutions is placed in the nebulizer reservoir, then the aerosol droplets will consist of a mixture of drug and radioactivity in proportions determined by their original concentrations in the reservoir. Assuming that the drug and radionuclide are equally volatile, the amount of radionuclide detected in the lungs should reflect the amount of drug deposited

(Dashe *et al.*, 1974). This method is a very powerful one, since it permits deposition and clinical effects of drugs to be assessed simultaneously. The use of nebulizers for delivery of respiratory drugs will be discussed further in Chapter 9.

Nebulization of previously prepared particles

Solid particles generated by nebulizers may be inhaled immediately, or may, depending on their physical characteristics, be collected and stored for subsequent use. Yeates *et al.* (1974) aerosolized an aqueous solution of human serum albumin labelled with ^{99m}Tc using an ultrasonic nebulizer, and then heated the droplets to evaporate the water. The solid albumin spheres (MMD 1.1 μm, GSD 1.8) were then collected by impaction in a liquid bath. The microspheres could then be stored for periods up to 6 months, and very rapidly labelled with ^{99m}Tc when required, using a simple chemical procedure. Other types of previously prepared particles, labelled with ^{99m}Tc and delivered from nebulizers, have included anion resin particles (Bertrand and Puchelle, 1977) and erythrocytes (Matthys, 1980). By their natures, these two aerosols are a little large for penetration to the more peripheral parts of the lung (mean sizes approximately 8 μm), but are suitable for monitoring mucociliary clearance from central lung regions. These and other particles placed either in the nose or at the base of the trachea via a catheter or bronchoscope may be used to assess either nasal mucociliary clearance or tracheal mucus velocity, if their subsequent rate of removal is observed by a gamma camera.

Suspensions of previously prepared solid particles are also available commercially, often as 'kits' to provide easily-prepared radioaerosols for lung ventilation scanning. Human albumin microspheres are the most common type of preparation (Santolicandro and Giutini, 1979). The radionuclide label, usually ^{99m}Tc, is added shortly before the microspheres are nebulized. Various types of colloid may also be used, providing that the particle size is suitable. Monodisperse suspensions of polystyrene latex (PSL) and polyvinyl toluene (PVT) in size ranges 0.1 μm to 4 μm may also be obtained. Labelling of PSL particles with ^{51}Cr has been achieved by emulsion polymerization of chromium acetylacetonide dissolved in styrene monomer (Hinrichs *et al.*, 1978). Beginning with 1.099 μm diameter PSL microspheres, particles of 1.4 μm count median diameter, labelled with ^{51}Cr, were produced, having GSD 1.2, and a very slow leaching rate (<0.2 per cent per day). A suspension of these particles may be aerosolized using a nebulizer. The concentration of particles must be sufficiently low to ensure that the majority of droplets contain only single particles.

Particles of fused clay, insoluble in body fluids and labelled with nuclear fission fragments, have been useful for measurement of alveolar clearance from the lung, a process that takes place over a period of many months (Newton *et al.*, 1980). Relatively long-lived radionuclides are therefore required. The labelling method generally utilizes the cation exchange properties of montmorillonite clay, which is first ground and suspended in water. Labelling is performed by packing exchange sites in the clay with sodium after some preliminary chemical processing, and the radionuclide cation is then exchanged with sodium in the clay. Nebulized clay particles are passed in an air stream through an oven at 1000°C, and the clay particles are fused into spheres with the label firmly bound. The radionuclides ^{85}Sr (half-life 65 days) and ^{88}Y (half-life 107 days) are particularly useful for long-term retention measurements in volunteer subjects (Bailey *et al.*, 1982).

Spinning disc generator

Principles

A spray of fairly uniform droplet size is formed when liquid is fed onto the centre of a rapidly rotating disc (May, 1949; Walton and Prewett, 1949). The liquid spreads over the disc surface as a film and flows to the edge of the disc where it accumulates until the centrifugal force acting upon it exceeds the retaining force of surface tension. At this point the liquid is flung off tangentially, and forms a spherical droplet.

If d = droplet diameter, R = disc radius, ω = angular velocity of the disc, and T and ρ are the liquid surface tension and density respectively, then it may be assumed that as the droplet leaves the disc, the product of the droplet mass and the accelerating force is proportional to the product of surface tension and droplet size, i.e.,

$$\frac{\pi d^3 \rho}{6} \times \omega^2 R \propto T \times d$$

Therefore

$$d \propto \frac{1}{\omega}\sqrt{\frac{T}{R\rho}}$$

Hence droplet size decreases as the angular velocity of the disc increases. The constant of proportionality in the above equation depends primarily upon the design of the disc, and in particular upon the sharpness of its edges. The term 'disc' is really a misnomer—the device is usually 'cone' or 'top' shaped, and is a few centimetres in diameter.

In order to produce particles small enough for inhalation, disc speeds exceeding 10^4 revolutions per minute (166 Hz) are required. Although motor-driven discs may

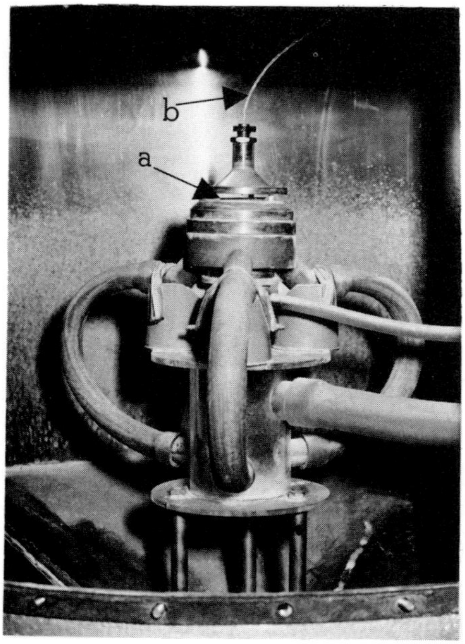

Figure 4.4 The spinning disc generator. The disc (a) is caused to rotate by compressed air, while a radioactive solution or suspension is supplied to its centre via a feed tube (b). Droplets are flung off the disc by centrifugal force. The tubing below the disc controls the air supply as well as the removal of small unwanted 'satellite' droplets

be used, compressed air is usually employed as a driving force in order to attain such speeds (*Figure 4.4*). The air usually impinges upon grooves cut obliquely in the underside of the disc. The liquid for aerosolization is supplied to the disc by some type of constant flow device, such as a peristaltic pump or constant rate syringe injector.

In addition to the primary droplets, secondary 'satellite' droplets are also formed. These are typically 1/4 of the diameter of the primary droplets, and are formed from the filament of liquid between the primary droplet and the disc at the moment of separation. They are formed at the rate of 3 or 4 per primary droplet, and usually comprise less than 10 per cent of the atomized liquid mass if the rate of liquid feed is less than 1 ml min^{-1}. Primary and satellite droplets are easily separated, since the latter have relatively little inertia and are projected only a short distance from the disc compared to the primary droplets.

Spinning disc generators are most frequently used to produce aerosols of solid inert materials, firmly labelled with gamma-emitting radionuclides. Solvents which readily evaporate after aerosolization are chosen—these may be aqueous solutions, or organic solvents such as xylene. The disc is usually housed within a large airtight tank, and the solvents evaporate as the droplets settle under gravity. The residue of solid radioaerosol particles is then characterized by a diameter d_s, related to the original droplet size (d) by the formula

$$d_s = (C/\sigma)^{1/3}d$$

where C and σ are solute concentration and density respectively. Aerosolization of a unit density 0.1 per cent solution would yield solid particles one tenth the size of the original liquid droplets. Varying the solute concentration offers a simple and convenient method for changing particle size. Most spinning disc generators are used to produce solid particles with mean diameters ranging from 1 μm to 30 μm. The GSD is typically 1.1, but will depend upon a number of factors, including the evenness of wetting of the disc surface and the closeness of the liquid feed needle to the disc centre. Some doublet or triplet particles may be formed owing to confluence of droplets.

The solid particles may be inhaled from the tank directly, or may be collected for subsequent re-nebulization by impaction in ethanol (Foord *et al.*, 1978), by drawing them onto a filter of appropriate pore size (Philipson, 1973), or by allowing them to settle onto the tank base.

Labelling procedures

A variety of solid radioaerosols has been manufactured by the spinning disc generator, as listed in *Table 4.3*. The labelling procedures fall broadly into three categories. Firstly, the test material is chemically labelled with radionuclide, and is then dissolved in a volatile solvent. After spinning, the solvent evaporates, leaving a solid radioaerosol. Secondly, a suspension of very fine particles of the test substance is mixed with the radiolabel, and spheres of the appropriate size are produced by correctly setting the disc speed. The spheres are tagged by the label by the process of physical inclusion. Thirdly, non-radioactive spheres are manufactured by the disc, and are subsequently made radioactive by irradiation in a nuclear reactor or cyclotron. Examples of these three techniques will be considered in detail.

TABLE 4.3. Radioaerosols generated by the spinning disc method, for use in studies of aerosol deposition or mucociliary clearance

Aerosol material	*Radiolabel*	*Authors*
Polystyrene	^{51}Cr	Booker *et al.*, 1967
	^{99m}Tc	Few *et al.*, 1970
	^{82}Br, ^{131}I	Black and Walsh, 1970
	^{11}C*	Philipson *et al.*, 1970
Teflon	^{99m}Tc	Camner *et al.*, 1971
	^{18}F*	Camner and Philipson, 1971
	^{51}Cr	Philipson *et al.*, 1975
	^{111}In	Camner and Philipson, 1978
	^{198}Au	Svartengren *et al.*, 1981
Iron oxide	^{7}Be, ^{51}Cr, ^{59}Fe, ^{141}Ce, ^{234}Th	Albert *et al.*, 1964
	^{198}Au, ^{99m}Tc	Lippmann and Albert, 1969
	^{99m}Tc	Hass *et al.*, 1976
Lucite	^{7}Be, ^{51}Cr, ^{59}Fe, ^{95}Zr-^{95}Nb	Albert *et al.*, 1964

*following cyclotron irradiation

Few *et al.* (1970) described a method for labelling polystyrene particles with ^{99m}Tc, and this method is now in widespread use. Polystyrene is an inert material, insoluble in body fluids, but easily dissolved in some organic solvents. A ^{99m}Tc generator is eluted with saline to give sodium pertechnetate ($Na^{99m}TcO_4$). After adjusting the pH, a drop of tetraphenylarsonium chloride is added, and the mixture is passed through a phase-separating filter paper together with chloroform. The filtrate contains about half the initial radioactivity, as tetraphenylarsonium pertechnetate, dissolved in the chloroform. This is evaporated to dryness, and the residue, together with a few milligrams of polystyrene is dissolved in xylene and methyl isobutyl ketone. After spinning, the xylene rapidly evaporates, leaving small insoluble polystyrene spheres, firmly labelled with ^{99m}Tc. The methyl isobutyl ketone serves to retard evaporation of xylene on the disc surface, which would result in accumulation of polystyrene residue and a reduction in monodispersity. Black and Walsh (1970) produced monodisperse polystyrene particles over a wide range of sizes, labelled with ^{82}Br or ^{131}I using a spinning disc generator. Labelled particles were manufactured using xylene solutions of ^{82}Br-labelled polymerized 3-bromostyrene or ^{131}I-labelled iodinated polystyrene, respectively. Labelled polystyrene particles below 1 μm diameter could not be made with the spinning disc however, but were obtained by the emulsion polymerization of ^{131}I-labelled 2,4-iodostyrene, the size being controlled by the number of polymerization stages.

Techniques for labelling iron oxide (Fe_2O_3) and lucite particles are not dissimilar. Albert *et al.* (1964) made particles of these materials, with sizes ranging from 1 μm to 8 μm, firmly labelled with a variety of radionuclides (*Table 4.3*). A spinning disc generator was used to atomize either iron oxide sol, or lucite in a xylene-acetylacetone solution. Labelling of iron oxide was achieved by addition of radionuclide in a carrier-free form to the sol, and labelling of lucite by chelating the radionuclides with acetylacetone to the lucite solution. Hass *et al.* (1976) labelled iron oxide microspheres with ^{99m}Tc following reduction of the iron oxide using stannous chloride in a nitrogen atmosphere.

Techniques for labelling Teflon (fluorinated ethylene propylene) may be rather different however. Teflon is a very useful substance for making test aerosols, since it is completely inert, and may be labelled by a variety of radionuclides. It is available commercially as a fine suspension of 0.1 to 0.2 μm grains in water. Radioaerosol particles may be produced by spinning a mixture consisting of Teflon, ethanol and a $^{99m}TcO_4$ residue. The ethanol evaporates after spinning and particles of the appropriate size are formed, depending upon the disc speed, and are loose agglomerations of many fine Teflon grains. The label is incorporated into the particles by physical inclusion. The particles must be collected, usually on a silver filter, and then heated at 240°C to seal the label inside the particles. The particles are then re-suspended for nebulization. Using the radionuclide ^{99m}Tc, specific activities >3.7 MBq mg^{-1} (100 μCi mg^{-1}) are obtainable (Camner *et al.*, 1971).

Labelling of Teflon or polystyrene can be accomplished by manufacturing non-radioactive particles using the techniques described above, and then inducing radioactivity by placing them in a beam of radiation in a cyclotron. Polystyrene particles, labelled with ^{11}C (specific activity approximately 3.7 MBq mg^{-1} (100 μCi mg^{-1})) have been obtained by irradiation in a 50 MeV proton beam. Radioactive ^{11}C is formed from stable ^{12}C in the polystyrene by the reaction (Philipson *et al.*, 1970)

$$p + {}^{12}C \rightarrow {}^{11}C + p + n$$

No significant quantities of other radionuclides are induced by this technique. Proton irradiation of Teflon produces not only ^{11}C, but also ^{18}F, by the reaction (Camner and Philipson, 1971)

$$p + {}^{19}F \rightarrow {}^{18}F + p + n$$

^{11}C has a half-life of 20 minutes, and ^{18}F 110 minutes, so that only ^{18}F remains in any quantity after a few hours. Specific activities of approximately 370 kBq mg^{-1} (10 μCi mg^{-1}) may be attained. Although the radionuclide labels are short-lived, the aerosols have been used for short-term studies. It is, of course, essential that a cyclotron should be close at hand.

Leaching

Leaching or dissociation of the radiolabel from insoluble particles may occur, and this must be assessed as part of the development of any new radioaerosol technique. The amount of leaching which occurs, and the rate at which this takes place are of particular importance if medium or long-term measurements are to be made of radioaerosol retention in the lung, since radiolabel which dissociates from the particles will be rapidly absorbed via the airway surfaces and carried away by the systemic circulation. Leaching may be assessed *in vitro* or *in vivo*. Particles securely wrapped in filter paper may be immersed in water for set periods of time, and any radioactivity appearing in the water is assumed to have leached from the particles. Alternatively the particles may be suspended in liquid and then centrifuged—radioactive material lost from the particles remains in the supernatant. Paper chromatography techniques may also be used to separate bound and free radiolabels. *In vivo* assessment of leaching involves collection of urine for 24 or 48 hours after particle inhalation. If no radioactive material has been lost from the insoluble particles, then no radioactivity will appear in the urine.

When the label is chemically bound to the test aerosol, leaching is generally very small. For polystyrene particles labelled with ^{99m}Tc, about 4 per cent of radioactivity is leached from the particles after 3 hours in saline, with the loss falling to less than 1 per cent in 24 hours thereafter (Few *et al.*, 1970). Labelling methods based on physical inclusion may involve greater losses however, since molecules of the label on the outside of the particles are likely to be loosely bound, even after heating. Leaching is particularly high in the first half-hour after irradiation, and it may be necessary to wash the particles in order to remove loosely bound radionuclide before the particles are used. When labelling is achieved by cyclotron irradiation, losses resulting from leaching are small, since the label is firmly bound—usually by covalent bonding—to the test material.

A system for radioaerosol production using the spinning disc technique

We have developed a spinning disc generator for the production of gamma-labelled aerosols, and their subsequent administration to patients in a controlled manner (*Figure 4.5*). The disc (A) is 2.5 cm in diameter, and following evaporation of solvents may be used to produce particles in the respirable range when the disc rotates at about 3×10^4 revolutions per minute. The smaller unwanted 'satellite' particles are carried under the rim of the disc and away to an exhaust (B). The disc is driven by a high pressure air supply (C), from a hospital air line, and a fine control maintained by means of a regulating valve (D). A connection from the air supply is fed to a mercury-in-glass manometer (E) and the pressure of mercury used as an index of disc speed. Liquid is supplied via a fine needle to the disc centre at a rate of about 1 ml min^{-1} by means of a motor-driven constant-rate syringe injector (F). The whole system is enclosed in an airtight brass tank (G) approximately 60 cm

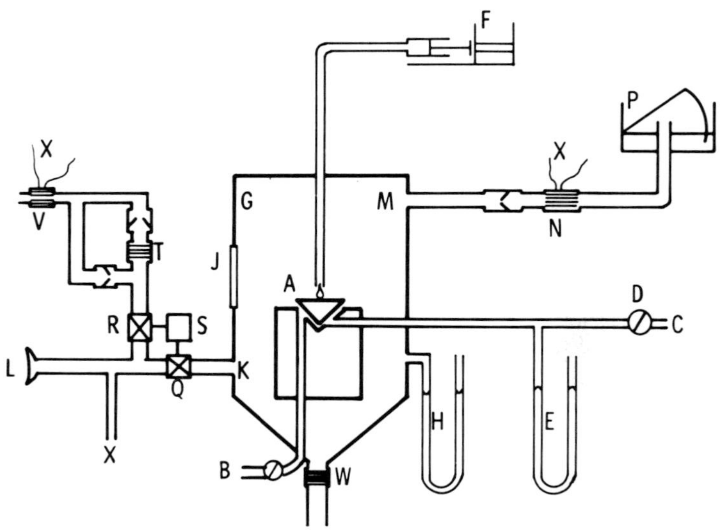

Figure 4.5 Diagrammatic representation of a system for the generation of monodisperse radioaerosols by the spinning disc method and their administration to human subjects. A = spinning disc, B = satellite exhaust, C = high pressure air supply, D = regulating valve, E = mercury manometer, F = constant rate syringe injector, G = airtight tank, H = water manometer, J = perspex window, K and M = air outlet and inlet, L = mouthpiece, N and V = pneumotachygraphs, P = Krogh spirometer, Q and R = valves to control inhalation and exhalation, S = delay unit, T = Martindale filter for exhaled air, W = filter for particle collection, X = connections to pressure transducers

in height and 40 cm in diameter, surrounded on all sides by 2 mm lead to act as radiation shielding for ^{99m}Tc. Air tightness can be checked by recording the fall in pressure inside the tank, using a water-in-glass manometer (H). A removable perspex window (J) in the side of the tank allows access to the disc for cleaning and maintenance.

In order to administer the aerosol to patients, two extra connections are made to the tank. The first (K) is connected to a mouthpiece (L) through which the patient inhales, while air enters the tank through the second connection (M), replacing the inhaled air. This air inlet is connected in series with a pneumotachygraph (N), which is used to measure the flow-rate of inspired air, and to a Krogh spirometer (P) used to limit inhalation to any required volume (usually 450 ml) by means of preset electrical contacts. Inhalation and exhalation are carried out through a system of solenoid valves. The inlet valve (Q) is initially open and the outlet valve (R) closed, so that the subject inhales air, containing the dispersed aerosol, from the tank. The inhalation is automatically terminated when the Krogh spirometer automatically closes the inlet valve at the preset inspired volume. A delay unit (S), preset to function after the required breath-holding pause, subsequently opens the outlet valve, following which the subject exhales. A Martindale filter (T) placed beyond the outlet valve can be used to assess the quantity of radioaerosol exhaled. Mouth pressure during breath-holding may be recorded by a pressure transducer and displayed together with inhalation flowrate on an ultra-violet recorder. A removable addition to this system enables the subject to breathe room air at a known rate through a second pneumotachygraph (V). The solenoid valves may be subsequently operated so that the subject inhales radioaerosol from the tank before being switched back to the room air supply. This permits a small bolus of aerosol to be delivered to the subject at a predetermined lung volume.

If required, the particles may be collected by drawing the air in the tank through a filter (W) of appropriate pore size, using a vacuum pump. This technique has been used in the production of ^{99m}Tc-labelled Teflon particles, which are subsequently stabilized by heating and are then placed in pressurized metered dose inhalers (Newman *et al.*, 1981). These particles are then used to assess pressurized aerosol deposition. In the case of polystyrene particles, collection of particles and their subsequent re-nebulization would also have the merit of avoiding the necessity for inhaling solvent vapour such as xylene directly from the tank, although patients seldom find the xylene unpleasant and this substance does not retard mucociliary clearance in the concentration normally used (Booker *et al.*, 1967). Collection and re-nebulization of particles also enables a more precisely known quantity of radioactivity to be administered than direct inhalation from the tank.

Sophisticated additions to the spinning disc system could involve several liquid feeds to the disc centre, so that by adjusting the solute concentration and by using various radionuclide labels in different liquid feeds, a variety of radioaerosols of differing particle size could be produced, without changing the operating conditions of the generator.

Using the system described above, monodisperse particles of polystyrene, labelled with ^{99m}Tc by the technique of Few *et al.* (1970), are inhaled directly from the tank as they settle under gravity. The rate of removal of the particles from the lungs is used as an index of mucociliary clearance (Chapter 6). Polystyrene particles with mean diameters 2 μm to 10 μm have been manufactured. Particles with a mean diameter 5 μm have a standard deviation 0.8 μm (geometric standard deviation,

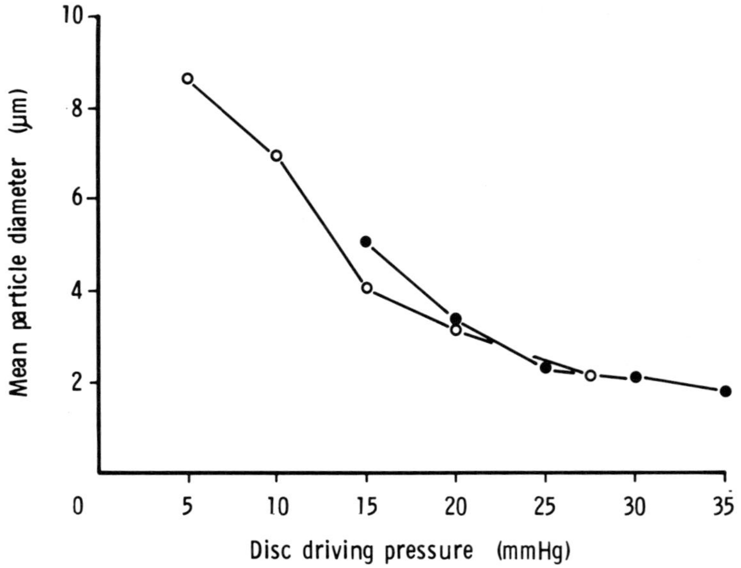

Figure 4.6 Mean particle size as a function of spinning disc air driving pressure. Data are shown for a 2.5 cm disc with a 0.2 per cent solution of polystyrene in xylene (open circles, from Few *et al.*, 1970) and for a 0.1 per cent suspension of Teflon in ethanol (closed circles, from Newman, 1982)

GSD, 1.15). The mean diameters of polystyrene and Teflon particles, generated by this system, are shown in *Figure 4.6*, as functions of the disc driving pressure. The particle size varies inversely with the air pressure, but it is difficult to make particles smaller than about 2 µm, since above 25 mmHg increases in pressure produce relatively small reductions in particle size.

Other techniques for making monodisperse radioaerosols

Condensation generators

Droplets in a narrow size range (GSD approximately 1.10) can be obtained by controlled condensation of organic vapours. The material to be aerosolized is first heated in a boiler at a temperature between 100 and 200°C, and the vapour produced is mixed with nucleation centres. These nuclei are produced by an electric spark or by heating a wire coated with an organic salt such as NaCl or AgCl. The mixture is then passed into a condensation chimney where the vapour cools and condenses onto the nuclei to form monodisperse droplets (Sinclair and La Mer, 1949). Droplet size depends upon the vapour concentration (and hence upon heating temperature) and also upon nuclei concentration.

Wilson and La Mer (1948) used this type of generator to produce an aerosol of glycerol, which was condensed onto radioactive ^{24}NaCl nuclei. With this aerosol they performed some of the earliest studies of regional deposition in the lung. Aerosols comprising oils which do not undergo hygroscopic growth within the lung may be manufactured by the condensation technique, and are particularly useful for deposition studies. A modified condensation generator was used by Smaldone *et al.* (1979) for assessment of aerosol deposition during exhalation at flow-limiting segments. A 1 μm diameter aerosol with a GSD of 1.3 was formed by condensing di-2-ethyl-hexyl sebacate oil vapour onto ^{99m}Tc-labelled human serum albumin particles.

Vibrating orifice generator

A highly monodisperse aerosol may be produced using the vibrating orifice generator. Liquid is forced through an orifice at a constant flow rate, generally using a constant flow syringe injector, and fragments into droplets. If the orifice is vibrated by a piezoelectric crystal, then the droplets are uniform in diameter, being produced at the rate of one droplet per cycle. GSD's of 1.01–1.03 are attainable, with the mean particle size ranging from 0.5 to 50 μm, depending upon the oscillation frequency (Marple and Rubow, 1980). Auxiliary air is usually supplied to prevent droplet coagulation. The vibrating orifice generator may be used to nebulize both solutions and suspensions, but has been used only rarely in radioaerosol studies.

Pressurized aerosols

Pressurized aerosol canisters (Sanders, 1970) which derive their driving force from propellants at high pressure, are so well known that it is surprising that they have been seldom used for radioaerosol generation. The chief reason for this is probably the technical problems associated with loading the radioactive material into the canister. The propellants are in the gaseous phase at room temperature and atmospheric pressure so that the canisters cannot be opened under normal laboratory conditions. The propellants cannot be dispensed unless they are either cooled or compressed.

There are basically two types of pressurized aerosol canister—the continuous spray (*Figure 4.7a*), used widely to deliver an enormous range of consumer products, and metered dose sprays (*Figure 4.7b*) which are used to administer various drugs for treatment of respiratory diseases (Chapter 9). The latter device delivers the contents of a small metering chamber (25, 50 or 100 μl volume) each time the canister is pressed, and up to 400 metered doses are available. There are two formulations which can be used with either continuous or metered dose sprays. The material to be atomized can be either a suspension of solid particles in the propellant, together with a surface active agent to prevent agglomeration, or a solution mixed uniformly with a cosolvent and the propellants. The best known propellants are the chlorofluorocarbons, a mixture of the volatile chlorofluorocarbon 12 and the less volatile chlorofluorocarbons 11 and 114 being used to obtain the desired spray characteristics. Inside the canister, the vapour and liquid phases are always in equilibrium, and the vapour pressure (that is, the pressure exerted by the molecules of the vapour phase) is a constant for a given propellant at a given temperature. Hence the driving pressure is constant throughout the life of the canister.

Spray formation is a 2 phase process, consisting of an initial rapid 'flashing' of some of the propellants followed by a slower secondary evaporation phase. The spray consists of large, rapidly moving propellant droplets comprising the suspension or solution to be atomized, and these neither evaporate nor slow down completely until they have travelled at least 20 cm from the canister. Consequently,

(a)

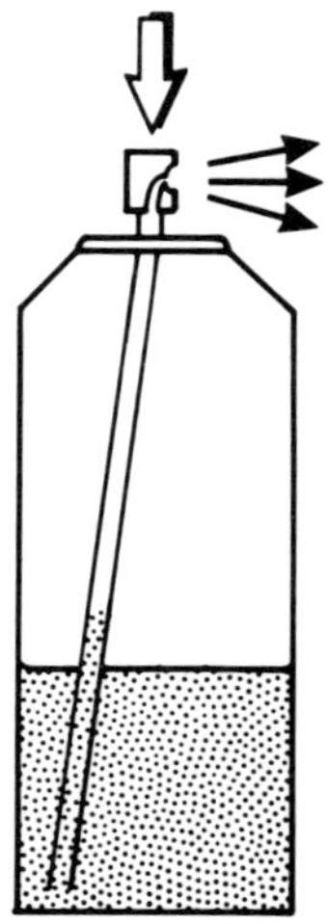

(b)

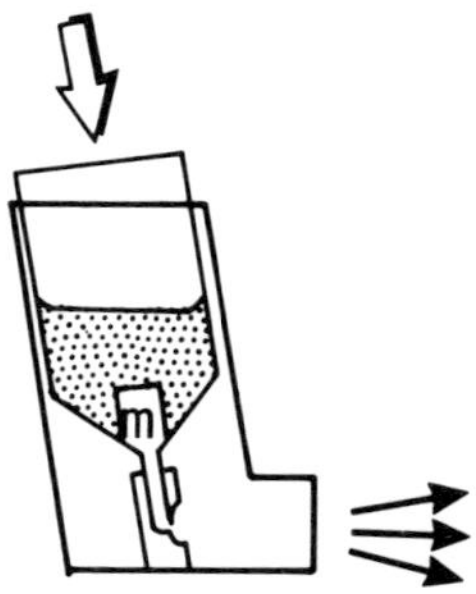

Figure 4.7 Pressurized aerosol canisters delivering continuous sprays (a) and metered doses (b). The latter delivers the contents of a metering chamber (m) each time it is pressed

pressurized aerosols fired directly into the oropharynx impact there almost entirely, and few penetrate to the lungs. Pressurized aerosol delivery systems have a potential use for radioaerosol delivery, providing that care is taken to minimize oropharyngeal losses. Various designs of reservoir or holding chamber (Chapter 9), designed to slow down and contain the aerosol cloud, could be useful in this respect. A pressurized aerosol canister could be used to store a solution or suspension labelled with a relatively long-lived radionuclide, and the radioaerosol could then be produced on demand. Such a system could at least in theory be used, with appropriate refinements to ensure an optimal aerosol size, to produce aerosols for lung ventilation scanning.

Radioaerosol studies using pressurized delivery systems have to date been confined to measurements of the deposition of hair spray aerosols and metered dose bronchodilator or steroid aerosols. Swift *et al.* (1979) labelled a commercially available brand of hair spray which consisted chiefly of methyl alcohol and propellants. A quantity of ^{99m}Tc was extracted into methyl ethyl ketone and injected into the canister under pressure. After thorough shaking of the canister, the radionuclide was incorporated into droplets subsequently released from the canister, which were sprayed into a booth prior to inhalation.

'Cold-fill' techniques have been used to add radioactive materials to metered dose aerosol canisters. If the canisters are cooled below −30°C, then the propellants remain in the liquid phase at atmospheric pressure, and the canisters may be opened safely. Either solid radioactive particles previously prepared using a spinning disc generator (Newman *et al.*, 1981) or radioactive solutions (Dolovich *et al.*, 1981) may be added, simulating suspension or solution aerosol formulations. As in the case of nebulizers, drugs labelled with ^{3}H have been administered from metered dose inhalers, primarily to assess pharmocokinetics, but studies with gamma-labelled drugs have been limited owing to the lack of suitable labels for the beta-adrenergic bronchodilators. Crystals of the anticholinergic agent ipratropium bromide have been labelled with ^{77}Br, and inhaled from metered dose canisters (Short *et al.*, 1981). The particle size was similar to that of the commercially available drug and the radionuclide was incorporated into the chemical structure of the drug itself.

Dry powder inhalers

Respiratory drugs may also be delivered as dry powders (Chapter 9). Specially designed breath-actuated inhalation devices are used, two designs of which are shown diagrammatically in *Figure 4.8*. In the earliest type of device (the 'Spinhaler', upper figure), a gelatin capsule containing sodium cromoglycate powder is mounted into a rotor upon which are several small fan blades. The capsule must be pierced by two small needles by sliding the outer casing of the inhaler relative to the inner casing. When the patient inhales, the capsule rotates rapidly and the powder is emptied from the capsule by the inhaled airstream. In a more recently introduced and simpler device (the 'Rotahaler', lower figure), the capsule is mounted in the far end of the inhaler, and is broken in half by twisting the outer and inner parts of the inhaler relative to one another. As before, the inhaled airstream draws the drug powder from the capsule.

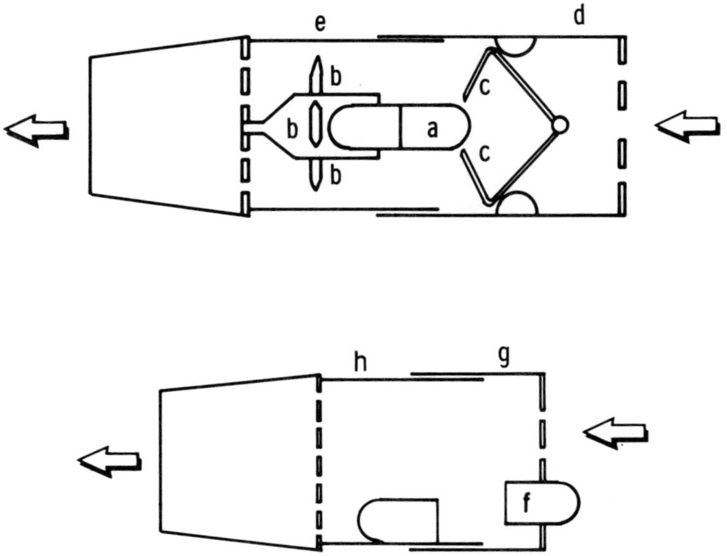

Figure 4.8 Dry powder inhalers. Two designs are shown, with the direction of air flow shown by arrows. Upper figure: a = capsule, b = fan blades, c = piercing needles, d = outer casing, e = inner casing. Lower figure: f = capsule, g = outer casing, h = inner casing

As in the case of pressurized canisters, dry powder devices have been neglected as a source of radioaerosols. Again this is surprising since this type of device offers potentially a simple, inexpensive alternative to more sophisticated devices such as the spinning disc generator. The major difficulty is probably that of ensuring particles small enough for inhalation. In practice, many large agglomerates are formed as the capsules empty, particularly if large lactose carrier particles are placed in the capsules in addition to the drug. Oropharyngeal deposition predominates, and few particles reach the lungs. However, a dry powder inhaler was used recently as a source of radioaerosol for mucociliary clearance studies (Ross *et al.*, 1979). A powder in the respirable range was obtained by crushing ^{99m}Tc-labelled sulphide colloid and was shown by electron microscopy to yield particles in the range between 0.02 and 5 μm. The powder was placed in a 'Spinhaler' capsule and inhaled. Clearance of the colloid particles from the lungs by the mucociliary mechanism was then measured.

Radiation dosimetry

Aerosol deposition patterns can be measured accurately using radiolabelled particles, and as little as 370 kBq (10 μCi) of gamma-emitting material may be required to give an adequate number of radioactive counts. Radiation doses will in general be greatest for insoluble radioaerosols which remain *in situ* in the alveolated zones, and for those radionuclides which emit beta rays as part of their decay scheme. The dose will depend upon the effective half-life of the radionuclide used—this quantity takes into account both physical decay and biological clearance of the radionuclide from the target organ. Insoluble radioaerosol particles deposited in the alveoli will probably be present for periods greatly in excess of the physical half-life of the radionuclide, and the dose received by this region of the lungs will be proportional to the physical half-life. Insoluble particles located on the conducting airways are cleared more rapidly, but their rate of removal may also be slow compared to the physical half-life of the radionuclide in the case of short-lived isotopes such as ^{11}C, ^{18}F and ^{99m}Tc.

Radiation dose from insoluble gamma-labelled aerosols used in clinical studies has been estimated by various workers, and results are summarized in *Table 4.4.* The radiation dose varies according to the radionuclide used, but ^{99m}Tc, which has a short half-life and which chiefly emits gamma rays, gives rise to particularly low doses. Although some beta rays are emitted in the ^{99m}Tc decay scheme, they are of

TABLE 4.4. Estimates of absorbed radiation dose to the lung (μGy) from deposition of 370 kBq (10 μCi) of radionuclide firmly labelled to insoluble particles

Radionuclide	*Dose* (μGy)	*Author*
^{99m}Tc	23	Pavia, 1973
^{99m}Tc	65	Philipson, 1977
^{99m}Tc	47	Short *et al.*, 1979
^{99m}Tc	21	Newman, 1982
^{99m}Tc	50	Foord *et al.*, 1978
^{51}Cr	1500	Foord *et al.*, 1978
^{11}C	90	Philipson, 1977
^{18}F	300	Philipson, 1977

very low abundance, and the dose which they produce is negligible. Approximately 12 per cent of all ^{99m}Tc disintegrations occur with the emission of internal conversion electrons ranging in energy from 120 to 140 keV, and the local absorption of these charged particles contributes approximately half the total radiation dose. Estimates of the dose to the lungs from ^{99m}Tc-labelled insoluble aerosols vary according to the assumptions made regarding particle distribution in the lungs, but all estimates indicate doses less than that received annually from 'background' radiation (approximately 1000 μGy, Coggle, 1971). Furthermore, they are smaller than the dose received during the course of a single chest x-ray (approximately 400 μGy, Advisory Committee on Biological Effects of Ionizing Radiation, 1977). Although the doses listed in *Table 4.4* are small, higher estimates may be made if the particles are assumed to be distributed only on the larger conducting airways, or if the dose to cells immediately in contact with the particles is calculated.

Insoluble material delivered to the conducting airways is cleared by the mucociliary escalator and is subsequently swallowed, so that the gastrointestinal tract then becomes the region irradiated by radioaerosol particles. However, these particles are passing through the gut, and are unlikely to remain stationary for a long period of time, at least in the small intestine. The doses received by the gastrointestinal tract from ^{99m}Tc-labelled insoluble particles are therefore small, and are comparable to or smaller than those received by the lung.

References

ADVISORY COMMITTEE ON BIOLOGICAL EFFECTS OF IONIZING RADIATION (1977). US Environmental Protection Agency

ALBERT, R.E., PETROW, H.G., SALAM, A.S. and SPIEGELMAN, J.R. (1964). Fabrication of monodisperse lucite and iron oxide particles with a spinning disc generator. *Health Phys.*, **10**, 933–940

ASMUNDSSON, T., JOHNSON, R.F., KILBURN, K.H. and GOODRICH, J.K. (1973). Efficiency of nebulizers for depositing saline in human lung. *Am. Rev. Respir. Dis.*, **108**, 506–512

BAILEY, M.R., FRY, F.A. and JAMES, A.C. (1982). The long-term clearance kinetics of insoluble particles from the human lung. In *Inhaled particles V*. Edited by Walton, W.H. Oxford; Pergamon Press, pp. 273–289

BERTRAND, A. and PUCHELLE, E. (1977). Mesure de la clearance muco-ciliare des bronches proximales chez le bronchitique chronique. *Path. Biol.*, **25**, 623–627

BLACK, A. and WALSH, M. (1970). The preparation of ^{82}Br and ^{131}I labelled polystyrene microspheres with diameters 0.1–30 μm. *Ann. Occup. Hyg.*, **13**, 87–100

BOOKER, D.V., CHAMBERLAIN, A.C., RUNDO, J., MUIR, D.C.F. and THOMSON, M.L. (1967). Elimination of 5μ particles from the human lung. *Nature*, **215**, 30–33

CAMNER, P. and PHILIPSON, K. (1971). Production of 7μ monodisperse fluorocarbon resin particles tagged with ^{18}F. *Int. J. Appl. Radiat. Isot.*, **22**, 349–353

CAMNER, P. and PHILIPSON, K. (1978). Human alveolar deposition of 4μ Teflon particles. *Arch. Environ. Health*, **36**, 181–185

CAMNER, P., PHILIPSON, K. and LINNMAN, L. (1971). A simple method for nuclidic tagging of monodisperse fluorocarbon resin particles. *Int. J. Appl. Radiat. Isot.*, **22**, 731–734

COGGLE, J.E. (1971). *Biological effects of radiation*. London; Wykeham Publications, p.129

DASHE, C.K., PONTO, R.A., GANAPES, C.H., DRAGE, C.W. and KRONENBERG, R.S. (1974). The distribution of nebulized isoproterenol and its effect on regional ventilation and perfusion. *Am. Rev. Respir. Dis.*, **110**, 293–300

DOLOVICH, M., RUFFIN, R.E., ROBERTS, R. and NEWHOUSE, M.T. (1981). Optimal delivery of aerosols from metered dose inhalers. *Chest*, **80**, Supplement, 911–915

FEW, J.D., SHORT, M.D. and THOMSON, M.L. (1970). Preparation of ^{99m}Tc labelled particles for aerosol studies. *Radiochem. Radioanal. Lett.*, **5**, 275–277

FOORD, N., BLACK, A. and WALSH, M. (1978). Regional deposition of 2.5–7.5μ diameter inhaled particles in healthy male non-smokers. *J. Aerosol Sci.*, **9**, 343–357

FRANCIS, R.A., AGNEW, J.E., SUTTON, P.P., PAVIA, D. and CLARKE, S.W. (1981). Ventilation imaging with easily prepared ^{99m}Tc aerosols. *Nucl. Med. Comm.*, **2**, 203–208

HASS, P.J., LEES, P.S. and LOURENÇO, R.V. (1976). Tagging of iron oxide particles with ^{99m}Tc for use in the study of deposition and clearance of inhaled particles. *J. Nucl. Med.*, **17**, 122–125

HINRICHS, R.J., KENOYER, J.L., PHALEN, R.F. and CROCKER, T.T. (1978). Labelling of monodisperse polystyrene microspheres with tightly bound ^{51}Cr. *Am. Ind. Hyg. Assoc. J.*, **39**, 570–575

ISITMAN, A.T., MANOLI, R., SCHMIDT, G.H. and HOLMES, R.A. (1974). An assessment of alveolar deposition and pulmonary clearance of radiopharmaceuticals after nebulization. *Am. J. Roentgenol.*, **120**, 776–781

JONES, J.G., MINTY, B.D., LAWLER, P., HULANDS, G., CRAWLEY, J.C.W. and VEALL, N. (1980). Increased alveolar epithelial permeability in cigarette smokers. *Lancet*, **1**, 66–68

KELLY, J.D. (1981). Choice of radionuclides for scintigraphy. In *Radionuclide imaging in drug research*. Edited by Wilson, C.G., Hardy, J.G., Frier, M. and Davis, S.S. London; Croom Helm Ltd., pp.39–59

KOTRAPPA, P., RAGHUNATH, B., SUBRAMANYAM, P.S.S., RAIKAR, U.R. and SHARMA, S.M. (1977). Scintigraphy of lungs with dry aerosol—generation and delivery system. *J. Nucl. Med.*, **18**, 1082–1085

LIPPMANN, M. and ALBERT, R.E. (1969). The effect of particle size on the regional deposition of inhaled aerosols in the human respiratory tract. *Am. Ind. Hyg. Assoc. J.*, **30**, 257–275

LITT, M. and SWIFT, D. (1972). The Babington nebulizer: A new principle for generation of therapeutic aerosols. *Am. Rev. Respir. Dis.*, **105**, 308–310

MARPLE, V.A. and RUBOW, K.L. (1980). Aerosol generation concepts and parameters. In *Generation of aerosols and facilities for exposure experiments*. Edited by Willeke, K. Ann Arbor; Ann Arbor Science Publishers Inc., pp. 3–29

MATTHYS, H. (1980). Beta receptor agonists. In *Progress in respiration research*, Vol. 14. Edited by Herzog, H. Basel; S. Karger, pp. 186–195

MAY, K.R. (1949). An improved spinning top homogeneous spray apparatus. *J. Appl. Physics*, **20**, 932–938

MERCER, T.T. (1981). Production of therapeutic aerosols: Principles and techniques. *Chest*, **80**, Supplement, 813–818

NEWMAN, S.P. (1982). Studies of inhaled therapeutic pressurised aerosols in man: Patterns of deposition and bronchodilator effect. University of London Ph.D. Thesis, Royal Free Hospital School of Medicine

NEWMAN, S.P., PAVIA, D., MORÉN, F., SHEAHAN, N.F. and CLARKE, S.W. (1981). Deposition of pressurized aerosols in the human respiratory tract. *Thorax*, **36**, 52–55

NEWTON, G.J., KANAPILLY, G.M., BOECKER, R.B. and RAABE, O.G. (1980). Radioactive labelling of aerosols; generation methods and characteristics. In *Generation of aerosols and facilities for exposure experiments*. Edited by Willeke, K. Ann Arbor; Ann Arbor Science Publishers Inc., pp. 399–425

PAVIA, D. (1973). Studies of the mucociliary clearance of the human lung with particular reference to the effects of tobacco smoke. University of London Ph.D. Thesis, School of Hygiene and Tropical Medicine

PHILIPSON, K. (1973). On the production of monodisperse particles with a spinning disc. *J. Aerosol Sci.*, **4**, 51–57

PHILIPSON, K. (1977). Monodisperse labelled aerosols for studies of lung clearance. University of Uppsala Ph.D. Thesis, Faculty of Science

PHILIPSON, K., CAMNER, P. and SVEDBERG, J. (1970). Tagging 7μ monodisperse polystyrene particles with ^{11}C. *Int. J. Appl. Radiat. Isot.*, **21**, 639–641

PHILIPSON, K., LINNMAN, L., HELLSTROM, P.A. and CAMNER, P. (1975). Labelling properties of ^{51}Cr in monodisperse Teflon particles. *Health Phys.*, **28**, 621–622

ROSS, I.T.H., WALLACE, J.C. and WAITE, D. (1979). A simplified method of monitoring mucociliary transport. *Br. J. Radiol.*, **52**, 968–971

SANDERS, P.A. (1970). *Principles of aerosol technology*. New York; Van Nostrand Rheinhold, pp. 3–7

SANTOLICANDRO, A. and GIUTINI, C. (1979). Patterns of deposition of labelled monodispersed aerosol in obstructive lung disease. *J. Nucl. Med. Allied Sci.*, **23**, 115–127

SHENFIELD, G.M., EVANS, M.E., WALKER, S.R. and PATERSON, J.W. (1973). The fate of nebulized salbutamol administered by intermittent positive pressure respiration to asthmatic patients. *Am. Rev. Respir. Dis.*, **108**, 501–505

SHORT, M.D., DOWSETT, D.J., HEAF, P.J.D., PAVIA, D. and THOMSON, M.L. (1979). A comparison between monodisperse ^{99m}Tc labelled aerosol particles and ^{81m}Kr for the assessment of lung function. *J. Nucl. Med.*, **20**, 194–200

SHORT, M.D., SINGH, C.A., FEW, J.D., STUDDY, P.R., HEAF, P.J.D. and SPIRO, S.G. (1981). The labelling and monitoring of lung deposition of an inhaled synthetic anticholinergic bronchodilating agent. *Chest*, **80**, Supplement, 918–921

SINCLAIR, D. and LA MER, V.K. (1949). Light scattering as a measure of particle size in aerosols. *Chem. Rev.*, **44**, 245–267

SMALDONE, G.C., ITOH, H., SWIFT, D.L. and WAGNER, H.N. (1979). Effect of flow-limiting segments and cough on particle deposition and mucociliary clearance in the lung. *Am. Rev. Respir. Dis.*, **120**, 747–758

SVARTENGREN, M., WIDTSKIÖLD-OLSSON, K., PHILIPSON, K. and CAMNER, P. (1981). Retention of particles on the first bifurcation and the trachea of rabbits. *Bull. Europ. Physiopathol. Respir.*, **17**, 87–91

SWIFT, D.L., ZUSKIN, E. and BOUHUYS, A. (1979). Respiratory deposition of hair spray aerosol and acute lung function changes. *Lung*, **156**, 149–158

WALTON, W.H. and PREWETT, W.C. (1949). The production of sprays and mists of uniform drop size by means of spinning disc type sprayers. *Proc. Phys. Soc. (B)*, **62**, 341–350

WASNICH, R.D. (1976). A high frequency ultrasonic nebulizer system for radioactive aerosol delivery. *J. Nucl. Med.*, **17**, 707–710

WILSON, I.B. and LA MER, V.K. (1948). The retention of aerosol particles in the human respiratory tract as a function of particle radius. *J. Ind. Hyg. Toxicol.*, **30**, 265–280

WOLLMER, P., BARR, M.M. and FAZIO, F. (1980). Clinical ventilation imaging with ^{113m}In aerosol. *J. Nucl. Med. Allied Sci.*, **24**, 215–220

YEATES, D.B., WARBISH, A. and ASPIN, N. (1974). Production of ^{99m}Tc labelled albumin microspheres for lung clearance studies and inhalation scanning. *Int. J. Appl. Radiat. Isot.*, **25**, 578–580

Chapter 5

Aerosol contributions to the investigation of lung structure and ventilatory function

John E. Agnew

Introduction

Information about lung structure and function may be derived from several forms of aerosol measurement. Gas mixing in the lungs can be assessed by looking at how many inhaled particles are recovered in a subsequent exhalation. But if a breath-hold pause is imposed between inspiration and expiration fewer particles are recovered, and inferences about airspace dimensions may be drawn from the extent to which particle recovery falls. Deposition patterns visualized with radioaerosols can be used to illustrate localized effects resulting from changes in airway calibre. Radioaerosol images can alternatively be used to map out the distribution of lung ventilation.

For all these aerosol applications, adequate control of inhalation conditions is mandatory. Gas mixing studies require particles with minimal probability of deposition within the lung. Loss of particles from the tidal volume can then be primarily attributed to bulk (non-diffusive) gas mixing, with the aerosol simply acting as a non-diffusible gas. The aerosol 'probe' for estimating airspace dimensions is based on the idea that deposition during a breath-hold pause will quantitatively depend on how far the particles settle under gravity before coming into contact with an airspace wall. This requires particles small enough to escape deposition by impaction during inspiration or expiration, but large enough to settle appreciable distances during a breath-hold pause of manageable length.

Radioaerosol imaging is sometimes performed with rather larger particles giving significant impaction in narrowed airways. Obstruction of the large airways characteristically increases deposition in the perihilar region with diminished particle penetration towards the lung periphery. Deposition abnormalities may also be demonstrated in subjects with small airways dysfunction but no evidence of large airways obstruction. Ventilation imaging, however, requires small radioaerosol particles. If losses by impaction in the large airways are insignificant, particle penetration to the lung periphery will then reflect the distribution of lung ventilation. Such particles thus can act as substitutes for radioactive gases in clinical ventilation imaging. Diagnostic imaging of pulmonary embolism requires the ability to demonstrate that ventilation is preserved in localized zones of absent perfusion. This can now be achieved by radioaerosol imaging.

The three main sections of this chapter look firstly at using inert, non-radioactive particles to study gas mixing and airspace dimensions, secondly at the way in which radioaerosol deposition patterns relate to airways obstruction, and then, thirdly, at the pros and cons of radioaerosol ventilation imaging in clinical practice.

Gas mixing and airspace dimensions

Early aerosol work on gas mixing in normal subjects looked at particle concentrations in tidally expired air after a sequence of tidal aerosol inhalations followed by one of particle-free air (Altshuler *et al.*, 1959). All inspirations and expirations were equal in volume. If no particle exchange took place between tidal and reserve (resident) air, then no airborne particles would have remained in the lungs after each cycle of inspiration plus expiration. Hence air expired after the inspiration of particle-free air would itself have been particle-free. But, in fact, particles were detectable even in the first fraction of this expirate. By only half-way through expiration, their concentration had risen to some 5–12 per cent of the inspired concentration (Altshuler *et al.*, 1959). This experimental work provided notable evidence that particle transfer does occur from tidal to reserve air, *and* that particles of the size in question (0.4 μm diameter) can readily remain airborne within the lung for two (or more) respiratory cycles. Plots of aerosol concentration against volume expired during the course of the first expiration after inhalation of particle-free air showed distinct inter-subject variability.

Because of their small size, the particles used for these gas mixing studies had diffusion constants about a million times smaller than those of respiratory gases. This means a Brownian movement displacement of about 10 μm per second as against about 6 mm for an oxygen molecule (Altshuler *et al.*, 1959). Transfer of such particles between tidal and reserve air cannot therefore appreciably occur by diffusion. Instead it represents the interchange of small gas volumes between the tidal and the reserve volumes. This may conveniently be called bulk transfer.

More recent aerosol work on gas mixing has often been based on a single breath inhalation technique. Typically a single 500 or 1000 ml inhalation containing a constant concentration of aerosol particles is followed by an exhalation of at least twice as great a volume. If neither particle deposition nor transfer from tidal to reserve air were to occur the concentration profile of the exhaled air would be that indicated by the dashed line in *Figure 5.1*—namely, the expired concentration would remain equal to the inspired concentration until the volume expired reached that initially inspired, and then would fall to zero. The continuous line indicates a more realistic profile that might be expected if loss and mixing were minimal. This should be contrasted with the dotted curve depicting the form of exhalation profile to be expected (Muir, 1967) with a diffusible tracer; for instance an insoluble gas such as argon. The continuous line profile implies very low concentrations in the reserve air while the dotted line (diffusible gas) profile implies a considerable concentration in the reserve air.

Some results actually obtained with the single breath technique are summarized in *Table 5.1*. They indicate particle recoveries of between 80 and 88 per cent in the tidal volume, and total recoveries (tidal plus reserve air) of distinctly less than 100 per cent. Incomplete total recovery may result from deposition losses or from particle transfer into volumes not exhaled in a maximum exhalation. Given some uncertainty about which may be the true cause, it is sensible to express tidal to

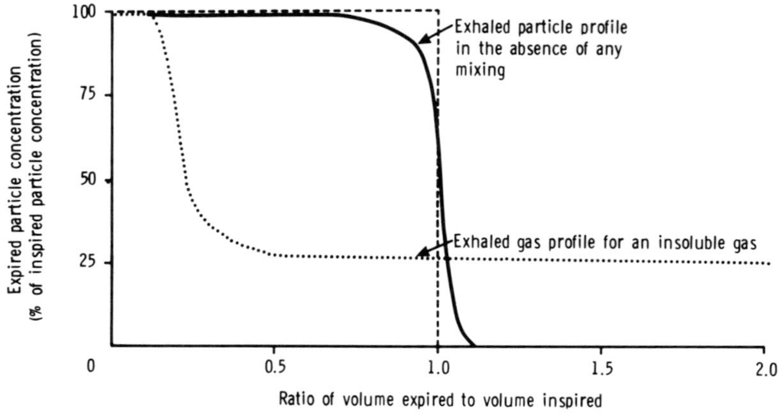

Figure 5.1 Aerosol particle concentration in expired air after inhalation of a single breath of uniform particle concentration. The continuous curve indicates the idealized profile to be expected in the absence of bulk gas mixing

reserve transfer in terms of the percentage of particles recovered which are recovered in the reserve air. Effectively this answers the question, 'Of all the particles accounted for, what percentage is demonstrably within the reserve air volume?' Under all the experimental conditions covered by *Table 5.1*, this transfer figure lies in a relatively narrow range: namely 9 to 12 per cent. Roughly similar values are obtained using 1 μm instead of 0.5 μm particles (Taulbee *et al.*, 1978), and with inhalation from lung volumes greater than FRC (Davies *et al.*, 1972). The data in *Table 5.1* demonstrate that neither flow rate nor volume inhaled have any detectable effect on mixing. Results obtained by Muir (1967) and by Muir *et al.* (1971), have also emphasized the unimportance of flow rate to mixing efficiency in normal subjects.

Exhaled aerosol particle distribution for normal subjects and patients with airflow obstruction are depicted in *Figure 5.2*. Despite several differences in technique, the normal profiles obtained by Gebhart *et al.* (1981) agree well with the mean normal profile reported earlier by Muir (1970). The width of the shaded band in the figure bears witness to a considerable degree of normal inter-subject variability, as in the earlier work of Altshuler *et al.* (1959).

The aerosol profile shown (*Figure 5.2*) for patients with airways obstruction relates to patients with severe obstruction (mean FEV_1 : 27 per cent of predicted).

TABLE 5.1. Recovery of half-micron particles during the first exhalation after single breath aerosol inhalation from FRC in normal subjects

Inhalation flow rate ($\ell\ min^{-1}$)	7.5	15	15	20	30	60
Volume inhaled (ml)	500	500	1000	625	1000	1000
% recovery in tidal air	81	86	80	82	85	88
% recovery in tidal + reserve air	91	94	89	92	93	98
Reserve air particles as % of total recovery	11	9	10	12	9	11
Reference	(a)	(a)	(b)	(c)	(a)	(a)

Key to references: (a) Taulbee *et al.* (1978), (b) Gebhart *et al.* (1981), (c) Davies *et al.* (1972).
Particle density ≃ 0.9 g cm^{-3}

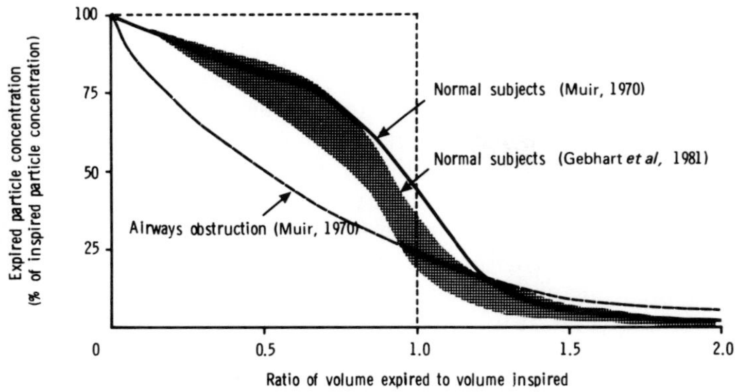

Figure 5.2 Experimental data on aerosol particle concentrations in exhaled air after single breath inhalation

Studies in patients with varying degrees of airways obstruction (FEV_1 : 12–99 per cent predicted) demonstrated a distinct correlation between percentage aerosol recovery in the tidal volume and percentage predicted FEV_1 (Muir, 1970). Patients with airways obstruction also showed lower total recovery than normal subjects; this was partly attributed to the limited expiratory reserve of the patients (Muir, 1970). Given that 2 or 3 times the inspired volume may even in normal subjects have to be exhaled before the exhaled particle concentration approximates to zero (Muir, 1967; Davies *et al.*, 1972; Gebhart *et al.*, 1981) patients with obstruction may not be able to achieve the manoeuvre required. This is an important practical limitation on using the technique for quantitative assessment of mixing in such patients. Even with 0.5 μm particles some deposition by impaction is likely to occur in narrowed airways. A measurement of recovery in the tidal volume alone cannot therefore constitute an adequate index to mixing, because it reflects the combined effects of increased mixing and increased deposition. Thus, the evidence that bulk transfer is increased in airways obstruction really rests on the observation of higher than normal exhaled particle concentrations at high expired volumes, as shown by the data of Muir (1970) in *Figure 5.2*.

Aerosol studies of gas mixing are better able to say that bulk transfer from tidal to reserve air does occur, than to say *where* it occurs. Mixing within the large airways could result from turbulent airflow or from secondary airflow patterns. If turbulence were an important factor, then presumably high inspiratory flow rates would tend to enhance mixing. This does not in practice occur. Recent modelling work on gas transport has emphasized that a complex interdependence of convection and diffusion at asymmetric branch-points of the airways may cause substantial non-uniformity of lung ventilation (Engel, 1983). Any complete description of tidal to reserve gas transfer in the lung—and of the adequacy of the aerosol technique for investigating it—would have to take this into account. Transfer must moreover, tend to be enhanced by any asymmetry of alveolar expansion and contraction (Cinkotai, 1974; Taulbee *et al.*, 1978). Further development of the aerosol technique for investigating gas mixing probably therefore requires very sophisticated modelling of aerosol dynamics in the lung, and an attempt to marry such modelling to existing models of gas transport in the lung.

Mixing and deposition

A few aerosol recovery studies have given further data about the relationship of recovery to airways obstruction, in terms of the combined effects of bulk transfer and particle deposition. Total recovery measured by Palmes *et al.* (1971) in an exhaled volume equal to twice the inhaled volume, amounted to only 77 ± 8 per cent (mean ± SD) in patients with bronchitis plus emphysema, as against 90 ± 3 per cent in normal subjects. This work was carried out with particles of 0.5–0.6 μm diameter as part of a study (discussed later in this chapter) also concerned with estimating airspace dimensions; inhaled volume in the normal subjects was 1000 ml but in the bronchitic patients ranged between 500 and 950 ml. Later results with essentially the same technique (but an inhaled volume of 1000 ml in all subjects) also demonstrated significantly decreased recovery in bronchitic as against non-bronchitic coal miners (Hankinson *et al.*, 1979). Miners with pinhead (type p) pneumoconiosis had lower recovery than those with micronodular (type q) pneumoconiosis; miners who smoked gave lower recoveries than those who did not (Hankinson *et al.*, 1979).

Recovery of 1 μm particles during tidal breathing at rest and while exercising was measured by Love and Muir (1976) using a steady state instead of a single breath technique. Recovery in the tidal volume related significantly to a test of small airways function ($MEF_{50-75\%}$, the forced expiratory flow rate in the third quarter of FVC) in a population of 58 working coal miners. Non-smoking miners tended to give an exhaled aerosol profile similar to that obtained for normal subjects with the single breath technique. 33 out of 42 smokers gave however either 'intermediate' or 'concave' profiles, the latter being associated with lower overall recovery and tending towards the 'airway obstruction' profile obtained with the single breath technique. These results might, as the authors comment, be caused by increased mixing or by enhanced deposition in proximal airways.

The 'aerosol probe'

The aerosol method for assessing airspace dimensions within the lung is sometimes referred to as the 'aerosol probe'. It is based on a very simple extension of the single breath aerosol mixing technique. If a breath-hold pause is imposed between inspiration of the aerosol and expiration of the breath to be analysed, time is available for the airborne particles to move within lung airspaces under the influence of gravity. Those particles which reach the wall of an airspace will be deposited on that wall. They will therefore fail to be recovered in the subsequent exhalation. The probability of a particular particle suffering deposition will be governed by how quickly it falls under the influence of gravity *and* how far it has to fall. The former is simply a question of its terminal settling velocity (Chapter 3) dependent on its aerodynamic diameter. The distance it has to fall is simply the vertical distance from its initial position at the start of the breath-hold pause to the airspace wall directly below.

On the average, such vertical distances will reflect the overall dimensions of the airspaces containing the aerosol. However as aerosol recovery is less than 100 per cent even without a breath-hold pause (*Table 5.1*), use of the 'aerosol probe' requires measurement of the *extra* loss of particles attributable to gravitational settling during the pause. Experimental measurements have generally been based not on a single duration of pause but on a series of different length pauses because

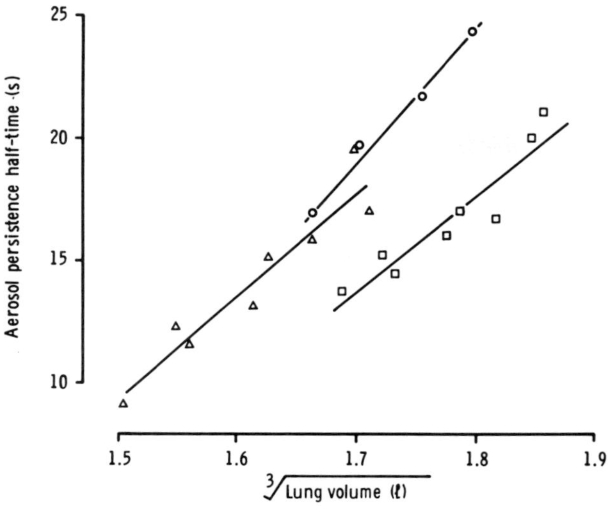

Figure 5.3 Data from Palmes *et al.* (1971) on the relationship of aerosol persistence to lung inflation. The results shown are from three different subjects (triangle, circle and square symbols). The choice of the cube root of lung volume for the horizontal axis is discussed in the text

of the finding that aerosol recovery decreases exponentially with the duration of the pause (Palmes, 1973). Results are often expressed in terms of the half-time of aerosol persistence in the lung under breath-holding conditions. Persistence simply means the probability of remaining airborne, i.e. being exhaled rather than being deposited, and is suitably characterized by its half-time because of its exponential decrease with time.

Obviously, the degree of lung inflation at which the breath is held must have an important influence on the results obtained. This has been investigated by Palmes *et al.* (1971), some of their data being summarized in *Figure 5.3.* Because the technique used was an inhalation of 1 ℓ and (after the pause) an exhalation of 2 ℓ, the lowest lung volume which could be studied was 2 ℓ above residual volume. For each subject, changes in aerosol persistence half-time were proportional to changes in the degree of lung inflation. This is illustrated in *Figure 5.3*, where the variable used to characterize lung inflation is the cube root of lung volume. The reason for choosing this variable is that experimental studies have shown airway dimensions to vary in proportion to the cube root of lung volume as inflation changes (Klingele and Staub, 1971; Hughes *et al.*, 1972).

The aerosol data can be seen to be consistent with this proportionality. In the original report by Palmes and colleagues (1971) persistence half-time was plotted against lung volume rather than its cube root; this in fact gives fractionally higher correlation coefficients for two subjects, fractionally lower for the third. The problem is that the range of lung volumes which can be studied is small as a subsequent exhalation of 2 ℓ is required. Hence the technique cannot really determine whether airspace dimensions genuinely change in proportion to lung volume or to the cube root of lung volume. Neither method of plotting gives regression lines passing through the origin.

What the results of Palmes *et al.* (1971) importantly demonstrate is that *changes* in aerosol persistence are proportional to *changes* in lung inflation. As with gas mixing studies, inter-subject differences are apparent. But there is a sensitive response to carefully controlled changes of airway dimension.

Extensive studies by Lapp *et al.* (1975) have also shown that the technique can give reproducible results in normal subjects. Breath-holding after inspiration of a 1.0 ℓ aerosol volume was at a volume approximately 0.2 ℓ below total lung capacity (TLC) and was followed by a 2.0 ℓ exhalation. Within-subject variability of the persistence half-time was assessed for 7 subjects studied 5–6 times each over a period of nearly two years; coefficients of variation ranged from 7.7 to 11.5 per cent. Calculated mean airspace diameters however covered a very wide range—from about 0.3 to 0.8 mm—and correlated only poorly with age, height or lung volume (Lapp *et al.*, 1975). The good reproducibility of the technique must however imply that it could be applicable to following within-subject changes over a length of time.

Aerosol probe findings in lung disease

Obviously the wide inter-subject variability reported for normal subjects is a drawback when considering application of the method to patients with abnormal lungs. A limited amount of work has however been carried out on patients with emphysema and on coal miners with pneumoconiosis. Two out of five patients classified by Palmes *et al.* (1971) as emphysematous but not bronchitic showed a substantial increase in aerosol persistence half-time, giving values of 43 and 50 s as against the normal range of approximately 23–25 s. This was taken to reflect loss of alveolar walls and enlargement of airspaces in regions accessible to the inhaled aerosol. In other instances emphysema might, as pointed out by the authors, affect only poorly or non-ventilated airspaces to which the aerosol particles would be unable to gain access. In such cases a falsely normal half-time would be recorded, reflecting aerosol handling in unaffected airspaces within the better ventilated lung zones. Results in patients suffering from bronchitis in association with emphysema were disappointing in that none of the nine patients studied were able to manage the 1 ℓ inhalation, breathhold, 2 ℓ exhalation manoeuvre (Palmes *et al.*, 1971). They were therefore (as already noted) studied at lower inhalation volumes (but with exhalation volumes twice that inhaled). Use of low inhalation volumes is likely to bias the results by tending to reflect aerosol persistence in more proximal airways. Grossly prolonged persistence (half time >50 s) was however detected in two instances, and probably did result from airspace enlargement due to emphysema.

Analysis of the 'aerosol probe' recovery function

Even with normal subjects, easily able to perform the manoeuvre required, results obtained with a 1000 ml aerosol inhalation must reflect lung dimensions at varying depths within the lung. As pointed out by Gebhart *et al.* (1981), the initial part of the 'recovery function' (a plot of recovery against the duration of the breath-hold pause) will tend to reflect the fate of particles in the smallest airways filled with aerosol while the later readings on the plot will tend to be influenced by particles in larger airways. They therefore recommend using the slope of the first phase of the recovery function as a means of estimating the diameters of the smallest airways filled with aerosol. Other authors have however taken the slope of the whole recovery function arguing that a volume of 1000 ml is so much greater than the conducting airways volume (of the order of 200 ml) that the half-time obtained will be determined predominantly by the dimensions of peripheral airspaces (Palmes *et al.*, 1971). For particles of 0.55 μm diameter a simple equation (Lapp *et al.*, 1975) may be used to estimate airspace dimensions:

$$\text{Airspace diameter} = 0.027 \times \text{half-time}$$

This gives a diameter in mm, for a half-time expressed in seconds, $0.027\,\text{mm}\,\text{s}^{-1}$ being the terminal settling velocity of the particles (Lapp *et al.*, 1975). The mathematical analysis of recovery functions is presented in more detail by Gebhart *et al.* (1981), who also discuss the optimum particle size for investigating airspace dimensions. Their conclusion is that monodisperse aerosols of aerodynamic diameter within the range of 1 to 1.5 μm should be ideal. These, having greater settling velocities, will give shorter half-times than the smaller particles used in earlier studies but should suffer negligible loss owing to impaction on inspiration and expiration. This suggestion is dependent on inhalation being slow and may not apply to patients with airways obstruction.

The bolus 'aerosol probe'

In order to provide information more specific to particular depths within the lung, bolus techniques are appropriate (Palmes *et al.*, 1973; Heyder, 1983). Rather more complicated equipment is required than for uniform labelling of the inspired volume. In the apparatus used by Palmes *et al.* (1973) an aerosol bolus was followed by a preset volume of particle-free air. The more recent procedure of Heyder (1983) permits insertion of an aerosol bolus into the inspirate at any stage of inhalation. This approach is illustrated diagrammatically in *Figure 5.4.* Aerosol boli of almost rectangular profile were achieved with very rapid increase of particle concentration from zero to its maximum value when the aerosol valve was opened and an equally rapid fall to zero when the valve was closed (Heyder, 1983). The exhaled particle profiles illustrate a considerable dispersion of particle concentrations although maximum concentrations in exhaled air correspond volumetrically

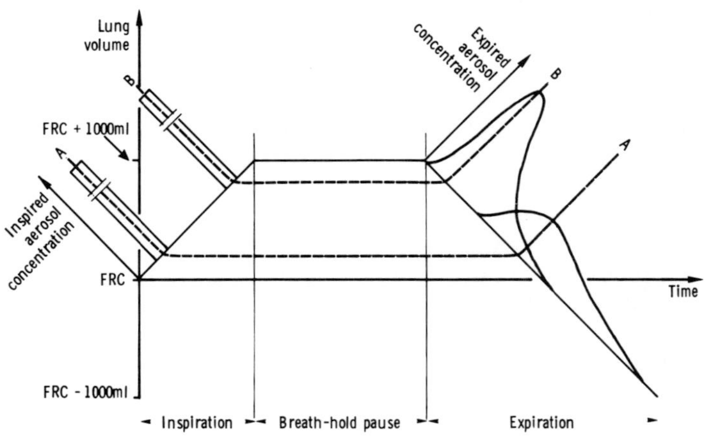

Figure 5.4 Schematic illustration of bolus 'aerosol probe' technique based on Heyder (1983). Bolus 'A' is inspired early in inspiration and therefore exhaled late in expiration. Bolus 'B' is inhaled late in inspiration and therefore recovered early in expiration. Boli such as 'A' exhaled late in expiration suffer much more dispersion than boli such as 'B' exhaled earlier

to the mid-point of the inhaled bolus (*Figure 5.4*). The more deeply a bolus was inhaled the greater was the dispersion of the bolus subsequently exhaled. This is illustrated by the much flatter exhaled profile for bolus A (*Figure 5.4*) inhaled early in inspiration than for bolus B inhaled much later in inspiration. The increase of dispersion with depth confirms earlier measurements on aerosol bolus dispersion by Muir *et al.* (1971). There is however some evidence that with a larger bolus volume, peak expired particle concentration may occur earlier in expiration than the volume corresponding to the mid-point of the inhaled bolus (Muir *et al.*, 1971). Considerations of bolus dispersion imply that however carefully inhalation conditions are controlled, some doubt must remain as to the exact depth of the particles within the lung during the breath-hold pause. This applies even when considering only volumetric depth within the lung. Matters become more complicated still when attempting to relate measured dimensions to airway models such as that of Weibel (1963)—a challenge nevertheless taken up both by Palmes *et al.* (1973) and by Heyder (1983). Data obtained by Heyder (1983) are, in *Figure 5.5*, compared

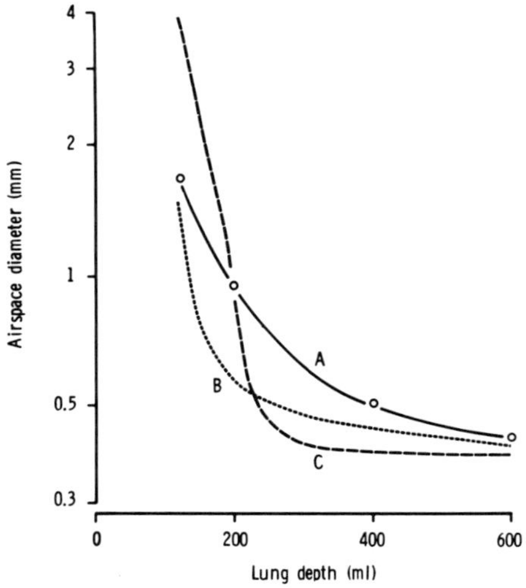

Figure 5.5 Airspace diameters at different lung depths: comparison between experimental data of Heyder (1983), curve A, and anatomical model data tabulated by Weibel (1963), curve B, and by Yeh and Schum (1980), curve C

with anatomical model data from two sources. Because airway dimensions depend on the degree of lung inflation, the anatomical model data have been scaled to the estimated mean lung volume of the subjects studied experimentally. This scaling was based on the simple—and possibly erroneous—assumption that the volume of each airway generation should change in direct proportion to the change in total lung volume, and that the diameter of each generation should change in proportion to the change in the cube root of total lung volume.

A volume of 60 cm^3 was attributed to oral cavity, pharynx plus larynx (Heyder, 1983). The model curves of *Figure 5.5* are based on taking lung volume as 1000 ml above the mean value measured for FRC (i.e. a mean lung volume of 3.95 ℓ). The figure illustrates close agreement between experimental and model data. In doing so, it bears witness to the potential power of the 'aerosol probe' for *in vivo* investigation of lung dimensions. Some 'smearing-out' of the experimental relative to the model data is inevitable. Two causes exist for this: (a) that bolus dispersion tends to spread its response over several generations, and (b) that the lung is not really symmetrical. In fact, the 'aerosol probe' may well reflect a realistic range of airspace dimensions at a given volumetric depth that cannot be obtained from symmetrical airway models. Experimental-model comparisons reported by Palmes *et al.* (1973) over volume depths of 200 to 800 ml resemble those shown in *Figure 5.5* although with slightly higher experimental values—probably reflecting the higher degree of lung inflation used (200 ml below TLC, giving a mean lung volume of 6.1 ℓ).

Summary of aerosol applications in the assessment of gas mixing and of airspace dimensions

Gas mixing studies with aerosols have provided important quantitative evidence of the contribution that bulk transfer makes to the mixing of gases within the lung. Although some problems affect performance and interpretation of these studies in patients with airways obstruction, there appears to be a substantial increase of bulk gas transfer in such patients. The aerosol probe is important as a non-invasive method of assessing airways dimensions. The technique can readily be repeated, giving reproducible data, but inter-subject variability is high. Increased airspace dimensions in patients with emphysema can be assessed only if the airspaces in question are accessible to the aerosol. Aerosol probe results in normal subjects concur well with airway model data.

Radioaerosol deposition in relationship to airways obstruction

In patients with airways obstruction aerosol deposition patterns will depend on the distribution of ventilation and on the sites of obstruction. Naturally these two factors interrelate. But the influence of airway narrowing on the distribution of ventilation need not be the same as its direct influence on sites of aerosol impaction. Adequate ventilatory flow is moreover a pre-requisite for aerosol to reach any particular lung zone irrespective of airway calibre.

Ventilation and obstruction: effects on particle deposition

Some basic ideas may be illustrated by a simple two-compartment model (*Figure 5.6*). This represents two lung zones X and Y ventilated from a large airway A via bronchial pathways B_X and B_Y. In the absence of any obstruction to either pathway, equal ventilatory flow is assumed to reach X and Y. Aerosol particles used for studying deposition patterns are generally inhaled at relatively low inhalation flow rates—say, with average flow rates in the range of 15 to 35 ℓ min^{-1}. For such flow rates the distribution of inhaled air normally depends in roughly equal measure on airways resistance and lung compliance (Milic-Emili, 1977). For patients with lung disease, changes in either compliance or resistance will affect the distribution of ventilation.

Compliance changes within either X or Y unaccompanied by any resistance changes in B_X or B_Y (*Figure 5.6*) will tend to cause asynchronous filling of the two zones X and Y. This implies changing flow rates in both B_X and B_Y. To take an extreme example, suppose that a completely sequential pattern of lung filling occurs during the course of a maximal inspiration from residual volume (RV)—with region X completely filling first and then, after that, region Y. Suppose also that the total time taken for inspiration is the same as that which would have been

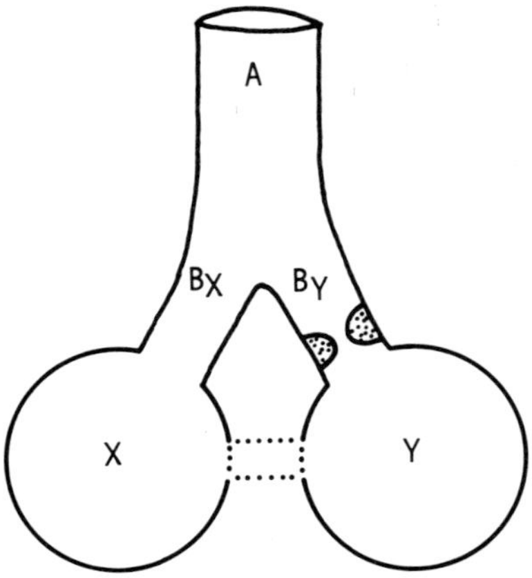

Figure 5.6 Two compartment model. Lung zones X and Y are assumed to receive equal ventilation when bronchial pathway B_Y is unobstructed. (A, parent airway; B_X and B_Y, bronchial pathways; X and Y, lung zones subtended by, respectively, B_X and B_Y). Broken lines indicate possibility of collateral communication between X and Y

required for parallel (synchronous) filling of X plus Y. The asynchronous filling pattern means that all the airflow passing through A (*Figure 5.6*) passes on through B_X alone during the first half of inspiration but through B_Y alone during the second half of inspiration. The synchronous filling pattern by contrast means that the airflow through A is divided equally between B_X and B_Y throughout the course of inspiration. Aerosol transit velocities through B_X will therefore be twice as great in the former (asynchronous) situation as in the latter (synchronous) case. The same is true for B_Y. Impaction probabilities for aerosol particles are (Chapter 3) approximately proportional to the linear velocity of the airstream carrying them. Thus in this, admittedly extreme, example, asynchronous filling would double particle deposition by impaction in *both* the bronchial pathways (B_X and B_Y). Hence it is clearly possible for compliance changes in the distal lung to increase aerosol deposition in more central airways. The extra deposition does not necessarily indicate specific sites of obstruction. This is important because reports in the literature differ as to whether central airways aerosol deposition reflects obstruction in large airways (Chopra *et al.*, 1979b) or in peripheral airways (Dolovich *et al.*, 1976). It may, in fact, result from either. It is also important that pressure-volume characteristic changes need only occur in a small fraction of lung units to give rise to asynchronous filling of the lung (Fukuchi *et al.*, 1980).

Complete obstruction to pathway B_Y (*Figure 5.6*) without any compensatory change in flow through the parent airway A will likewise double linear velocities in B_X. This too will double aerosol impaction in B_X. Again the sites of extra deposition, being within the patent bronchial pathway, are not *at* the site of obstruction. Macklem and colleagues (1973) have drawn attention to the insidious role such diversion of deposition sites can play when the deposited particles are irritant substances as opposed to inert test particles. Once obstruction is established, inspired air is directed through the least affected airways which are thereby exposed to an increased concentration of deposited irritant. Using a two-compartment model of obstruction, Macklem and colleagues (1973) also demonstrated that dense gases can penetrate much more deeply into the lungs than lighter gases; they therefore inferred that small aerosol particles (i.e. those with low probabilities of impaction and sedimentation) will tend to penetrate more deeply than would be suggested by simple (volume-based) calculations. Nevertheless it seems unlikely that such particles should penetrate better than gases through collateral ventilation channels; some will be deposited in B_X and others within X before the possibility of penetration to Y arises.

Partial obstruction of one bronchial pathway—the situation actually illustrated in *Figure 5.6*—has two different effects on aerosol deposition. The first, analogous to that occurring with complete obstruction, is extra deposition in the fully patent pathway (B_X) owing to increased airflow via that route. The second is localized aerosol impaction in the region of the obstruction itself caused by increased linear velocities. If the obstruction is severe, the first effect will predominate. But if it is relatively slight, thereby causing little diversion of ventilatory airflow, the second will generally predominate. Partial obstruction affecting both bronchial pathways (B_X and B_Y) will enhance aerosol impaction in each. Uniform constriction of the large airways can thereby give the patterns of central deposition readily recognized in patients with chronic bronchitis or asthma.

Such deposition roughly corresponds to the large airways bronchoconstriction pattern modelled in *Figure 3.9* (Chapter 3). In fact model calculations of aerosol impaction probabilities generally tend to show maximum deposition at about the fourth and fifth airway generations (Gerrity *et al.*, 1979). At moderate inspiratory flow rates, these are also the sites of maximal viscous airflow resistance (Pedley *et al.*, 1970). Bronchoconstriction of these airways will thus have a particularly strong effect both on the resistive element controlling the distribution of airflow and on localized patterns of aerosol deposition.

Responsiveness of radioaerosol images to airways obstruction

Radioaerosol particles of up to 3 or 4 μm aerodynamic diameter inhaled at low to moderate flow rates tend to give an even distribution of lung radioactivity in normal subjects. Slightly enhanced deposition may be seen in hilar or perihilar regions but in general the images closely resemble those obtainable with a radioactive gas such as ^{133}Xe or ^{81m}Kr. In patients with airways obstruction, radioaerosol images are almost always abnormal. Depending on the particle size and inhalation flow rate used, they may appear very much more 'abnormal' than those seen with radioactive gases.

The major clinical application of radioaerosol lung imaging is—in combination with perfusion imaging—for the diagnosis of pulmonary embolism (Fazio *et al.*, 1982). The requirements are just the same as for the widespread use of radioactive gases (^{133}Xe and ^{81m}Kr in particular) for this purpose. The ventilation imaging agent should be physically suitable for gamma camera imaging. It should ideally also be appropriate for combined use with a ^{99m}Tc-labelled perfusion agent. Its crucial role is to demonstrate whether or not ventilation is preserved in localized zones of impaired perfusion. To fulfil this role, a radioaerosol must mimic radioactive gas. It must give only minimal local deposition at large airways sites so that the bulk of the particles are available as tracers for the ventilation of peripheral zones. Deposition in the lung periphery must be high enough to permit good visualization of all ventilated peripheral zones. Relative to the physical factors affecting deposition discussed in Chapter 3 this implies small particles, slow inhalation and, if possible, a post-inspiratory breath-hold pause. The importance of slow inhalation is illustrated in *Figure 5.7*. Obtained with large (5 μm) particles, this depicts (left-hand image) relatively even deposition in a normal subject at low flow rate but a 'bronchogram' appearance (right-hand image) when flow rate was doubled.

The requirements outlined for an aerosol ventilation imaging agent naturally differ from those appropriate to detecting localized changes in airway calibre. They also differ from those appropriate to depositing particles on the conducting airways for a mucus clearance test. Nevertheless a number of reports on varying aerosol techniques have tried to suggest that the technique in question is suitable both for ventilation imaging and for detecting obstruction. This can be true up to a point. A particular technique may be able to give good ventilation images in subjects with normal lung function and images indicative of airways obstruction in patients with diminished lung function. This is not however the clinical requirement for patients suspected of having pulmonary embolism. Several recent reports have therefore rightly concentrated on achieving radioaerosol images which are as *insensitive* as possible to the effects of airways obstruction. This should really include being as

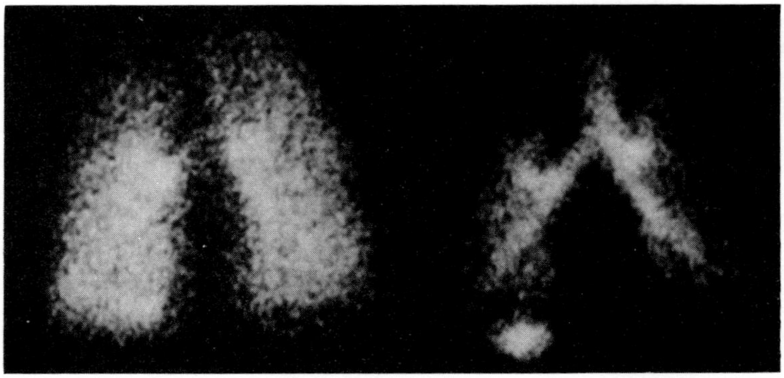

Figure 5.7 Effect of inhalation flow rate on radioaerosol images in a normal subject. The particles used were 5 μm diameter polystyrene spheres labelled with ^{99m}Tc. On one occasion (left) these were inhaled at a mean flow rate of 21 ℓ min^{-1}; on the other occasion (right) mean flow rate was 43 ℓ min^{-1}; alveolar deposition fell from 71 to 31 per cent.

insensitive as possible to those effects (considered in the discussion of *Figure 5.6*) which may tend to enhance perihilar deposition even when the larger bronchi are unobstructed.

The following sections of this chapter therefore look first at radioaerosol applications where sensitivity to airways obstruction is desirable, then at quantitative analysis of lung radioaerosol penetration in relationship to airways obstruction and then only after that at radioaerosol imaging for pulmonary embolism. The sections relating to pulmonary embolism are concerned with clinical requirements, choice of technique and the achievement of minimal sensitivity to airways obstruction.

Radioaerosol images in airways obstruction

Radioaerosol images in COAD (chronic obstructive airways disease) are characterized by the presence of irregular 'hot' and 'cold' spots and, often, by excessive perihilar deposition (Ramanna *et al.*, 1975; Lin and Goodwin, 1976; Santolicandro and Giuntini, 1979; Adiseshan, 1982; Garg *et al.*, 1983). Images obtained with 5 μm particles are illustrated in *Figures 5.8* and *5.9*. One classification scheme for

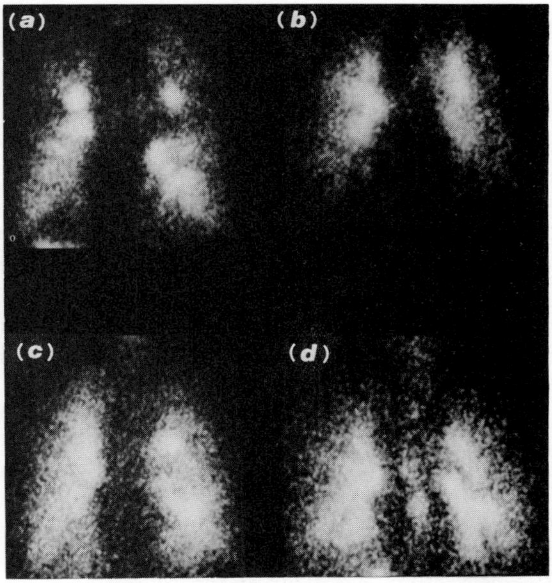

Figure 5.8 Radioaerosol images (5 μm particles) in patients with mild to moderate airflow obstruction (FEV_1: 52–84 per cent predicted; MMFR 17–76 per cent predicted. (a) and (b) chronic bronchitis, (c) and (d) asthma

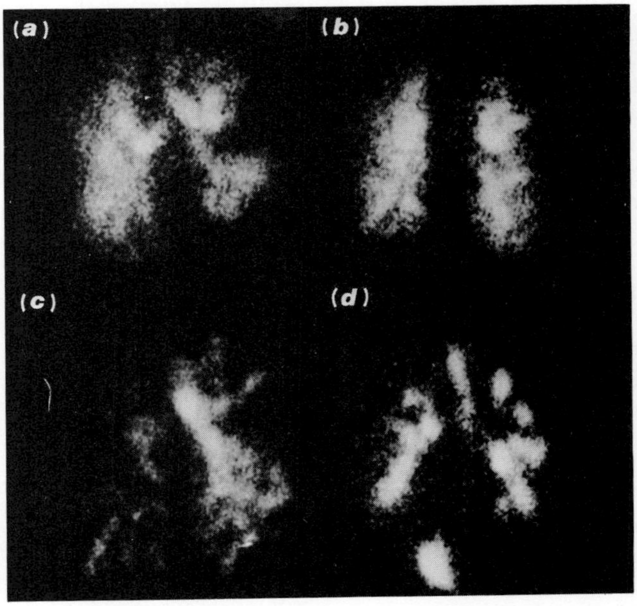

Figure 5.9 Radioaerosol images (5 μm particles) in patients with severe airflow obstruction (FEV_1, 25–49 per cent predicted; MMFR 9–20 per cent predicted. (a) and (b) chronic bronchitis, (c) emphysema, (d) asthma

aerosol images in airways obstruction (Taplin and Chopra, 1978) categorizes images as either:

Type A: 'excessive deposition of activity in the major airways'

or

Type B: 'excessive central deposition plus regions of poor aerosol penetration to the lung periphery'.

Both categories emphasize the importance of increased perihilar deposition. Type A image patterns were typically found in subjects with minor abnormalities on lung function testing whereas type B images were associated with moderate to severe impairment of lung function (Taplin and Chopra, 1978). When large particles are used, grossly abnormal deposition patterns may occur (*Figure 5.8*) in patients with only moderate impairment of lung function.

Chronic bronchitis may give 'hot' spots quite close to the lung periphery (Santolicandro and Giuntini, 1979; Greening *et al.*, 1980; Hayes, 1980). They roughly correspond to zones of well preserved ventilation as detected by ^{81m}Kr ventilation imaging (Fazio *et al.*, 1978b). The most obvious interpretation therefore is that they represent high particle deposition in a bronchial pathway 'B_X' (*Figure 5.6*) when obstruction to 'B_Y' is relatively severe.

Compared with chronic bronchitis, less study has been made of radioaerosol images in asthma. The predominant defect seen in stable asthma appears to be enhanced perihilar deposition with reduced peripheral visualization, i.e. a 'type B' pattern (Chopra *et al.*, 1979b). As assessed by blind marking, central deposition even in asymptomatic asthma is significantly ($p < 0.01$) greater than in normal non-smoking control subjects (Agnew *et al.*, 1982a). In acute asthma, Itoh *et al.* (1977) have reported localized 'hot' spot patterns similar to those seen in some patients with chronic bronchitis; these may also be seen in stable asthmatics (*Figures 5.8* and *5.9*).

Radioaerosol images in bronchial carcinoma tend to show a localized 'hot' area at or near the site of obstruction when a main or lobar bronchus is partially obstructed (Itoh *et al.*, 1976). Partial or complete obstruction of a segmental bronchus gives rise to a segmental zone of decreased deposition (Itoh *et al.*, 1976). Radioaerosol imaging might therefore sometimes be a useful preliminary to bronchoscopy, but is unable (Itoh *et al.*, 1976) to localize the site of obstruction in patients with concomitant COAD, because of the multiple irregularities generally seen.

Several articles have claimed that radioaerosol imaging might be useful for the early detection of developing airways obstruction. This concept is based partly on work showing a high incidence of aerosol image abnormalities in rather mixed populations of subjects and partly on quantitative analyses (discussed later in this chapter) comparing radioaerosol lung penetration in smokers to that in non-smokers. Little attention has however been paid to the logistics of applying radioaerosols widely in any 'screening' role. Procedures involving radiation should, of course, only be used for such a purpose if any available alternatives are obviously inferior *and* if the procedure in question can be shown to be effective. Neither criterion has in fact been satisfactorily met. An increasing range of 'conventional' lung function tests may now be considered for screening purposes (Becklake and Permutt, 1979). Moreover, comparison of radioaerosol images and lung function data in a random group of subjects from a population study of COAD (Tashkin *et al.*, 1979) attributed high *sensitivity* to radioaerosol imaging (84 per cent) but unacceptably poor *specificity* (62 per cent), i.e. an inappropriately high (for screening purposes) proportion of 'false positive' images in normal subjects. The judgements of *sensitivity* and *specificity* were based on clinical examination, respiratory questionaire and a range of lung function tests, and so cannot be totally accurate. Nevertheless they confirm widespread practical doubt that radioaerosol imaging could be used for early detection of airways obstruction.

Sensitivity to the early stages of developing airways obstruction implies sensitivity to dysfunction of the small airways. Of relevance to this is a study carried out by Chopra *et al.* (1979b) in patients with stable asthma. It looked at the effects of (a) inhaled and (b) subcutaneous terbutaline on radioaerosol images, ^{133}Xe images and lung function tests. The relative responsiveness of the two forms of imaging to the two modes of terbutaline administration led to the suggestion that it was ^{133}Xe imaging, not aerosol imaging, which acted as a sensitive indication of small airways obstruction. The radioaerosol images, by contrast, were judged to show a sensitive response to large airways obstruction (Chopra *et al.*, 1979b).

Quantitative analysis of radioaerosol lung penetration

Two alternative approaches have been widely used. The first—applicable only to insoluble particles—is the use of retention at 24 hours as a measurement of 'alveolar deposition'. The second is to assess peripheral relative to perihilar radioactivity from a gamma camera radioaerosol view.

Measurement of alveolar deposition has been discussed in Chapter 3 and plays a vitally important role in the assessment of tracheobronchial mucus clearance (considered in later chapters). Extensive studies have shown that alveolar deposition is very variable in normal non-smoking subjects and even more so in smokers (Lippmann, 1977). A marked overlap occurs between smokers and non-smokers. The variability of normal alveolar deposition may well substantially arise from considerable inter-subject differences in airway dimensions, as evidenced by the 'aerosol probe' results discussed earlier in this chapter.

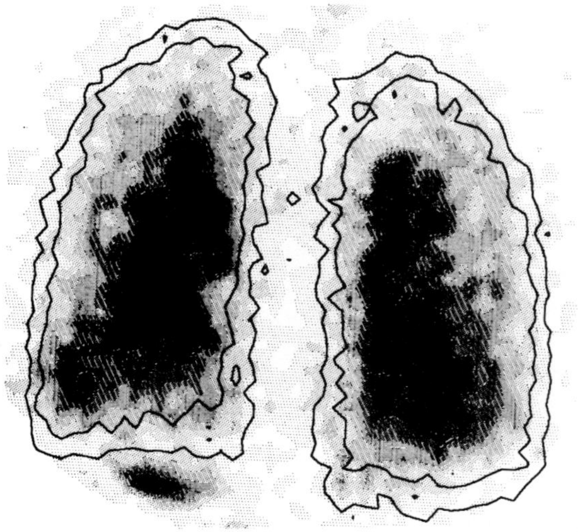

Figure 5.10 Aerosol image aligned with ^{81m}Kr contours. The contour lines shown represent 15 and 30 per cent respectively of the maximum ^{81m}Kr count in any one computer matrix cell (data collected in the form of a 64 × 64 matrix)

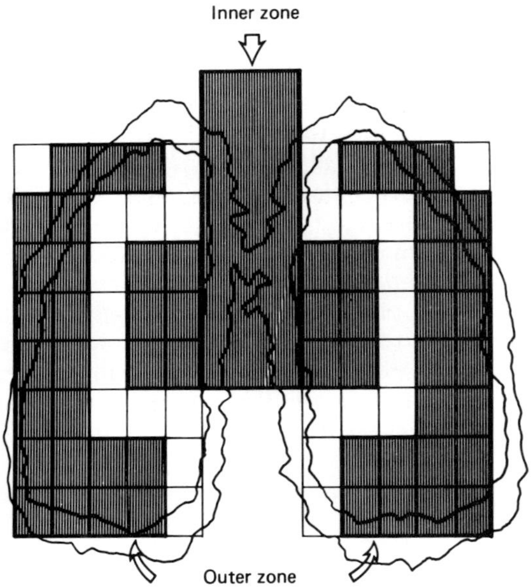

Figure 5.11 Zones used for calculating penetration index. These are defined within a simple 5 × 8 matrix fitted to the ^{81m}Kr contours for each lung—a different subject from *Figure 5.10*

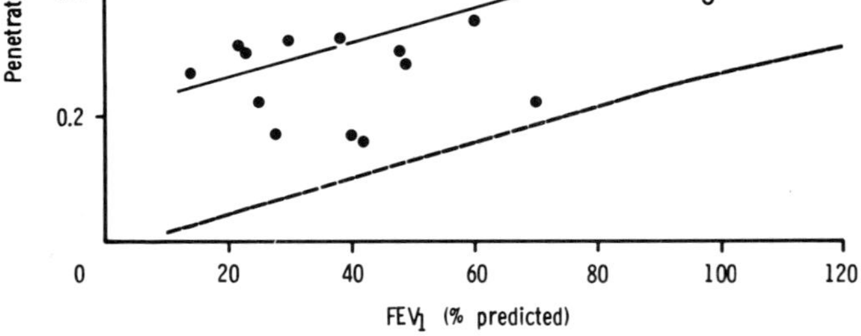

Figure 5.12 Relationship of penetration index to per cent predicted FEV_1: filled-in symbols are used for patients with chronic bronchitis, open symbols for normal control subjects. Data were obtained with 5 μm ^{99m}Tc particles; mean inhalation flow rates were 40–45 ℓ min^{-1}. (The continuous line is the regression line calculated for all subjects; the dashed lines indicate 95 per cent confidence limits for individual observations)

One method of analysing gamma camera data is illustrated in *Figures 5.10* and *5.11*. The radioaerosol image is first aligned with a ^{81m}Kr ventilation image (*Figure 5.10*). Penetration index is then calculated as the outer to inner zone radioactivity ratio for radioaerosol divided by the same ratio for ^{81m}Kr gas (Agnew *et al.*, 1981b) using the zones defined in *Figure 5.11*. Correction for background radioactivity is required when administered activities are low. A penetration index value of approximately unity implies that the radioaerosol penetrates approximately as well to the peripheral zone as the short-lived radioactive gas. ^{81m}Kr, in fact, has a half-life of only 13 s and so provides images of ventilation rather than of lung volume (Fazio and Wollmer, 1981).

A penetration index based on comparing aerosol to ^{81m}Kr images hence describes aerosol distribution relative to the effectiveness with which inner and outer zones (*Figure 5.11*) are ventilated. It does not however give precise information about the location of the deposited radioaerosol particles: radioactivity detected in the peripheral zone may correspond to particles on small conducting airways or to particles in the acini.

Several reports have shown this or similar forms of penetration index to correlate well with lung function tests. *Figure 5.12* illustrates one example. It is based on 20 patients with chronic bronchitis and 6 non-smoking normal subjects who inhaled 5 μm particles under closely similar conditions (with, in particular, mean inhalation flow rates in the range of 40–45 $\ell\,min^{-1}$). Although the correlation between penetration index and FEV_1 is highly significant, there is clearly marked overlap between bronchitic and normal subjects and a wide scatter of individual values about the regression line. For patients with FEV_1 about 35 per cent predicted the 95 per cent confidence limits are equivalent to variations of approximately ±70 per cent about the mean penetration index of 0.3.

Studies in a larger subject population ($n = 80$) at lower flow rates (15–35 $\ell\,min^{-1}$) have also shown strong correlation ($p < 0.001$) between FEV_1 and penetration index (Agnew *et al.*, 1981a) and a wide spread of individual readings. A significant correlation between $\dot{V}_{max}25$ (maximum flow rate with 25 per cent FVC to be expired) and penetration index was also seen (Agnew *et al.*, 1981a). However assessment of the data in terms of partial correlation coefficients (penetration index as the '*y*-variable', FEV_1 and $\dot{V}_{max}25$ as the two '*x*-variables') shows penetration index in that subject population to depend significantly ($p < 0.001$) on FEV_1 but *not* $\dot{V}_{max}25$. A very strong ($p < 0.001$) correlation between penetration index (radioaerosol relative to ^{81m}Kr) and FEV_1 was also reported by Greening *et al.* (1980) using heterodisperse particles of 1.2 μm mass median diameter in 8 normal volunteers plus 20 patients with chronic bronchitis.

Using small particles from a nebulizer plus settling bag system, Garg *et al.* (1983) investigated the relationship between aerosol image scores (assessed by two observers) and lung function measurements (including FEV_1/FVC and MMFR) in 5 non-smokers, 21 smokers and 12 patients with COAD. Re-assessing their data in terms of partial correlation coefficients also suggests that aerosol results correlate significantly ($p < 0.001$) with 'large airways function' (i.e. FEV_1/FVC) but not with 'small airways function' (i.e. MMFR).

Thus overall loss of airway calibre, as reflected in diminished FEV_1, readily reduces radioaerosol lung penetration over a range of particle sizes and inhalation flow rates. This is a natural consequence of the various mechanisms (already considered) whereby changes in airflow velocities or airways calibre can enhance perihilar deposition. In this context, it is important to note that small airways dysfunction can in practice be associated with diminished penetration even when large airways function tests, such as FEV_1, remain normal. Dolovich *et al.* (1976) reported reduced outer to inner zone ratios in smokers compared to non-smokers and furthermore showed a very significant ($p < 0.01$) reduction in *aerosol penetrance index*, the mean level of this index in smokers being approximately half that recorded in non-smokers. *Penetrance* is a more complicated index than *penetration* being calculated as the number of particles in the outer zone at 24 hours divided by the number initially present in the inner zone (and adjusted by a volume correction factor, derived from ^{135}Xe imaging, to correct for differences in regional lung volume). The critical difference between *penetrance* and *penetration* in fact lies in using outer zone alveolar deposition rather than outer zone total deposition as the numerator of the index. The radioactive particles used by Dolovich *et al.* (1976) consisted of ^{131}I-labelled albumin which may (Sanchis *et al.*, 1972) to some extent be transported by mechanisms other than mucociliary transport or cough. If these include any contribution from lung permeability mechanisms (Chapter 8), distinction between smokers and non-smokers would thereby be enhanced as permeability is much greater in smokers than in non-smokers (Jones *et al.*, 1980). Recent support for the findings of Dolovich *et al.* (1976) has come in a report by Chamberlain *et al.* (1983) using 0.8 μm heterodisperse ^{99m}Tc sulphur colloid particles. At two different breathing rates, significantly more perihilar deposition occurred in smokers than in non-smokers. Other studies comparing penetration index in smokers and non-smokers have however found no difference, or even slightly higher penetration in the smokers than in the non-smokers (Greening *et al.*, 1980; Agnew *et al.*, 1981b; Fazio *et al.*, 1982; Hannan *et al.*, 1982; Foster *et al.*, 1983). Reduced penetration index in smokers is thus obviously not a universal finding applicable to all aerosol techniques. In subjects with asymptomatic asthma, small airways dysfunction has been shown to relate to diminished penetration in that penetration index correlated significantly ($p < 0.05$) with 'mean small airways function', 'MSAF' (the mean of percentage predicted MMFR and percentage predicted $\dot{V}_{max}25$) but *not* with FEV_1 (Agnew *et al.*, 1982a).

Several quantitative indices of radioaerosol distribution other than penetration index or penetrance have been proposed. In normal non-smokers, *skew* and *kurtosis* values, derived from histogram analysis of radioaerosol images, correlated both with FEV_1 and MMFR; the strongest ($p < 0.001$) correlation was that between skew and MMFR (Garrard *et al.*, 1981). This demonstrates that minor changes in small airways calibre within a population of normal subjects can have a detectable effect on radioaerosol deposition patterns. A different form of histogram analysis has compared radioaerosol and ^{81m}Kr distributions within a single 5 × 8 matrix representing each lung (Agnew *et al.*, 1981b and 1982a). *A distribution index* calculated on this basis correlated significantly ($p < 0.01$) with 'mean small airways function' (Agnew *et al.*, 1982a).

Summary of airways obstruction effects

Overall, it is clear from a range of published reports that radioaerosol images can readily be affected by airways obstruction. Image abnormalities—reduced penetration in particular—will often relate to impaired FEV_1 values. Under some circumstances, small airways dysfunction may also be an important determinant of the aerosol image. These findings stem from the basic physics of aerosol deposition. Narrowing of the large airways directly enhances deposition within them by increasing linear airflow velocities and thereby increasing the probabilities of particle impaction. This will particularly accentuate deposition in those bronchi corresponding to the peak of the deposition curves calculated for anatomical models of the airways (Chapter 3). Small airways dysfunction may be associated with changed patterns of flow in the major bronchi. These changed patterns will also tend to enhance perihilar deposition, which may therefore represent a response to either large or small airways dysfunction. Localized hot spots in more peripheral zones can result from flow being diverted from the most to the least obstructed bronchial pathways. Such hot spots may occur in chronic bronchitis or in asthma.

Ventilation imaging with radioaerosols

Textbooks of nuclear medicine describe the combined role of ventilation plus perfusion imaging in the diagnosis of pulmonary embolism. The procedure is important because pulmonary embolism is both common and treatable. Pulmonary embolism cannot however be reliably diagnosed on clinical grounds nor by means of simple radiology. Thus diagnosis rests on $\dot{V}/\dot{Q}$ (ventilation/perfusion) imaging unless resort is made to angiography.

$\dot{V}/\dot{Q}$ imaging

Typically, pulmonary embolism gives rise to multiple well defined defects on the perfusion image. These may be lobar or segmental; often they affect both lungs (Biello *et al.*, 1979; Fazio and Wollmer, 1981). Airways obstruction and infection can both however give similar patterns of defective perfusion. Thus whilst a normal perfusion pattern is generally relied on to exclude the diagnosis of pulmonary embolism, abnormal patterns of perfusion have to be considered non-specific. The key factor to interpretation is that defects actually due to obstruction or infection will also appear as defects on ventilation imaging. Those due to embolism will almost always show well-preserved ventilation. An example of a large perfusion defect in a lung region where ventilation remains normal is illustrated in *Figure 5.13*.

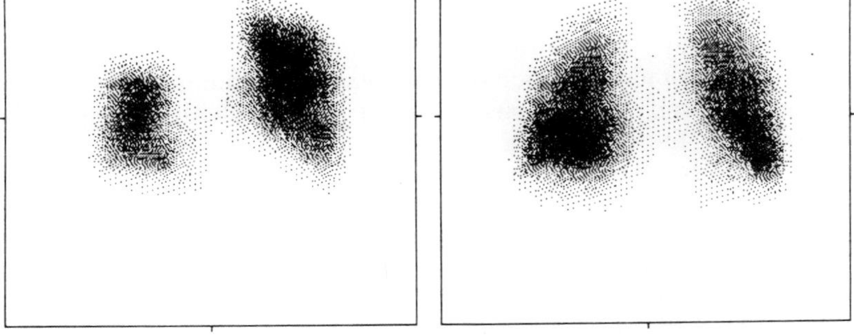

Figure 5.13 Illustration of $\dot{V}/\dot{Q}$ 'mismatch'. The perfusion image (left) shows a substantial defect at the right apex. The ventilation image, obtained with ^{99m}Tc-DTPA aerosol particles, shows normal ventilation

$\dot{V}/\dot{Q}$ 'mismatch' (poor perfusion, good ventilation) constitutes effective evidence of pulmonary embolism. Other possible causes of such $\dot{V}/\dot{Q}$ 'mismatch' do exist but they are rare and can generally be predicted on clinical or radiological grounds (Li *et al.*, 1978). Examples are arterial malformation, drug abuse, radiotherapy treatment and, in a few instances, carcinoma of the bronchus. Isolated small (subsegmental) zones of 'mismatch' are generally considered not to provide reliable evidence of pulmonary embolism (McNeil, 1976; Biello *et al.*, 1979; Neumann *et al.*, 1980; Fazio and Wollmer, 1981; Kotlyarov and Reba, 1982; Secker-Walker, 1983). This is particularly the case if they coincide with lung opacities on the chest X-ray.

Pulmonary angiography constitutes the standard against which $\dot{V}/\dot{Q}$ imaging may be judged but is an invasive procedure involving some risk for the patient. If, on clinical grounds, patients are selected for angiography after $\dot{V}/\dot{Q}$ imaging, selection will inevitably—as pointed out by Biello *et al.*, 1979—be biased towards patients in whom the $\dot{V}/\dot{Q}$ imaging procedure failed to give a definite answer, i.e. those with 'indeterminate' images. Comparisons with angiography have however been of great value in leading to the concept that reports on abnormal $\dot{V}/\dot{Q}$ patterns should be categorized as showing low, intermediate or high probabilities of pulmonary embolism (McNeil, 1976; Biello *et al.*, 1979; Neumann *et al.*, 1980). Criteria differ for assigning images to the various categories. 'Intermediate' probability to Biello *et al.* (1979) implies a single moderate-sized $\dot{V}/\dot{Q}$ mismatch with no corresponding abnormality on the conventional chest radiograph. They estimate this to correspond to a 33 per cent probability of angiographically demonstrable embolism. A moderate-sized defect is defined as 25–75 per cent of segmental volume and a large defect as greater than 75 per cent of segmental volume. 'High' probability would require at least one large or two moderate-sized zones of $\dot{V}/\dot{Q}$ mismatch. This they estimate to correspond to a 92 per cent probability of angiographically demonstrable embolism. Some differences between their approach to $\dot{V}/\dot{Q}$ interpretation and the earlier $\dot{V}/\dot{Q}$ reporting strategy of McNeil (1976) are discussed by Biello *et al.* (1979). Stringent criteria for issuing 'high-probability' reports are also advocated by Neumann *et al.* (1980). They, and other authors, stress that accurate $\dot{V}/\dot{Q}$ reporting additionally requires a good quality chest radiograph taken on the same day as the $\dot{V}/\dot{Q}$ images.

As a clinical procedure, it is highly desirable that both perfusion and ventilation imaging should be performed within hours of each other. Firstly, this is to achieve a diagnosis with minimum delay and inconvenience to the patient. Secondly, it is to avoid interpretation being complicated by the possibility of regional lung function changes occurring between the two procedures, a factor of particular relevance in patients with unstable airways obstruction.

Perfusion imaging is almost always based on ^{99m}Tc-labelled albumin macroaggregates or microspheres given intravenously. These are efficiently trapped in precapillary lung vessels, thereby giving images quantitatively proportional to regional blood flow. The fraction of precapillary vessels thus micro-embolized is small and so involves no hazard. The value of taking views in 4–6 different projections should be stressed. Quite substantial perfusion defects may be missed if only one or two views are recorded. Posterior oblique views may be more valuable than laterals because of a better relationship to segmental anatomy. They also avoid the cross-talk ('shine-through') from the contralateral lung which handicaps interpretation of lateral views.

Many centres perform ventilation imaging with a radioactive gas, usually either

^{133}Xe or ^{81m}Kr (Alderson and Line, 1980; Fazio and Wollmer, 1981). The low gamma-ray energy (81 keV) of ^{133}Xe unfortunately tends to give images weighted towards the more superficial zones of the lung. This is a drawback for comparing with ^{99m}Tc (141 keV) images. A gradual build-up of absorbed ^{133}Xe in blood and in the chest wall makes it difficult to obtain satisfactory views in more than one projection. By contrast, ^{81m}Kr (191 keV) has almost ideal properties for use with ^{99m}Tc (Fazio *et al.*, 1978a). It can be detected without interference from the slightly less energetic ^{99m}Tc radiation yet has an almost identical dependence of detection efficiency on source depth within the body. Its very short half-life (13 s) avoids any build-up of background radioactivity in blood or tissue, and in addition means that simply switching off the ^{81m}Kr supply makes it possible to record a further ^{99m}Tc image without any interference from ^{81m}Kr radiation. The short half-life also means that ^{81m}Kr images are essentially images of ventilation rather than of lung volume (Fazio and Wollmer, 1981). The disadvantages of ^{81m}Kr are expense and limited availability. It has to be supplied in the form of a generator containing its parent nuclide ^{81}Rb which is produced in a cyclotron and has a half-life of only 4.6 h. A generator can thus be used only on the day of its manufacture.

Increasing interest has therefore developed in radioaerosols for ventilation imaging. This stems partly from the drawbacks of gas techniques, and partly from a realization of the advantages aerosols have to offer. The crucial requirements for aerosol ventilation imaging are

(a) that the particles should be small enough to reach the lung periphery without undue impaction in large airways *en route*, and
(b) that a satisfactory method should be set up for using the radioaerosol technique in combination with ^{99m}Tc perfusion imaging.

Radioaerosols for ventilation imaging

The transition involved in going from particles suitable for assessing airways obstruction (or mucus clearance) to those suitable for ventilation imaging is illustrated in *Figure 5.14.* The left-hand image was obtained in a patient with severe airways obstruction a few minutes after the start of a mucociliary clearance test. The monodisperse particles used had a 5 µm aerodynamic diameter and were inhaled at about 30 ℓ min^{-1}. Central hyperdeposition is apparent with scattered 'hot spots' throughout the lung fields. By contrast a far more even spread of radioaerosol is seen in the centre image obtained in the same patient but with much smaller particles (mass median aerodynamic diameter <0.8 µm, GSD ≃ 2.5). The small particles used were ^{99m}Tc labelled DTPA (diethylenetriamine pentaacetic acid) inhaled from a nebulizer plus settling bag system (Francis *et al.*, 1981). The important thing in achieving an even distribution was the smallness of the particles. Their distribution is closely similar to that of ^{81m}Kr gas (in the same patient) shown in the right-hand section of the figure.

Figure 5.15 illustrates another comparison between the small ^{99m}Tc-DTPA particles (left) and ^{81m}Kr (right)—again in a patient with chronic bronchitis. Definition of the lung periphery as a whole, and of the mid-zone defect in particular, is equally good with both agents.

When debating whether or not to choose an aerosol ventilation imaging technique for clinical use there are, of course, drawbacks to consider. Firstly, it is obviously important to avoid large particles and high inhalation flow rates,

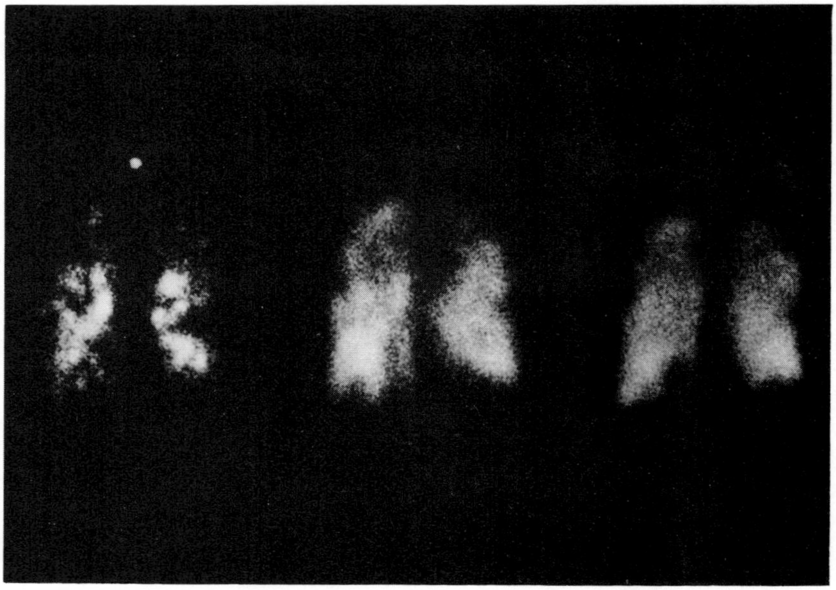

Figure 5.14 Ability of small radioaerosol particles to give a satisfactory ventilation image in severe chronic bronchitis (FEV_1 35 per cent predicted, MMFR 16 per cent predicted). The left-hand image was obtained with monodisperse 5 μm particles, the centre image with heterodisperse particles of less than 0.8 μm MMAD and the right-hand image with ^{81m}Kr gas; all are posterior images

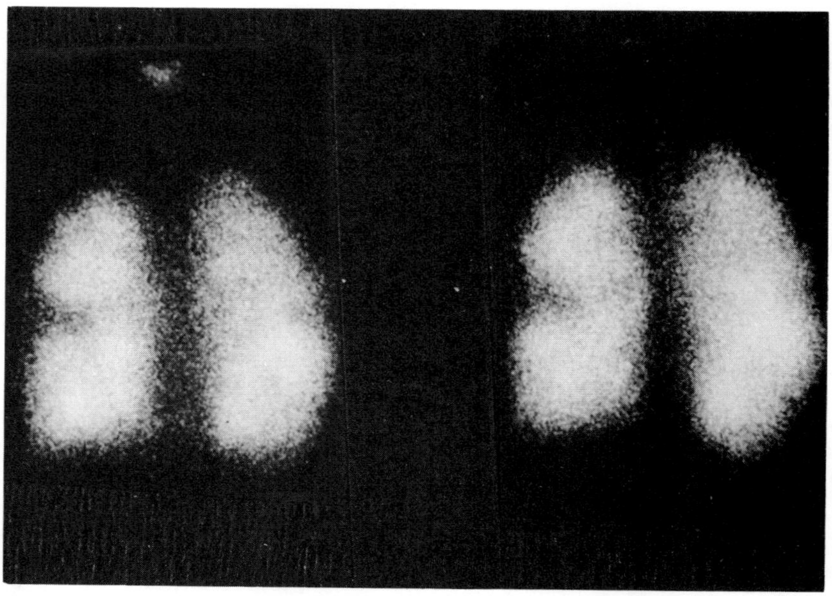

Figure 5.15 Similarity of ^{99m}Tc-DTPA aerosol image (left) and ^{81m}Kr image (right) in a patient with chronic bronchitis (FEV_1 37 per cent predicted, MMFR 24 per cent predicted); posterior images

TABLE 5.2. Aerosols for $\dot{V}/\dot{Q}$ imaging

Type of radioaerosol particle	*Particle diameter* (μm)*	*Generator system*	*$\dot{V}/\dot{Q}$ procedure*	*References*
^{99m}Tc colloid or DTPA	<2 μm	Nebulizer + 3 ℓ settling bag	1. Perfusion (low dose) 2. Ventilation (standard dose)	Taplin and Chopra, 1978 Chopra *et al.*, 1979a and 1979b; Hayes, 1980
^{113m}In albumin	<2 μm (85%)	Nebulizer + 50 ℓ settling bag	1. Perfusion 2. Ventilation } readily distinguished by different radionuclide energies	Wollmer *et al.*, 1980; Fazio *et al.*, 1982
^{99m}Tc DTPA	<2.1 μm (95%)	Nebulizer + 25 ℓ settling bag	1. Ventilation (low dose) 2. Perfusion (standard dose)	Francis *et al.*, 1981 Agnew *et al.*, 1982b + 1982c
^{99m}Tc DTPA	—	Nebulizer + heating chamber	1. Ventilation 2. Two-hour delay 3. Perfusion	Adiseshan, 1982
^{99m}Tc DTPA	—	Nebulizer + 2 settling bags	1. Ventilation 2. 4–6 hour delay 3. Perfusion	Godart *et al.*, 1982
^{99m}Tc-albumin	2 μm (monodisperse)	Pre-prepared, re-aerosolized from ethanol solution	—	Hannan *et al.*, 1982

*Percentage figures given in brackets relate to percentage of total inhaled radioactivity carried by particles of stated size.

particularly in patients with airways obstruction. Secondly, it is important to evaluate radiation hazards to the patient if excessive localized areas of high deposition occur and to staff performing the test if radioactive particles may accidentally be released into the laboratory atmosphere. Thirdly, it is difficult to devise an ideal technique for use in partnership with ^{99m}Tc perfusion imaging. On chemical (and availability) grounds ^{99m}Tc itself is often chosen as the aerosol label. If so, it then has to be differentiated from the ^{99m}Tc used for perfusion imaging. This may be done (as discussed later in the present chapter) either by allowing a long interval between the two procedures or by using much greater radioactivity for one than for the other (so that activity remaining from the first procedure can be 'swamped out' by that given for the second). A high energy nuclide, ^{113m}In, offers an alternative aerosol label although with an energy (393 keV) too high for satisfactory comparison with ^{99m}Tc.

Table 5.2 attempts to summarize some radioaerosol techniques proposed for clinical ventilation imaging in conjunction with perfusion imaging.

Preparation of small particles

Most of the aerosol methods in *Table 5.2* rely on gravitational settling to eliminate large particles from the heterodisperse range delivered by Venturi-action jet nebulizers. These nebulizers are inexpensive and readily available; they can be used to nebulize any convenient form of radioactive solution. The settling bag, once filled, constitutes a large volume radioactive source, which should be surrounded by shielding, particularly if high radioactivity levels are used. It acts as a reservoir from which the patient can inhale at will, in contrast to continuous generation systems in which nebulization has to be interrupted while the patient breath-holds and exhales, or alternatively some means has to be found for safe collection of the aerosol generated at these stages of the respiratory cycle.

Several possibilities other than the settling bag exist for eliminating large particles from nebulizer outputs. The parallel-plate separator relies on gravitational settling from aerosol travelling horizontally between parallel plates of very narrow vertical separation (Minty *et al.*, 1981). The ball-bearing separator relies on impaction from aerosol travelling through a matrix of closely packed steel ball-bearings or glass beads (Royston and Minty, 1983). Two forms of 'virtual separator' equipment have been described by Suzuki *et al.* (1982). The 'virtual separator' relies on the inability of large particles to follow abrupt changes in airflow direction, but instead of being allowed to impact they are carried forward with a small fraction of the airstream while the main bulk of the airstream, carrying with it the smaller particles, is deflected through a sharp angle. 'Modifier A' consisting of a virtual separator plus an impactor was able to produce particles of MMD 1.1–1.4 μm from three commercially available nebulizers driven at 15 ℓ min^{-1} (Suzuki *et al.*, 1982). 'Modifier B', selecting out fine particles by means of the virtual separator, was able to produce particles of MMD 0.4–0.8 μm from five commercial nebulizers driven at 7 or 15 ℓ min^{-1} (Suzuki *et al.*, 1982).

Thus techniques are available for obtaining small particles from nebulized radioactive solutions. Particles as small as 0.5 μm diameter will give minimal total deposition in the lung—hence the application found by particles of this size for the gas mixing studies considered earlier. Appreciable periods of breath-holding are therefore indicated in order to ensure that most of the inhaled radioactivity in any breath is not lost from the lung in the subsequent exhalation. Particles of about

2 μm diameter represent the largest acceptable size and even so can give significant hot spots resulting from impaction in large airways (Greening *et al.*, 1980). Fast inhalation should be avoided for particles larger than about 1 μm.

The aerosol techniques outlined in *Table 5.2* mostly rely on ^{99m}Tc-DTPA particles produced by a jet nebulizer. Studies by Waldman *et al.* (1982) have shown chemical instability in ^{99m}Tc-DTPA particles produced by an ultrasonic nebulizer, but no evidence of any such instability in particles from a jet nebulizer, even after being allowed to 'age' for 10 minutes. Extensive use has been made of ^{99m}Tc-DTPA for renal investigations, and large doses of DTPA salts have been used as a therapeutic agent (with no evident ill-effects) for the partial removal of accidentally inhaled plutonium. Clearance of ^{99m}Tc-DTPA from the lungs, by alveolar permeability mechanisms discussed in Chapter 8, helps to lessen the radiation dose to the lungs. It also lessens the ventilation 'background' left in the lungs if a perfusion test is to follow.

Perfusion or ventilation imaging first?

Clinically it is logical to perform perfusion imaging first. If the perfusion images are normal, pulmonary embolism is effectively excluded and there is no point in proceeding to the ventilation procedure. A valuable saving in time, effort and radiation dose may thus be obtained. But several of the procedures outlined in *Table 5.2* are based on ventilation preceding perfusion—the illogical order. This arises from practical difficulties implicit in using the same radionuclide (^{99m}Tc) for both procedures. Given that same-day imaging of perfusion and ventilation represents an important objective, distinction between the two procedures requires very different ^{99m}Tc activities for the two or a fast clearance of the agent given first. This has to be the ventilation agent because ^{99m}Tc perfusion agents are cleared only slowly from the lungs.

Hayes (1980) argues for lowering the perfusion dosage and raising the ventilation dose so that perfusion may precede ventilation. Suggested activities are 500 μCi (18.5 MBq) for perfusion and 3 mCi (111 MBq) for ventilation. This procedure has been in very regular use for a long time and offers easy assessment of ventilation 'filling-in' defective zones on the perfusion image (Hayes, 1980). In expert hands it is clearly practicable and effective. It obviously merits consideration for any centre where many patients are likely to have normal perfusion images. However for centres lacking experience in handling radioactive aerosols a disadvantage is that high activities have to be nebulized (suggested activity in the nebulizer is 30 mCi (1.11 GBq) in a 3 ml volume). Accidental release of airborne particles could contaminate equipment and might represent some hazard to personnel in the vicinity. Inadvertently fast inhalation by the patient could lead to high deposited activity in the oropharynx or on the large airways, raising the possibility of high localized radiation dosage.

To varying extents, the procedures involving DTPA aerosol ventilation prior to perfusion imaging benefit from lung clearance of DTPA before the start of perfusion imaging. Some 10 per cent of inhaled ^{99m}Tc-DTPA is likely to remain in the lungs after 4–6 h (Godart *et al.*, 1982). If this long an interval is allowed between the two procedures the DTPA residue will have negligible effect on the perfusion image. Alternatively the ventilation dose may be reduced so that perfusion imaging can be carried out immediately afterwards (Francis *et al.*, 1981). For centres lacking radioaerosol experience, this has the particular advantage of avoiding high nebulized activities. It must however imply longer imaging times (to achieve good counting statistics); and the rate of DTPA clearance from the lungs (discussed below) may thereby become a more important factor.

A distinction between 'perfusion first' and 'ventilation first' approaches is that the former need only demonstrate 'filling-in' by the ventilation agent of a previously demonstrated perfusion defect, i.e. a zone where no perfusion radioactivity is present. The latter approach, 'ventilation first', has to be able to demonstrate whether or not a perfusion defect exists at a site where (depending on activity levels and time interval) appreciable ventilation agent radioactivity may remain.

The various aerosol-based $\dot{V}/\dot{Q}$ procedures currently available each have their own particular advantages. Differing local needs and skills should dictate the choice made in any particular imaging department.

Clearance rate of soluble particles

Reference has already been made to the lung clearance of soluble aerosolized substances, ^{99m}Tc-DTPA in particular, as a factor to consider in choosing an aerosol-based $\dot{V}/\dot{Q}$ procedure. Much more attention is paid in Chapter 8 to DTPA clearance as a measure of lung permeability but it is considered here in relation to ventilation imaging.

^{99m}Tc is obtained from a generator as sodium pertechnetate solution (i.e. with the ^{99m}Tc in the chemical form of the TcO_4^- ion). This solution can readily be nebulized but the deposited ^{99m}Tc tends to be cleared from the lungs rather too rapidly for routine imaging purposes; clearance half-times measured by Chopra *et al.* (1979a) in upper and lower lung zones of normal non-smokers ranged from 4.5

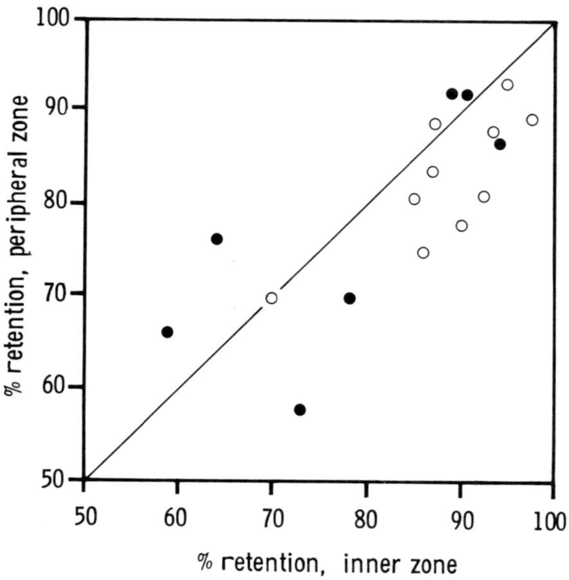

Figure 5.16 ^{99m}Tc retention following ^{99m}Tc-DTPA inhalation in peripheral lung zone (vertical axis) and inner lung zone (horizontal axis) over the length of time required to collect 4–5 lung images. Mean interval between images analysed was 16 min (range 9–26 min). Filled-in symbols are patients who were still current smokers; open symbols were ex-smokers or non-smokers

to 12.3 minutes. Clearance half-times for ^{99m}Tc-DTPA measured by the same authors ranged from 19 to 99 minutes in normal non-smokers but were significantly reduced in a group of 10 patients with systemic sclerosis (lowest values recorded being 8 minutes for the upper zone and 11 for the lower zone). Asymptomatic smokers show significantly faster ^{99m}Tc-DTPA clearance than non-smokers (Jones *et al.*, 1980; Minty *et al.*, 1981). Is clearance therefore so fast in some patients that multiple-view imaging will be impossible? There is also some evidence from animal studies that peripheral zone clearance may be faster than that from central airways (Oberdorster *et al.*, 1983). Does this imply rapidly diminishing peripheral visualization with ^{99m}Tc in humans? A partial answer to these questions is provided by *Figure 5.16*. This is based on work in which routine imaging in four projections (posterior, right and left posterior oblique and anterior views in sequence) was followed by a repeat posterior image used to check the amount of radioactivity remaining in outer and inner lung zones (Agnew *et al.*, 1982c). The mean interval between initial and repeat posterior images was 16 minutes. The lowest inner zone retention was 59 per cent, which was in a current smoker with a 14 minute interval between images. The lowest outer zone retention value was 58 per cent, in another current smoker, with a 16 minute interval between images. Overall, though, clearance rates from outer and inner zones were similar (*Figure 5.16*). This implies that visualization of the lung periphery does not tend to decrease rapidly during the time required for a routine sequence of images. (It also implies that permeability measured in a 'large airways' zone *may* be similar to that measured in a 'small airways plus alveoli' zone.) In practice it has generally been possible with the low-dose ^{99m}Tc-DTPA method to accumulate 4 views (200 000 counts each) within about 10 minutes from inhaling the aerosol (Agnew *et al.*, 1982c).

Radiation dose

A standard 2 mCi (74 MBq) ^{99m}Tc-macro-aggregated albumin dose given intravenously for perfusion imaging has been estimated to deliver about 800 mrad (8 mGy) to the lungs (DHSS, 1979). Standard ^{133}Xe and ^{81m}Kr ventilation procedures probably deliver lung doses (DHSS, 1979) of respectively 60 mrad (0.6 mGy) and 45 mrad (0.45 mGy). Aerosol doses will vary widely with different patterns of distribution and rates of clearance. A low aerosol activity of 500 μCi (18 MBq) has been estimated to deliver 291 mrad (2.9 mGy) to the lungs if spread uniformly throughout the lungs but cleared at a negligibly slow rate (Short *et al.*, 1979). This reduces to 233 mrad (2.3 mGy) if as small a proportion as 30 per cent of the aerosol is cleared with a half-time as long as 3 h (Short *et al.*, 1979). Very fast clearance of ^{99m}Tc-DTPA would reduce the lung dose to much lower levels but with the possibility of an appreciable dose to the kidneys, estimated as 150 mrad (1.5 mGy) for 500 μCi (18.5 MBq) given intravenously (DHSS, 1979). The importance of clearance rates to dose estimates is borne out by an estimate that ^{99m}Tc-DTPA aerosol will give several times less dose to the lungs than a ^{99m}Tc-colloid aerosol (Taplin and Chopra, 1978) simply because of the faster clearance obtained with DTPA. It should be emphasized that all dose estimates for aerosol imaging must be very approximate. Irregular deposition patterns will lead to an irregular distribution of radiation dose. To some extent, thickness of mucus in patients with chronic bronchitis will lessen the possibility of high localized dosage to basement membrance cells when deposition is concentrated in hot spots.

Quantitative comparison of radioaerosol and radioactive gas ventilation images

The overall lung penetration shown by several types of radioaerosol particle usable for ventilation imaging has been compared with that of ^{81m}Kr gas (Greening *et al.*, 1980; Agnew *et al.*, 1982b and 1982c; Fazio *et al.*, 1982; Hannan *et al.*, 1982). One such assessment is illustrated in *Figure 5.17* which compares the penetration of ^{99m}Tc-DTPA particles from a settling bag system (vertical axis) with that of ^{81m}Kr (horizontal axis). The majority of the data points lie close to the identity (45 degree) line. Lung function results were available for 21 of these patients. Five out

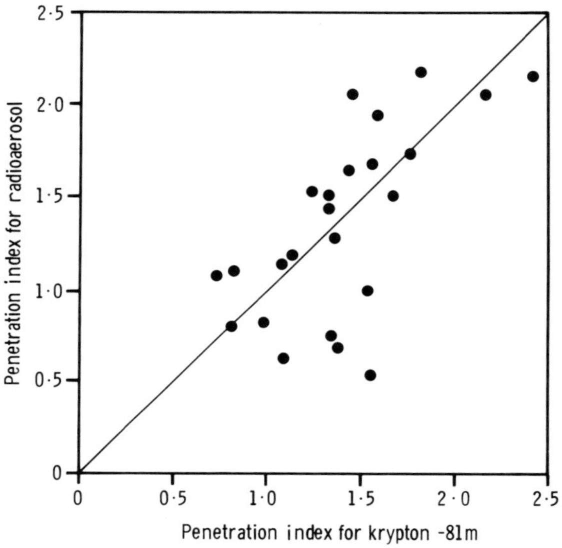

Figure 5.17 Penetration of ^{99m}Tc-DTPA particles (vertical axis) compared with penetration of ^{81m}Kr gas (horizontal axis) in 24 patients with varying degrees of airways obstruction. The ^{99m}Tc axis was, for this purpose, calculated as a simple outer-to-inner zone ratio (zones defined in *Figure 5.11*) and was not divided by the ^{81m}Kr index. The ^{81m}Kr index was also calculated as a simple outer-to-inner zone ratio

of the nine patients with FEV_1 less than 60 per cent predicted and MMFR less than 30 per cent predicted showed comparatively poor penetration of ^{99m}Tc relative to ^{81m}Kr but only in one instance was aerosol penetration less than 50 per cent of the ^{81m}Kr value (*Figure 5.18*). These results illustrate a degree of lung penetration similar to that reported by Fazio *et al.* (1982) and by Hannan *et al.* (1982). The former authors assessed penetration in 9 patients with chronic bronchitis (mean FEV_1 : 40 (SD 28) per cent predicted). Mean aerosol penetration relative to ^{81m}Kr was 0.63, with no individual value of less than 0.5. Visual inspection of these images prompted the comment that even in severe obstruction there was always 'detectable passage of particles to the lung periphery' (Fazio *et al.*, 1982). Mean penetration index in six patients with COAD studied by Hannan *et al.* (1982) was 0.69 (SD 0.21). The quantitative studies thus demonstrate that small aerosol particles can penetrate quite well to the lung periphery even in patients with chronic airflow obstruction.

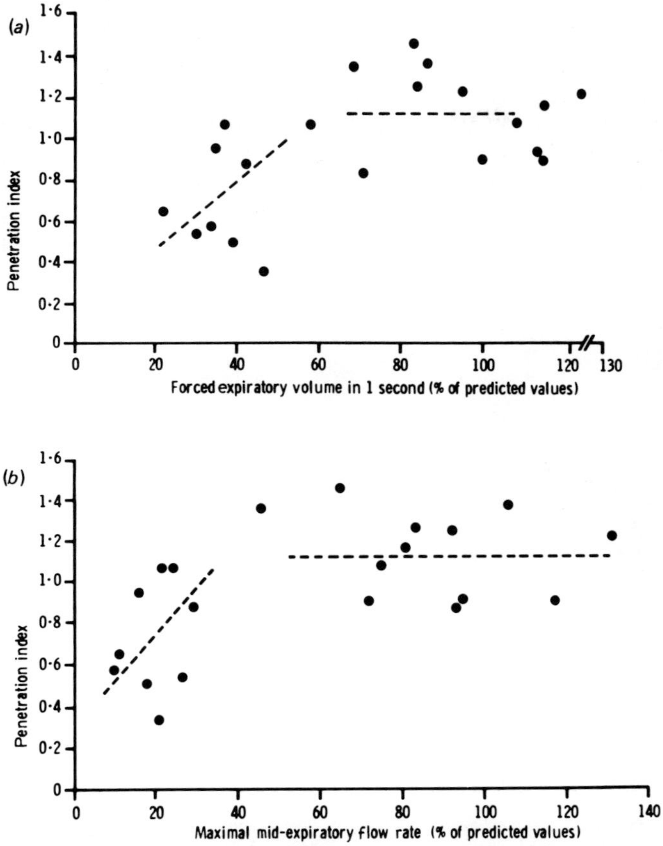

Figure 5.18 Penetration of ^{99m}Tc-DTPA aerosol relative to ^{81m}Kr gas in relationship to (a) per cent predicted FEV_1 and (b) per cent predicted MMFR. The penetration index shown (vertical axis) is the outer-to-inner zone ratio for ^{99m}Tc divided by that for ^{81m}Kr

Clinical effectiveness of aerosol-based $\dot{V}/\dot{Q}$ imaging

Same day $\dot{V}/\dot{Q}$ procedures, using aerosol particles for the ventilation image, have been adopted for regular use at several centres. ^{99m}Tc solutions for nebulization can readily be prepared by any nuclear medicine unit, are relatively inexpensive and can be made available any day of the week. Whether gas or aerosol is used for ventilation imaging, the diagnosis of pulmonary embolism should be made on the basis of at least one segmental or several subsegmental zones of $\dot{V}/\dot{Q}$ mismatch. Demonstration of ventilation in zones of such size should remain possible even when some loss of radioaerosol penetration occurs. *Figure 5.19* illustrates poor aerosol visualization of the lung periphery but yet good enough to demonstrate that, in this instance, ventilation matches perfusion. The increased central airways deposition of aerosol and the mottled patchiness of the perfusion image both result from chronic airflow obstruction. Likewise the aerosol ventilation image shown in *Figure 5.20* is of poorer technical quality than would, probably, have been obtained with ^{81m}Kr. Yet it is more than adequate to demonstrate a substantial zone of $\dot{V}/\dot{Q}$ mismatch in the left lung.

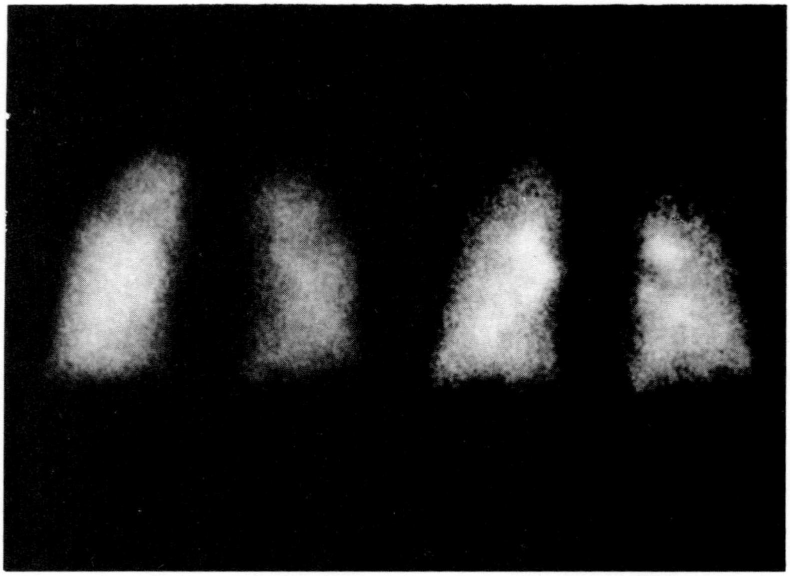

Figure 5.19 Routine diagnostic $\dot{V}/\dot{Q}$ imaging: perfusion image (left) compared with ^{99m}Tc-DTPA aerosol ventilation image (right); posterior images. Some central aerosol hyperdeposition is seen but penetration is adequate for peripheral visualization

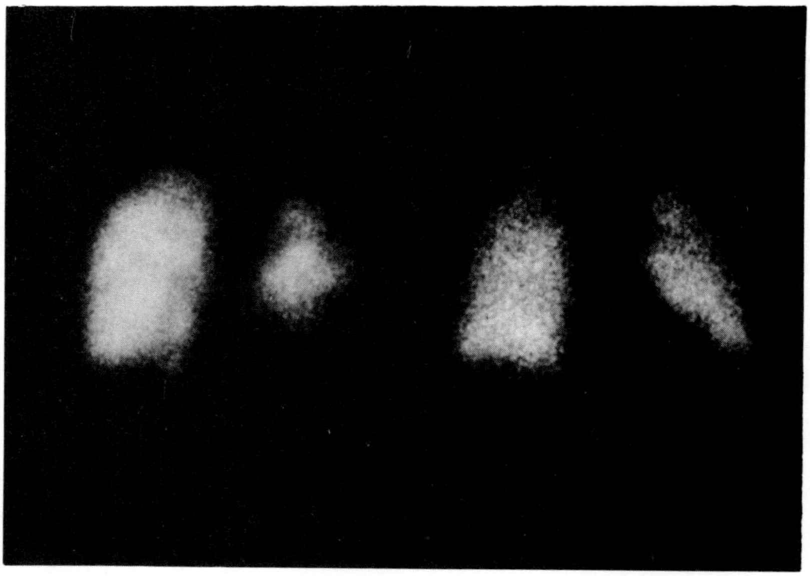

Figure 5.20 Routine diagnostic $\dot{V}/\dot{Q}$ imaging; example of $\dot{V}/\dot{Q}$ mismatch; anterior images. Perfusion image (left) shows substantial defect at left base but ^{99m}Tc-DTPA image (right) shows well-preserved ventilation in this region

Generally when radioaerosol penetration is poor, it can be *seen* to be poor. Thus images where central deposition is pronounced must be reported on with caution. This particularly applies if there appear to be matching $\dot{V}/\dot{Q}$ defects. A matching defect could arise if a moderate perfusion defect resulting from pulmonary embolism happened to coincide with a false 'ventilation defect' caused, in fact, by poor radioaerosol penetration.

The key point established by comparisons of $\dot{V}/\dot{Q}$ imaging with pulmonary angiography has been that V/Q reports should be phrased in terms of *probability*—low, intermediate or high. The criteria of Biello *et al.* (1979) were based on ventilation images obtained pre-perfusion with ^{133}Xe (usually only in one projection). The ability of radioaerosol (and ^{81m}Kr) readily to provide ventilation images in multiple projections may lead to some adjustment of the criteria for 'low', 'intermediate' or 'high' probability reports. Substitution of radioaerosol for gas ventilation imaging would however seem unlikely to change the value of a 'high' probability report. The fundamental defect is one of perfusion. The ventilation agent has to establish whether or not ventilation is preserved within the zone or zones in question. *Figures 5.13* and *5.20* illustrate that aerosol ventilation imaging can achieve this well; *Figure 5.15* illustrates an example of close matching between ventilation and perfusion images in a patient with a matched $\dot{V}/\dot{Q}$ defect. The quantitative results of *Figures 5.17* and *5.18* confirm the practical ability of aerosol imaging to act as a substitute for ^{81m}Kr.

Limited comparisons of ^{99m}Tc aerosol and ^{133}Xe ventilation imaging, together with ^{99m}Tc perfusion imaging, in patients subsequently undergoing angiography have shown the aerosol images to give better agreement than ^{133}Xe with the angiographic data (Alderson *et al.*, 1981; Ramanna *et al.*, 1981). It is nevertheless possible that poor aerosol penetration in a patient with severe airways obstruction might just occasionally lead to a 'low' probabiity report when ^{133}Xe or ^{81m}Kr imaging might have led to an 'intermediate' probability report. Given that the 'intermediate' report implies only a one in three probability of embolism (Biello *et al.*, 1979), the effective impact on patient management of a few 'intermediate' to 'low' changes must be open to debate. 'Intermediate' reports are perhaps to be expected in less than 10 per cent of patients seen (Neumann *et al.*, 1980), although this proportion must naturally depend on the clinical range of patients referred for $\dot{V}/\dot{Q}$ imaging. Two advantages of the radioaerosol approach are worthy of re-emphasis:

(a) the ability to obtain ventilation views in multiple projections (not easily possible with ^{133}Xe) and,
(b) ready availability throughout the week (not generally the case for ^{81m}Kr).

In addition, $\dot{V}/\dot{Q}$ comparisons based on using ^{99m}Tc for both procedures have the advantage that radiation absorption in the body and detection by the gamma camera are identical for the ventilation as for the perfusion images.

Summary of radioaerosol ventilation imaging for $\dot{V}/\dot{Q}$ analysis

In the diagnosis of pulmonary embolism, the function of an aerosol ventilation image is to demonstrate whether or not ventilation is preserved in lung zones where perfusion is absent. $\dot{V}/\dot{Q}$ mismatch (poor perfusion, good ventilation) implies a high probability of pulmonary embolism if the combined images show at least one segmental or several subsegmental regions of mismatch. Radioaerosol agents may readily be prepared for ventilation imaging but care must be taken to avoid large particles or fast inhalation. Images can be obtained in multiple projections.

Frequently, ^{99m}Tc is used as the radioactive label for both the aerosol ventilation agent and the perfusion imaging agent. Because it is clinically desirable to carry out both procedures on the same day, some means must be found to distinguish ventilation radioactivity from perfusion radioactivity. Several different approaches are available, based on differing levels of radioactivity for the two procedures and on allowing differing time intervals between the two.

Quantitative radioaerosol—^{81m}Kr comparisons have shown that radioaerosol particles can penetrate as well as ^{81m}Kr gas to the lung periphery in subjects with normal lung function. Even in patients with severe chronic airways obstruction, adequate visualization of peripheral zones can generally be obtained. Radioaerosol techniques can thus achieve effective ventilation imaging in clinical practice.

References

ADISESHAN, N. (1982). An improved technique for inhalation imaging. *Clin. Nucl. Med.*, **7**, 180–186

AGNEW, J.E., BATEMAN, J.R.M., PAVIA, D. and CLARKE, S.W. (1982a). Radioaerosol and ^{81m} krypton assessment of regional ventilation in asymptomatic asthma (abstract). *Thorax*, **37**, 235

AGNEW, J.E., BATEMAN, J.R.M., WATTS, M., PARAMANANDA, V., PAVIA, D. and CLARKE, S.W. (1981a). The importance of aerosol penetration for lung mucociliary clearance studies. *Chest*, **80** (Suppl.), 843–846

AGNEW, J.E., FRANCIS, R.A., PAVIA, D. and CLARKE, S.W. (1982b). Quantitative comparison of ^{99m}Tc-aerosol and ^{81m}Kr ventilation images. *Clin. Phys. Physiol. Meas.*, **3**, 21–30

AGNEW, J.E., FRANCIS, R.A., PAVIA, D. and CLARKE, S.W. (1982c). ^{99m}Tc-DTPA aerosol ventilation imaging: theoretical and practical assessment. In *Nuclear medicine and biology*. Edited by Raynaud, C. Paris; Pergamon Press, 2018–2021

AGNEW, J.E., PAVIA, D. and CLARKE, S.W. (1981b). Airways penetration of inhaled radioaerosol: an index to small airways function? *Eur. J. Respir. Dis.*, **62**, 239–255

ALDERSON, P.O. and LINE, B.R. (1980). Scintigraphic evaluation of regional pulmonary ventilation. *Semin. Nucl. Med.*, **10**, 218–242

ALDERSON, P.O., KOTLYAROV, E.V., LOKEN, M.K. and DELAND, F.H. (1981). A comparison of Xe-133 ventilation and Tc-99m aerosol inhalation imaging as aids to perfusion scanning in the scintigraphic detection of pulmonary embolism (abstract). *J. Nucl. Med.*, **22**, P42–P43

ALTSHULER, B., PALMES, E.D., YARMUS, L. and NELSON, N. (1959). Intrapulmonary mixing of gases studied with aerosols. *J. Appl. Physiol.*, **14**, 321–327

BECKLAKE, M.R. and PERMUTT, S. (1979). Evaluation of tests of lung function for 'screening' for early detection of chronic obstructive lung disease. In *The lung in the transition between health and disease*. Edited by Macklem, P.T., Permutt, S. New York; Marcel Dekker, 345–387

BIELLO, D.R., MATTAR, A.G., McKNIGHT, R.C. and SIEGEL, B.A. (1979). Ventilation-perfusion studies in suspected pulmonary embolism. *Am. J. Roentgenol.*, **133**, 1033–1037

CHAMBERLAIN, M.J., MORGAN, W.K.C. and VINITSKI, S. (1983). Factors influencing the regional deposition of inhaled particles in man. *Clin. Sci.*, **64**, 69–78

CHOPRA, S.K., TAPLIN, G.V., TASHKIN, D.P. and ELAM, D. (1979a). Lung clearance of soluble radioaerosols of different molecular weights in systemic sclerosis. *Thorax*, **34**, 63–67

CHOPRA, S.K., TAPLIN, G.V., TASHKIN, D.P., TREVOR, E. and ELAM, D. (1979b). Imaging sites of airway obstruction and measuring functional responses to bronchodilator treatment in asthma. *Thorax*, **34**, 493–500

CINKOTAI, F.F. (1974). Fluid flow in a model alveolar sac. *J. Appl. Physiol.*, **37**, 249–251

DAVIES, C.N., HEYDER, J. and SUBBA RAMU, M.C. (1972). Breathing of half-micron aerosols. I. Experimental. *J. Appl. Physiol.*, **32**, 591–600

DHSS (Department of Health and Social Security) (1979). Notes for guidance on the administration of radioactive substances to persons for purposes of diagnosis, treatment or research. London; HMSO

DOLOVICH, M.B., SANCHIS, J., ROSSMAN, C. and NEWHOUSE, M.T. (1976). Aerosol penetrance: a sensitive index of peripheral airways obstruction. *J. Appl. Physiol.*, **40**, 468–471

ENGEL, L.A. (1983). Gas mixing within the acinus of the lung. *J. Appl. Physiol.*, **54**, 609–618

FAZIO, F. and WOLLMER, P. (1981). Clinical ventilation-perfusion scintigraphy. *Clin. Physiol.*, **1**, 323–337

FAZIO, F., LAVENDER, J.P. and STEINER, R.E. (1978a). ^{81m}Kr ventilation and ^{99m}Tc perfusion scans in chest disease: comparison with standard radiographs. *Am. J. Roentgenol.*, **130**, 421–428

FAZIO, F., WOLLMER, P., LAVENDER, J.P. and BARR, M.M. (1982). Clinical ventilation imaging with In-113m aerosol: a comparison with Kr-81m. *J. Nucl. Med.*, **23**, 306–314

FAZIO, F., SANTOLICANDRO, A., SOLFANELLI, S., PALLA, A., FORNAI, E. and GIUNTINI, C. (1978b). Lung imaging following inhalation of technetium 99m-labelled microspheres: a comparison with the Krypton-81m ventilation technique. In *Clinical and experimental applications of Krypton 81m*. Edited by Lavender, J.P. London; British Institute of Radiology, pp. 130–140

FOSTER, W.M., LANGENBACK, E. and BERGOFSKY, E. (1983). Quantitation of lung mucus clearance in large and small airways of healthy smokers, as compared to non-smokers, identifies an early indicator of abnormal function (abstract). *Am. Rev. Respir. Dis.*, **127**, 165

FRANCIS, R.A., AGNEW, J.E., SUTTON, P.P., PAVIA, D. and CLARKE, S.W. (1981). Ventilation imaging with easily prepared ^{99m}Tc aerosols. *Nucl. Med. Commun.*, **2**, 203–208

FUKUCHI, Y., COSIO, M., MURPHY, B. and ENGEL, L.A. (1980). Intraregional basis for sequential filling and emptying of the lung. *Respir. Physiol.*, **41**, 253–266

GARG, A., GOPINATH, P.G., PANDE, J.N. and GULERIA, J.S. (1983). Role of radio-aerosol and perfusion lung imaging in early detection of chronic obstructive lung disease. *Eur. J. Nucl. Med.*, **8**, 167–171

GARRARD, C.S., GERRITY, T.R., SCHREINER, J.F., YEATES, D.B. (1981). Analysis of aerosol deposition in the healthy human lung. *Arch. Environ. Health*, **36**, 184–193

GEBHART, J., HEYDER, J. and STAHLHOFEN, W. (1981). Use of aerosols to estimate pulmonary air-space dimensions. *J. Appl. Physiol.*, **51**, 465–476

GERRITY, T.R., LEE, P.S., HASS, F.J., MARINELLI, A., WERNER, P. and LOURENÇO, R.V. (1979). Calculated deposition of inhaled particles in the airway generations of normal subjects. *J. Appl. Physiol.*, **47**, 867–873

GODART, G., ROBIENCE, Y.J., RICHEZ, M., DELWARTE, J. and RAVEZ, P. (1982). Labelled particles in comparison with radioactive rare gases for ventilation imaging. In *Nuclear medicine and biology*. Edited by Raynaud, C. Paris; Pergamon Press, 2530–2532

GREENING, A.P., MINIATI, M. and FAZIO, F. (1980). Regional deposition of aerosols in health and in airways obstruction: a comparison with krypton-81m ventilation scanning. *Bull. Eur. Physiopathol. Respir.*, **16**, 287–298

HANKINSON, J.L., PALMES, E.D. and LAPP, N.L. (1979). Pulmonary air space size in coal miners. *Amer. Rev. Respir.Dis.*, **119**, 391–397

HANNAN, W.J., EMMETT, P.C., AITKEN, R.J., LOVE, R.G., MILLAR, A.M. and MUIR, A.L. (1982). Effective penetration of the lung periphery using radioactive aerosols. *J. Nucl. Med.*, **23**, 872–877

HAYES, M. (for TAPLIN, G.V.) (1980). Lung imaging with radioaerosols for the assessment of airway disease. *Semin. Nucl. Med.*, **10**, 243–251

HEYDER, J. (1983). Charting human thoracic airways by aerosols. *Clin. Phys. Physiol. Meas.*, **4**, 29–37

HUGHES, J.M.B., HOPPIN, F.G. and MEAD, J. (1972). Effect of lung inflation on bronchial length and diameter in excised lungs. *J. Appl. Physiol.*, **32**, 25–35

ITOH, H., ISHII, Y., SUZUKI, T., YENEKURA, Y., MORITA, R. and TORIZUKA, K. (1977). Radioscintigraphy in the diagnosis of upper airway obstruction. *Radiology*, **123**, 135–140

ITOH, H., ISHII, Y., SUZUKI, T., HAMAMOTO, K., TORIZUKA, K., OYAMADA, H. and YONEYAMA, T. (1976). Inhalation scintigraphy with radioaerosols in bronchogenic carcinoma. *Radiology*, **119**, 623–636

JONES, J.G., MINTY, B.D., LAWLER, P., HULANDS, G., CRAWLEY, J.C.W. and VEALL, N. (1980). Increased alveolar epithelial permeability in cigarette smokers. *Lancet*, **2**, 66–68

KLINGELE, T.G. and STAUB, N.C. (1971). Terminal bronchiole diameter changes with volume in isolated, air-filled lobes of cat lung. *J. Appl. Physiol.*, **30**, 224–227

KOTLYAROV, E.V. and REBA, R.C. (1982). Diagnostic efficacy of ventilation/perfusion ($\dot{V}/\dot{Q}$) segmental equivalent concept in the diagnosis of pulmonary embolism. In *Nuclear medicine and biology*. Edited by Raynaud, C. Paris; Pergamon Press, 2052–2055

LAPP, N.L., HANKINSON, J.L., AMANDUS, H. and PALMES, E.D. (1975). Variability in the size of airspaces in normal human lungs as estimated by aerosols. *Thorax*, **30**, 293–299

LI, D.K., SELTZER, S.E. and McNEIL, B.J. (1978). $\dot{V}/\dot{Q}$ mismatches unassociated with pulmonary embolism: Case report and review of the literature. *J. Nucl. Med.*, **19**, 1331–1333

LIN, M.S. and GOODWIN, D.A. (1976). Pulmonary distribution of an inhaled radioaerosol in obstructive pulmonary disease. *Radiology*, **118**, 645–651

LIPPMANN, M. (1977). Regional deposition of particles in the human respiratory tract. In *Handbook of physiology: reaction to environmental agents*. Edited by Lee, D.H.K. *et al.* Bethesda, Ma.; The American Physiological Society, 213–232

LOVE, R.G. and MUIR, D.C.F. (1976). Aerosol deposition and airway obstruction. *Am. Rev. Respir. Dis.*, **114**, 891–897

MACKLEM, P.T., HOGG, W.E. and BRUNTON, J. (1973). Peripheral airway obstruction and particulate deposition in the lung. *Arch. Intern. Med.*, **131**, 93–97

McNEIL, B.J. (1976). A diagnostic strategy using ventilation-perfusion studies in patients suspect for pulmonary embolism. *J. Nucl. Med.*, **17**, 613–616

MILIC-EMILI, J. (1977). Ventilation. In *Regional differences in the lung*. Edited by West, J.B. New York; Academic Press, pp. 167–199

MINTY, B.D., JORDAN, C. and JONES, J.G. (1981). Rapid improvement in abnormal pulmonary epithelial permeability after stopping cigarettes. *Brit. Med. J.*, **282**, 1183–1186

MUIR, D.C.F. (1967). Distribution of aerosol particles in exhaled air. *J. Appl. Physiol.*, **23**, 210–214

MUIR, D.C.F. (1970). The effect of airways obstruction on the single breath aerosol curve. In *Airways Dynamics: Physiology and Pharmacology*. Edited by Bouhuys, A. Springfield, Ill.; C.C. Thomas, pp. 319–325

MUIR, D.C.F., SWEETLAND, K. and LOVE, R.G. (1971). Inhaled aerosol boluses in man. In *Inhaled particles III*. Edited by Walton, W.H. Old Woking; Unwin Bros., pp. 81–90

NEUMANN, R.D., SOSTMAN, H.D. and GOTTSCHALK, A. (1980). Current status of ventilation-perfusion imaging. *Semin. Nucl. Med.*, **10**, 198–217

OBERDÖRSTER, G., UTELL, M.J., WEBER, D.A., HYDE, R.W. and MORROW, P.E. (1983). Differential bronchial and alveolar deposition and absorption of ^{99m}Tc-DTPA (Diethylenetriamine pentacetic acid) aerosols (abstract). *Am. Rev. Respir. Dis.*, **127**, 167

PALMES, E.D. (1973). Measurement of pulmonary air spaces using aerosols. *Arch. Intern. Med.*, **131**, 76–79

PALMES, E.D., GOLDRING, R.M., WANG, C-S. and ALTSHULER, B. (1971). Effect of chronic obstructive pulmonary disease on rate of deposition of aerosols in the lung during breath holding. In *Inhaled particles III*. Edited by Walton, W.H. Old Woking; Unwin Bros., pp. 123–130

PALMES, E.D., WANG, C-S., GOLDRING, R.M. and ALTSHULER, B. (1973). Effect of depth of inhalation on aerosol persistence during breath holding. *J. Appl. Physiol.*, **34**, 356–360

PEDLEY, T.J., SCHROTER, R.C. and SUDLOW, M.F. (1970). The prediction of pressure drop and variation of resistance within the human bronchial airways. *Respir. Physiol.*, **9**, 387–405

RAMANNA, L., TASHKIN, D.P., TAPLIN, G.V., ELAM, D., DETELS, R., COULSON, A. and ROKAW, S.N. (1975). Radioaerosol lung imaging in chronic obstructive pulmonary disease: Comparison with pulmonary function tests and Roentgenography. *Chest*, **68**, 634–640

RAMANNA, L., WAXMAN, A., BRACHMAN, M., JULIEN, P., BERMAN, D., TANASESCU, D. and KOERNER, S. (1981). Scintigraphic determination of pulmonary embolism: the value of aerosol in indeterminate studies (abstract). *J. Nucl. Med.*, **22**, P92

ROYSTON, D. and MINTY, B.D. (1983). A cheap simple particle generation system for use with *in vivo* measurement of alveolar-capillary barrier permeability (abstract). *Am. Rev. Respir. Dis.*, **127**, 319

SANCHIS, J., DOLOVICH, M., CHALMERS, R. and NEWHOUSE, M. (1972). Quantitation of regional aerosol clearance in the normal human lung. *J. Appl. Physiol.*, **33**, 757–762

SANTOLICANDRO, A. and GIUNTINI, C. (1979). Patterns of deposition of labelled monodispersed aerosols in obstructive lung disease. *J. Nucl. Med. Allied Sci.*, **23**, 115–127

SECKER-WALKER, R.H. (1983). Respiratory Disease. In *Clinical nuclear medicine*. Edited by Maisey, M.N., Britton, K.E. and Gilday, D.L. London; Chapman and Hall, pp. 41–81

SHORT, M.D., DOWSETT, D.J., HEAF, P.J.D., PAVIA, D. and THOMSON, M.L. (1979). A comparison between monodisperse Tc-99m-labeled aerosol particles and Kr-81m for the assessment of lung function. *J. Nucl. Med.*, **20**, 194–200

SUZUKI, T., SWIFT, D.L., WAGNER, H.N. and PROCTOR, D.F. (1982). A new apparatus for generating hygroscopic radioactive aerosols for inhalation studies. *Eur. J. Nucl. Med.*, **7**, 474–479

TAPLIN, G.V. and CHOPRA, S.K. (1978). Inhalation lung imaging with radioactive aerosols and gases. *Prog. Nucl. Med.*, **5**, 119–143

TASHKIN, D.P., DETELS, R., COULSON, A.H., ROKAW, S.N. and SAYRE, J.W. (1979). The UCLA population studies of chronic obstructive respiratory disease II: Determination of reliability and estimation of sensitivity and specificity. *Environ. Res.*, **20**, 403–424

TAULBEE, D.B., YU, C.P. and HEYDER, J. (1978). Aerosol transport in the human lung from analysis of single breaths. *J. Appl. Physiol.*, **44**, 803–812

WALDMAN, D.L., OBERDOERSTER, G., DRAGO, S.R., UTELL, M.J., HYDE, R.W., WEBER, D.A. and MORROW, P.E. (1982). Chemical stability of Tc-99m DTPA (diethylenetriamine penta-acetic acid) after nebulisation and inhalation (abstract). *Aerosol Sci. Tech.*, **2**, 296

WEIBEL, E.R. (1963). *Morphometry of the human lung*. Berlin; Springer-Verlag

WOLLMER, P., BARR, M.M. and FAZIO, F. (1980). Clinical ventilation imaging with ^{113m}In aerosol. *J. Nucl. Med. Allied Sci.*, **24**, 215–220

YEH, H.-D. and SCHUM, G.M. (1980). Models of human lung airways and their applications to inhaled particle deposition. *Bull. Math. Biol.*, **42**, 461–480

Chapter 6

Lung mucociliary clearance

Demetri Pavia

Introduction

Mucociliary clearance is one of the lungs' non-specific, host defence mechanisms. This clearance mechanism together with alveolar clearance and cough helps to keep the lungs clean and sterile even when exposed to a polluted atmosphere. The beating action of the cilia propels the mucus overlying their tips onwards towards the epiglottis carrying with it trapped inhaled insoluble material plus any locally produced biological debris.

In the human lung cilia are to be found from the level of the trachea down to the terminal bronchioles. The length of the cilia is shorter in the peripheral compared to the proximal airways. There is some evidence suggesting that cilia beat slower in the distal compared to the proximal airways although the converse has also been reported and further studies are needed to clarify this point. The flow of mucus is fastest in the trachea and studies indicate that mucus flows at progressively slower rates in the more distal airways of the lungs. Clearance of mucus from the lungs by the cilia can be thought of in terms of an escalator with increasing speed the nearer it gets to the mouth. It has been suggested that this increase in the flow of mucus is necessary in order to handle (a) the secretions which are converging from airways with a total of cumulative circumference at the level of the terminal bronchioles of several metres to that of the trachea which is only of a few centimetres and (b) the excess secretions encountered en route and produced primarily by the submucosal glands which are mainly found in the cartilaginous airways. It has been postulated that a certain amount of re-absorption of lung secretions, primarily in the distal ciliated airways, must also be taking place. This hypothesis evolved in order to explain how the fluid load resulting from the convergence of thousands of bronchioles leading to the trachea does not give rise to 'long-jam' effects. Estimates of the quantity of mucus transported by the mucociliary escalator per 24 hours in man vary from 10 ml, from collections made at tracheostomy level of normal accident victims, to 100 ml by extrapolating to man from animal studies. However, it is not unusual for 200–300 ml of sputum to be collected from bronchitic patients during exacerbations.

For many years attention was focussed on the apparent viscosity of mucus (a non-Newtonian fluid) and its role in mucociliary clearance. Mucus however is viscoelastic in nature and the importance of the elastic component in mucociliary clearance has been highlighted in recent years (Chen and Dulfano, 1978). There appears to be a fairly large range of Newtonian viscosity but a small range of linear elastic modulus of sputum for its optimal transportability *in vitro*. If the sputum viscoelastic properties rise or fall below the optimal range then this would cause a reduction in its transportability by the cilia.

In its course from the terminal bronchioles to the oesophagus the mucus flow encounters a number of obstructions over which or past which it must flow (Hilding, 1957). Among these are the openings of the tributary bronchi, normally occurring squamous islands or areas of metaplasia, the squamous epithelium of the vocal cords and any other normal or abnormal areas that are devoid of cilia. At each bronchial opening and at the vocal cords the axial progress of the mucous flow ceases and mucus is caused to flow in two opposite directions. The efficiency with which these obstacles are surmounted depends on (a) the traction of the mucous layer which in turn depends on the viscoelastic properties of the mucus and (b) the relative activity of the cilia in the portion of the area in question and on the change in the direction of ciliary beat. Where there is comparative stasis of mucous flow then the possibility exists of prolonged action in such sites of carcinogenic substances contained in the ciliary stream. The suggestion has been made that the distribution of squamous-cell carcinoma in the respiratory tract bears a relationship with holdups in mucus flow.

Measurement of lung mucociliary clearance

Measurement of the efficiency of mucociliary transport in the lungs is achieved chiefly in two ways (Pavia *et al.*, 1980b). The first approach involves the actual measurement of the flow of mucus and the second the rate of removal of deposited inhaled aerosols yielding an index of mucus flow efficiency.

Mucus velocity

Measurement of the linear flow of mucus involves the timing of the movement of marker(s) placed on the mucus over a given distance.

There are essentially four techniques for measuring the velocity of mucus in the human lung although only one of these utilizes aerosols: the *cinefibrescopic technique* due to Sackner *et al.* (1973) makes use of Teflon discs (0.68 mm in diameter, 0.13 mm in thickness and weighing 0.13 mg) which are insufflated through the inner channel of a fibreoptic bronchoscope onto the tracheal mucosa in a circumferential distribution (*Figure 6.1a*). The movement of these discs is filmed and essentially the discs serve as markers of tracheal mucus transport. A measure of tracheal mucous velocity (TMV) is obtained by measuring the time taken for the discs to move a given distance. Usually the TMV value quoted is the mean of measurements made on 10–20 discs.

The radioisotopic technique utilizing a fibreoptic bronchoscope by Chopra *et al.* (1979) is based on the following principles. The length of the trachea is determined by means of a graduated fibreoptic bronchoscope. Two reference points, namely the larynx and the carina, are registered on a polaroid film from the display of a gamma camera by inserting a sealed plastic catheter tagged with say a 50 μCi of ^{99m}Tc source at its tip through the inner channel of the bronchoscope. A minute suspension (about 40 μl) of albumin microspheres 5–7 μm in diameter, numbering

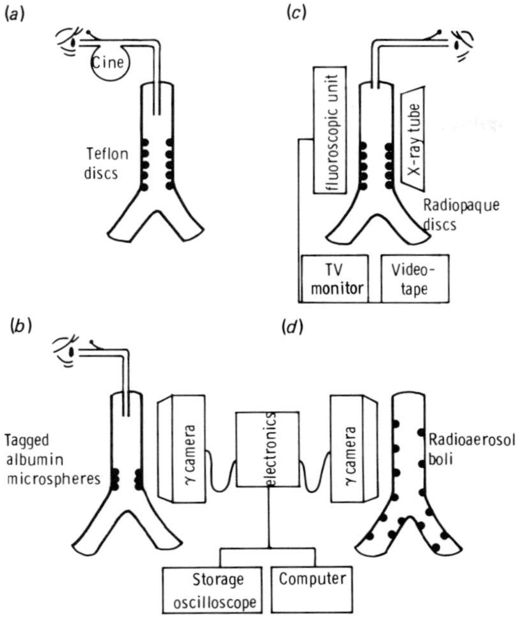

Figure 6.1 Schematic diagrams of techniques for measuring tracheal mucus velocity: (a) cinefibrescopic technique (b) radioisotopic technique utilizing a fibreoptic bronchoscope (c) roentgenographic technique (d) radioaerosol boli technique

approximately 50 000 and tagged with ^{99m}Tc is deposited on the mucosal surface at the lower end of the trachea via a catheter placed through the inner channel of the bronchoscope (*Figure 6.1b*). The movement of the microspheres towards the larynx serves as a marker of mucous movement. Sequential pictures of the microspheres in the trachea are taken at say 1 minute intervals over an observation period of 30–60 minutes, i.e. the time taken for the spheres to reach the larynx. Once again a measure of the average TMV is achieved by dividing the distance moved by the microspheres by the time taken.

The *roentgenographic technique* is a modification of the cinebronchofibrescopic method (Friedman *et al.*, 1977b). Teflon tape, coated with the radio-opaque substance bismuth trioxide, is fed into a specially designed punch which is attached to a source of compressed air on one side and to a fibreoptic bronchoscope on the other. When triggered, the punch produces individual discs which are blown through the inner channel of the bronchoscope into the trachea. The cephalad motion of these particles in the trachea is recorded with a fluoroscopic unit provided with image intensifier, television monitor and videotape (*Figure 6.1c*). A total of, say, 10 tracheal x-rays are taken at one minute intervals. Several discs are identified and the distance covered by each disc during the procedure is noted. From these measurements an average TMV is derived.

The *radioaerosol boli technique* due to Yeates *et al.* (1975) entails the inhalation of a radioaerosol with a suitable inhalation manoeuvre. Inspiring the radioaerosol from near total lung capacity with a high flow rate, the aerosol deposits mainly in local boli in the large airways. The boli transported up the trachea by ciliary action can be monitored and recorded using a gamma camera (*Figure 6.1d*) or a specially designed multidetector probe located over the trachea. The TMV can be measured from the distance moved by the boli in a given time.

The average values for TMV reported for healthy, non-smokers by the invasive-techniques, i.e. those techniques using a fibreoptic bronchoscope, are considerably higher (up to fivefold) than those obtained with the non-invasive radioaerosol boli technique. For example the cinebronchofibrescopic technique yields a mean ± SD TMV of 21.5 ± 5.5 mm min^{-1} (Santa Cruz *et al.*, 1974) while the radioisotopic technique utilizing a bronchoscope gives 15.5 ± 0.7 mm min^{-1} (Chopra *et al.*, 1979). By comparison, the radioaerosol boli method gives a mean ± SD TMV of 4.4 ± 1.3 mm min^{-1} (Yeates *et al.*, 1975). The intermediate, in terms of invasiveness, technique in which the bronchoscope is only inserted to the level of the vocal cords (Friedman *et al.*, 1977b) gives velocities (11.4 ± 3.8 mm min^{-1}) much nearer to those obtained by the non-invasive technique. The respiratory epithelium is fragile; simple contact by gauze, cotton swabs, aspiration and instrumentation has been shown to cause epithelial injury as well as an outpouring of secretions.

The discrepancies reported in the absolute values for TMV in non-smokers are not to be taken to reflect such a large inter-subject variability of this measurement but the influence of methodology used in obtaining them. Such discrepancies do not invalidate the use of each technique for studying the effect of specific factors on mucous clearance rates. The bronchoscopic techniques, although invasive, have several distinct advantages. For example, the short observation periods (a few minutes up to one hour) minimize artefacts resulting from coughing and permit repeated measurements within a short period of time. This means that if the acute effects of a drug on mucous flow were being investigated, a baseline run on the same subject could be performed on the same day. The marker(s) used in the bronchoscopic techniques can be precisely positioned thus yielding measurements of mucous velocity in an anatomically well defined region. However the use of the techniques has been restricted to the large airways and, in practice, mainly to the trachea although some reports have appeared of measurements in the main bronchi. It must be emphasized that results obtained from the trachea/main bronchi—or indeed often just from a portion of these airways—may give no indication of the mucociliary function from more distal ciliated airways. An indication of the transport rates beyond the main bronchi must be inferred from measurements of clearance of deposited radioaerosols from the lungs.

The radioaerosol technique for measuring lung mucociliary clearance

The radioaerosol technique is the most widely used method for obtaining an index of the efficiency of the lung mucociliary escalator. Albert and Arnett (1955) were the first to use inhaled radioaerosols for measuring lung mucociliary clearance in man. Their method entails the inhalation of an aerosol labelled unleachably with a gamma-emitting radionuclide. By monitoring the radioactivity, using external scintillation gamma counters, emanating exclusively from the subject's chest immediately after inhalation a measure can be made of the quantity of radioaerosol initially deposited within the lungs. With time after inhalation, counting shows a progressive loss of radioactivity from the lungs for two reasons: (a) physical decay of the radioisotope and (b) biological clearance of the deposited radioaerosol from the lungs. After subtracting background radioactivity from the recorded counts, it is an easy matter to correct for physical decay of the radioisotope knowing its physical half-life. The whole lung clearance curve has been described as comprising numerous phases. A whole lung clearance curve, such as the stylized version shown in *Figure 3.10*, can as a first approximation be thought of as being made up of two phases. The fast phase is taken to represent clearance of radioaerosol from the ciliated airways exclusively via the mucociliary escalator in health and in lung disease via the escalator and by coughing. The slower phase has generally been taken to represent alveolar clearance (*see* Chapter 8). By convention the fraction of radioaerosol remaining in the lungs after 24 hours is taken to represent material which has been deposited on non-ciliated airways. Subtracting this estimate of so-called 'alveolar deposition' from the preceding readings on the whole lung clearance curve results in a plot of 'tracheobronchial clearance', i.e. clearance of radioaerosol which was initially deposited on the ciliated airways.

Studies in healthy man, using longer lived radioisotopes than ^{99m}Tc ($T_{1/2}$ = 6 h), indicate that there is little change in the amount of radioaerosol present in the lungs at 24 compared to 48 and 72 hours after inhalation of radioaerosol (Camner and Philipson, 1978). This supports the 'working concept' that the 24 hour retention value is a good estimate of alveolar or perhaps more correctly non-ciliated airways deposition. The same is not necessarily true in lung disease where mucociliary clearance might be depressed. In some patients with airways obstruction substantial clearance of radioaerosol takes place between 24 and 48 hours after inhalation. In such studies, alveolar deposition would be overestimated on the basis of '24 hour retention in the lungs' with the consequence of *overestimating* the efficiency of the mucociliary escalator (*see* Chapter 3).

Various types of aerosols are being used to study LMC, the most commonly used being Teflon, polystyrene, iron oxide, erythrocytes, albumin and resin (*see* Chapter 4). Several gamma-emitting radioisotopes have been used to label these particles (*see* Chapter 4) with ^{99m}Tc being the most popular one. It is important that the particles be tagged unleachably with the radioisotope of choice so that when these particles are washed in the lung secretions there is no appreciable loss of activity from them over the period of time for which lung mucociliary clearance is being measured.

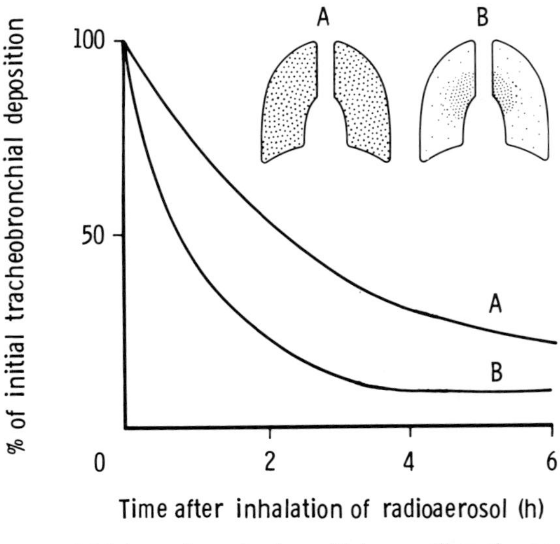

Figure 6.2 Schematic tracheobronchial mucociliary clearance curves arising from a predominantly proximal deposition of radioaerosol within the lungs (B) and from a diffuse radioaerosol deposition (A)

The rate of removal of deposited radioaerosols from the lungs is directly related to their initial site of deposition. In health and possibly in lung disease, particles deposited centrally in the lungs (B) will be cleared more quickly from the lungs by the mucociliary escalator than those particles which are deposited peripherally (A) because of the shorter transfer path and the progressive increase in mucous velocity from the peripheral airways to the trachea (*Figure 6.2*). The main factors that effect the deposition of inhaled aerosols in the lungs are (as discussed in Chapter 3): (a) the physical properties of the aerosol (b) the mode of inhalation of the aerosol and (c) the patency of the airways.

Measurement of initial deposition of radioaerosol

Because of the dependence of LMC rate on initial radioaerosol distribution within the lungs it is imperative, when using this technique, to ascertain the initial distribution of the radioaerosol within the lungs before any interpretation of the clearance curve is made. This can be achieved partly by mapping the initial distribution across the lungs using either a rectilinear gamma scanner or a gamma camera. With computing facilities a penetration index can be derived. Penetration index (as discussed in Chapter 5) is a ratio of peripheral to central deposition of radioaerosol within the lungs obtained from two regions of the lungs which have been arbitrarily defined. A high penetration index implies a high peripheral deposition and conversely a low penetration index suggests a predominantly central deposition. Alternatively, a measurement of lung retention after 24 hours indicates the fraction of the inhaled aerosol not deposited on the ciliated airways. A high 24 hour retention value (alveolar deposition) indicates a predominantly peripheral deposition of the radioaerosol within the lungs; a low alveolar deposition suggests a central deposition. In order to map the initial distribution of the radioaerosol a higher level of radioactivity is required compared to measurements of retention by means of scintillation counters alone. A high level of radioactivity (lung burden) results in a higher absorbed radiation dose to the volunteer subject.

Measurement of radioaerosol clearance

Monitoring clearance of radioactivity from the lungs has been achieved mainly by a widely collimated scintillation counter(s) or by gamma camera (Pavia *et al.*, 1980b). If a relatively high initial lung burden is acceptable ($>\sim 100\,\mu Ci$ of ^{99m}Tc) then the gamma camera, with an on-line computer for data processing, is the instrument of choice. Such a monitoring system in addition to yielding a measure of lung retention of tracer particles also has the added advantage of providing information regarding their distribution within the lungs. This permits estimates of clearance to be made from particular zones of the lungs, i.e. regional clearance. For medium doses of lung activity ($\sim 30\,\mu Ci$ of ^{99m}Tc) a single, suitably collimated scintillation counter located anteriorly and centrally to the chest will suffice for aerosol clearance measurements. However in order to minimize variations in geometrical counting efficiency, owing to the continuous re-distribution of the deposited radioaerosol within the lungs, it is better to use more than one detector. Investigators have used either two detectors, axially opposite to each other and located anteriorly and posteriorly to the chest or laterally, or a series of detectors arranged circumferentially around the subject's chest. For low doses of radioactivity ($\sim 1\,\mu Ci$ of ^{99m}Tc) a whole body scintillation counter within a well-shielded room can be used. The counter(s) used to measure lung retention must be collimated in such a manner that the field of view includes both lungs but excludes the stomach. The passage of radioactivity within the oesophagus on its way from the lungs to the stomach is rapid in relation to the time interval needed to make a measurement of lung retention at any given time.

The absorbed radiation dose to the lungs (*see* Chapter 4) from one lung mucociliary clearance investigation can be as low as ⅛–¼ of that received from a simple posterio-anterior chest x-ray to the equivalent of that received from one chest x-ray when using a gamma camera exclusively to monitor clearance and alveolar deposition. Informed, written consent should be obtained from the subjects prior to undertaking such studies. The approval of the Ethical Practices Committee of the institution where the studies are due to take place should be sought in all instances.

Only tracer amounts of an aerosol needs to be deposited in the lungs for a mucociliary clearance study. For example, less than 50 μg of polystyrene is required of which, in healthy subjects, perhaps 50 per cent will be removed from the lungs within 24 hours. In patients with airways obstruction because of reduced penetration to the periphery a greater proportion than that in health will be removed over the first 24 hours.

Analysis of radioaerosol clearance curves

The quantitative information derived from tracheobronchial clearance curves can take several forms. Some investigators favour the measurement of the time taken (T_{50}) to clear say 50 per cent of the tracer particles deposited on the tracheobronchial tree (*Figure 6.3a*). Others find it useful to measure the amount of tracheobronchial deposition retained at a given time, say at 2.0 and 6.0 hours after

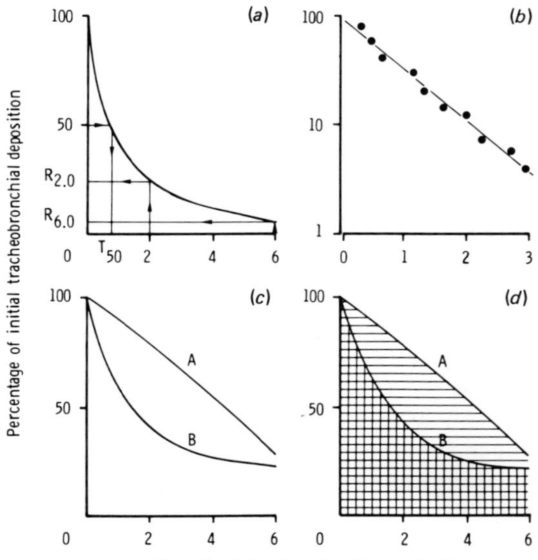

Figure 6.3 Ways of analysing the trachebronchial clearance curves: (a) time taken to clear 50 per cent (T_{50}) or amount retained (i.e. $R_{2.0}$) at a given time (i.e. 2 h) (b) fitting a regression line and measuring its slope (c) shape of curves (d) areas under curves

inhalation ($R_{2.0}$ and $R_{6.0}$) (*Figure 6.3a*); or conversely the amounts cleared over these time periods ($C_{2.0} = 100 - R_{2.0}$ and $C_{6.0} = 100 - R_{6.0}$). Often it is possible, usually over relatively short observation periods (say 0–1 or 0–3 hours), to express tracheobronchial clearance which has been plotted on semilogarithmic paper in terms of a linear regression (*Figure 6.3b*). The slope of this regression line which has been fitted to the observed data by the method of least squares is then used as an index of mucociliary clearance. Further, the shape of the clearance curves can also be a source of information regarding the efficiency of the mucociliary escalator. For example in *Figure 6.3c* the amount cleared by 6 hours is similar for curves A and B. However in the case of curve A clearance was at a slower rate. Another way of analysing the data would be to compare the areas under these two curves over the 6-hour observation period (*Figure 6.3d*).

Cough correction

Because of the long monitoring periods (1–8 hours) involved using some radioaerosol techniques, it is inevitable that some patients will cough even when instructed to avoid doing so. This is not necessarily a serious limitation of the technique. By careful monitoring of the patient throughout the tracheobronchial clearance observation period and by recording all coughs, collection of all sputum samples and counting of the radioactivity present in the sputum it is possible to estimate the proportion of tracheobronchial deposition that has been cleared by (a) productive coughing and (b) mucociliary transport (Agnew *et al.*, 1982). A correction for swallowed sputum has been proposed by Fazio and Lafortuna (1981) whereby any step-wise drops in radioaerosol clearance can be picked up with a gamma camera. Those drops which coincide with times of recorded coughing bouts are then added back to the clearance curves.

Generation and inhalation of radioaerosol

The administration of radioaerosols to humans should be carried out under carefully controlled conditions. The apparatus for the delivery of radioaerosols needs to be simple and reliable so as to enable the investigator to generate and deliver radioaerosols which will yield the desired deposition within the lungs. The spinning top generator (May, 1949) has been found to be by far the most versatile means of generating monodisperse aerosols. Such a generator is capable of producing aerosols of any desired mass median aerodynamic diameter (MMAD) in the range of 1–10 μm. Altering the size of the tracer particles is one means by which deposition within the lungs can be varied. The labelling of such tracer particles with various gamma-emitting radionuclides has already been described in Chapter 4.

The mode of inhalation of the tracer particles is the other parameter which can affect their deposition within the lungs. For the purposes of minimizing the variability in the measurement of mucociliary clearance between and within subjects it is important that the investigators should be able to control, in a strict manner, the mode of inhalation. *Figure 4.5* shows a system for generating and administering radioaerosols to humans for LMC studies.

Figure 6.4a is a schematic diagram of the lungs. The ciliated airways are depicted by generation 0 (trachea) to 16 (terminal bronchioles): the non-ciliated airways by generation 17 (respiratory bronchioles) to 23 (alveoli). The function of the mucociliary escalator is generally assessed in four ways. *Figure 6.4b* shows the tracer particles on the trachea/main bronchi and such a deposition is suited for yielding measurements of the mucous velocities in the trachea/main bronchi. *Figure 6.4c* shows the deposition of the radioaerosol to be predominantly central, perhaps over the first 4–6 airway generations. The clearance of such particles will result in an index of the efficiency of the mucociliary escalator from the proximal airways. *Figure 6.4d* shows a more uniform distribution of radioaerosol within the lungs. In order to label a representative number of the peripheral ciliated airways it is inevitable that a proportion of the tracer particles will deposit in essentially non-ciliated airways. The clearance curve derived from such a radioaerosol distribution will give an index of the efficacy of the whole escalator. *Figure 6.4e* shows a predominantly peripheral distribution of radioaerosol within the lungs and will result in an index of mucociliary clearance pertaining primarily to the peripheral ciliated airways (Lippmann *et al.*, 1981).

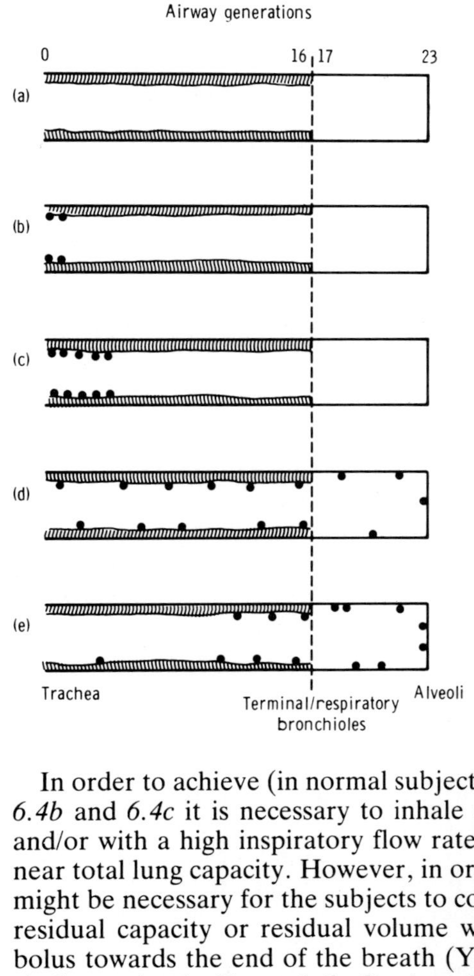

Figure 6.4 Schematic diagrams of different radioaerosol deposition patterns for assessing the efficiency of mucociliary transport

In order to achieve (in normal subjects) the deposition patterns shown in *Figures 6.4b* and *6.4c* it is necessary to inhale relatively large particles (MMAD >5 μm) and/or with a high inspiratory flow rate (>60 ℓ min^{-1}) with the breath taken from near total lung capacity. However, in order to achieve high inspiratory flow rates it might be necessary for the subjects to commence inspiration either from functional residual capacity or residual volume with the radioaerosol being delivered as a bolus towards the end of the breath (Yeates *et al.*, 1975) for a deposition pattern similar to that in *Figure 6.4b*. On the other hand, for the deposition pattern such as that shown in *Figure 6.4c* the radioaerosol might well be available throughout the inspiration manoeuvre.

For a more uniform pattern of deposition in the airways (*Figure 6.4d*) an aerosol with a MMAD in the range of 3–6 μm needs to be generated and inhaled from functional residual capacity with an inspiratory flow rate of less than 30 ℓ min^{-1}. The size of the breaths taken may be equivalent to those in tidal breathing (~500 ml). At the end of inspiration an adequate breath-holding pause will maximize the deposition of the aerosol at its furthest point of entry into the lungs. For example, for 5 μm MMAD aerosol with a settling velocity of 0.7 mm s^{-1}, a 3 seconds breath-holding pause will ensure deposition in all horizontal airways with diameters of 2 mm or less.

A predominantly distal deposition of radioaerosol (*Figure 6.4e*) is achieved with small particles, MMAD (in the range of 1–3 μm) and with a large breath taken at a low inspiratory flow rate (<20 ℓ min^{-1}) and followed with a relatively large breath-holding pause (e.g. 5–10 s).

Regional clearance

It is often useful when examining the effects of pharmacological agents, environmental pollutants or disease on lung mucociliary clearance to look for regional effects. One way of studying regional differences is to measure clearance from the lungs from a deposition pattern such as that shown in *Figure 6.4d* whilst at the same time observing (whenever possible) movement of radioaerosol boli through the trachea/main bronchi. The measurement of the trachea or main bronchi mucous velocities can then be taken as an index of large airways mucociliary function whilst clearance of particles from the lungs (tracheobronchial clearance) is taken to represent clearance from somewhat more distal ciliated airways. Furthermore in health at least, based on the assumption that the particles deposited nearer to the mouth will be the ones to be removed from the lungs first then one can interpret the initial part of the whole lung clearance curve as representing removal of radioaerosol deposited in the proximal airways and the latter part removal of radioaerosol from the distal ciliated airways (Sutton *et al.*, 1981).

Another way of looking at regional clearance will be to deposit particles as shown in *Figure 6.4c* on one day and a day or two later, when the residual radioactivity (if any) in the lungs has adequately decayed, monitor clearance from the peripheral airways using a deposition pattern similar to that shown in *Figure 6.4e*. Simultaneous observation of clearance from the proximal and peripheral regions is possible with the use of two gamma-emitting radionuclides for labelling the aerosols, e.g. ^{99m}Tc and ^{198}Au. The radionuclides should be chosen to have gamma rays with sufficiently differing energies for discriminatory counting purposes.

Yet another way of looking at regional clearance is by means of a gamma camera. It is important, after delineating the regions of interest, to be able to ascertain the proportion of the radioactivity signal that originates from particles deposited in non-ciliated airways for any one region. It is also important that account be taken of particles not only being cleared from the region of interest but of those entering the region (i.e. in transit) from neighbouring ones on their way to the trachea. One way of estimating alveolar deposition is to use a high lung burden and perform a 24 hour count using the gamma camera. Perhaps a simpler approximation will be to apportion the 24 hour whole lung deposition, obtained by scintillation counter(s), according to the signal obtained from the various regions of interest during a lung ventilation scan using radioactive ^{81m}Kr gas and a gamma camera. This allows regional clearance measurements to be made with the gamma camera over say a 6 hour observation period with moderate lung burdens (i.e. 20–30 μCi of ^{99m}Tc) (Agnew *et al.*, 1983).

If clearance from the proximal airways is to be studied (i.e. *Figure 6.4c*) then a gamma camera is necessary to monitor initial topographical distribution of the test radioaerosol. The use of scintillation counters only can never give reliable information about the initial deposition of the radioaerosol despite careful control of (a) the physical properties of the test aerosol and (b) their inhalation by the volunteer subjects.

Variability in the measurement of mucociliary transport

Variability in the measurement of a parameter can be expressed in terms of the coefficient of variation (COV = (mean/SD) × 100). A wide inter-subject variation is found regardless of the technique used to assess lung mucociliary function.

The variability, both between subjects (inter-) and within subjects (intra-), seen in the measurement of any one parameter of lung mucociliary clearance is the net result of the variation inherent within the experimental procedure and also that of the biological system. Yeates and co-workers (1982) have shown that the intra-subject variability of tracheobronchial mucociliary clearance can be apportioned equally between variances owing to (a) mucociliary transport and (b) deposition of radioaerosol within the airways. There are a few studies which suggest that the rate of mucociliary clearance might well depend to some extent on genetic factors. For example, tracheobronchial clearance tends to be more reproducible in monozygotic compared to dizygotic twins.

There is some evidence indicating that the inter-subject variability increases with the extension of lung pathology. From Lourenço *et al.* (1971 and 1972) data one can calculate the intersubject variability for the amount of tracheobronchial deposition cleared in 6 hours. Under identical experimental conditions this variability increases from a value of 17 per cent for healthy non-smokers to 27 per cent for asymptomatic smokers, to 40 per cent for patients with bronchiectasis. The intersubject variability for the measurement of mucous velocity in an anatomically well-defined airway, i.e. the trachea of healthy subjects, can vary from 57 per cent for the radioaerosol boli technique (Yeates *et al.*, 1981a) to approximately double that for the roentgenographic technique (Goodman *et al.*, 1978). This is somewhat surprising since the variability in the deposition of the tracer particles must be quite small.

It has also been suggested that an increase in the variation of otherwise similar tracheobronchial clearance curves about their mean following pharmacological intervention compared to placebo can be interpreted as an effect of the drug on the mucociliary escalator (Venizelos *et al.*, 1981).

Comment

The objective measurement of lung mucociliary transport provides an overall estimate of the effectiveness with which mucus is cleared from the lungs. It cannot, however, readily differentiate between clearance of mucus by cough and clearance via the mucociliary escalator. Furthermore, the measurement of mucociliary transport does not provide any evidence by which mechanism drugs and disease may effect the removal of mucus. A speeding or slowing of clearance by a drug may result from (a) an effect on ciliary beat frequency (b) changes in the biochemical and physical properties of lung secretions (c) changes in the volume of lung secretions (d) changes in the optimal thickness of the periciliary layer, or, from any combination of two or more of these factors. The techniques used for measuring LMC are however sensitive and are capable of demonstrating positive effects in trials with only a modest number of subjects, e.g. n = 10–12 (Pavia *et al.*, 1983a).

The remaining sections of this chapter contain a brief resume of the studies which have been carried out, primarily in man, in order to ascertain the effect of various physiological factors, environmental pollutants, disease and pharmacological agents on LMC.

Physiological factors

Age

In a study of the effects of long-term cigarette smoking in an aged healthy group of subjects we noted a weak inverse association between age and efficiency of lung mucociliary clearance (Pavia *et al.*, 1970). Two later studies have demonstrated, in a convincing way, the effects of age on mucociliary clearance. Using the roentgenographic technique, tracheal mucous velocities (TMV) in an elderly group of healthy subjects were reported to be on average 60 per cent less than those measured in a group younger by some 40 years on average (Goodman *et al.*, 1978). In another study (Puchelle *et al.*, 1979), the removal of radioaerosol from proximal airways was found to be decreased by some 35 per cent in an older group of healthy subjects (mean age: 53 years) compared to a younger group (age range: 21–37 years). However this association between age and clearance was found not to hold when 72 healthy, non-smoking adults (age range: 18–45 years) had their tracheal mucous velocities measured using the radioaerosol boli technique (Yeates *et al.*, 1981b).

Sex

One group commented in the early 1970s that all female subjects who had been studied by them up to that time appeared to have faster clearances than male subjects. These observations however have not been corroborated by studies from other laboratories which tend to show no differences in clearance rates between the two sexes.

Posture

In patients with excessive secretions posture appears to play a role in the rate of clearance of their lung secretions (*see* Chapter 7). For example, patients with cystic fibrosis show an enhanced TMV when they are placed in the 25 degrees head down position compared to when they are upright. Posture, on the other hand, does not appear to have an effect on mucociliary clearance in health. One group of investigators reported no difference in the TMV of normal subjects measured in the erect and supine positions. Yet another group of workers went so far as to measure TMV in healthy subjects while in the 25 degrees head down position and found no difference compared to those TMV's obtained with the subjects in the upright position. In our laboratory, tracheobronchial mucociliary clearance was measured in 10 healthy subjects whilst in one instance, they lay supine and were inactive during a 6 hour observation period and in another when they were in the upright position. No difference was detected as a result of this change in posture.

Circadian rhythm

In a controlled study, we measured clearance in 10 healthy volunteers with the 6 hour observations commencing either at midnight on one occasion or at mid-day on another. The subjects, whilst laying supine in both instances, abstained from food and drink and remained awake throughout both observation periods. No difference in clearance was noted between the two runs suggesting that there was no effect of circadian rhythm on LMC.

Sleep

We have investigated the effect of sleep on LMC in two separate studies. In the first, 10 healthy subjects were studied twice, on each occasion the observation period being 6 hours. Both observation periods commenced around midnight with the subject on one occasion remaining awake but supine and in the other being allowed to sleep under observation. A significant retardation in clearance was noted during the sleep period. Whether this was brought about by a slowing of ciliary beat frequency and/or a change in the amount and visco-elastic properties of lung secretions is not known. In the second study, a group of 10 asthmatics, known to have early morning wheeze and reduction in their peak expiratory flow rates, were studied. On one occasion the patients' LMC was measured during the day, whilst they were in the upright position and on another occasion whilst they were asleep at night. Once again a significant retardation in the clearance of lung secretions was noted whilst the patients were asleep. This retardation in clearance although of no clinical consequence in healthy subjects might well be of relevance in patients with airways obstruction. Such patients tend to have excess secretions which are removed at a slower rate than in health; any further slowing in clearance might account for nocturnal attacks of cough, sputum and wheeze. In all of the above studies the order of the two runs was randomly allocated thus removing any bias such as may arise from any learning effect.

Exercise

The effect of exercise such as brisk pedalling on a bicycle ergometer for half an hour compared with quiet breathing resulted in a significant enhancement of LMC in healthy, non-smoking subjects. In the same subjects, controlled eucapnic hyperventilation also resulted in increased mucociliary clearance, though to only 50 per cent of that achieved during exercise. This increase was attributed to either (a) a mechanical effect of increased lung movement or (b) an effect of the autonomic nervous system mediated via the parasympathetic pathway producing stimulation of airway glands and/or sympathetic stimulation of cilia owing to exercise-induced catecholamine release (Wolff *et al.*, 1977). However, we found that simple exercise such as performing routine duties within a hospital environment compared to relaxing (throughout the 6 hour observation period) did not have any effect on the rate of removal of lung secretions in healthy subjects.

Environmental pollutants

Inert particles

The effect on LMC of exposure to inert particulate matter has been investigated in healthy subjects (Camner *et al.*, 1973a). Twenty breaths of carbon particles (11 μm) at a concentration of 50 mg ℓ^{-1} resulted in an enhancement of LMC in proximal airways.

Sulphur dioxide and sulphuric acid

Sulphur dioxide is a major component of urban pollution. It has been shown to affect nasal mucociliary clearance in an adverse manner. Healthy, non-smoking subjects exposed to 5 ppm of SO_2 for 3 hours exhibited no effect on LMC except perhaps for a small transient speeding after 1 hour's exposure. Furthermore, exposure of healthy subjects whilst exercising to 5 ppm of SO_2 resulted in an increase of LMC over and above that achieved by exercise alone (Wolff *et al.*, 1975).

Submicronic sulphuric acid droplets are another ambient pollutant found in urban areas at atmospheric concentration of 10–20 μg m^{-3}. The effect on LMC of short-term inhalation by healthy humans of sulphuric acid (H_2SO_4) mist has been studied. The results indicate that H_2SO_4 mist inhalation, which primarily deposits in the peripheral airways, results in varying regional effects of clearance of lung secretions depending on dose. At high doses of H_2SO_4 (1000 μg m^{-3}) a pronounced transient slowing is observed to take place in the proximal and peripheral airways. On the other hand, at low doses (100 μg m^{-3}) there is a marked slowing of peripheral clearance but in this instance an acceleration of proximal clearance is noted (Lippmann *et al.*, 1981).

Urban factor

The effect of living in an urban environment on lung mucociliary clearance has been investigated. Fifteen pairs of non-smoking monozygotic twins in which one of each pair lived in the city of Stockholm and the other in a rural district had their LMC measured under identical conditions. On the average no difference was observed between the two pairs in the mucociliary clearance rates (Camner and Philipson, 1973).

Tobacco smoke

The histological changes noted in the respiratory tract of cigarette smokers coupled with the observed *in vitro* ciliotoxic effects of cigarette smoke has resulted in numerous studies seeking to establish the effects of cigarette smoke on lung mucociliary clearance in man.

Studies of the acute effects of cigarette smoking on LMC have yielded conflicting results together with the suggestion that the acute effects of smoking might well be different in various regions of the lung (Pavia *et al.*, 1980a). One study demonstrated that chain smoking for 2 hours had no adverse effect on TMV while another reported no effect on TMV as a result of smoking one cigarette. On the other hand, chain smoking for 2 hours in a third study showed an acceleration of tracheobronchial clearance from the proximal airways and a fourth study concluded that chain smoking 2–7 cigarettes gave rise to a transient increase of peripheral clearance. Our studies on 22 subjects who chain smoked 2–5 cigarettes showed a significant retardation in whole lung clearance, the effect being reversible soon after cessation of chain smoking (Pavia *et al.*, 1971). A further study claimed a speeding of peripheral clearance with an accompanied slowing of clearance from the proximal ciliated airways following chain smoking.

Studies of the long-term effects of tobacco smoking have shown on the whole an impairment of LMC (Camner, 1980). The effects on LMC of giving up smoking have been studied. It appears that in relatively asymptomatic smokers giving up the habit reverts their depressed LMC to normal values within three months of cessation of smoking. The LMC of bronchitic patients who gave up smoking one year or more prior to their assessment of LMC has been compared with those of a matched group of chronic bronchitics who were still smoking. No significant difference was found in the rates of removal of lung secretions between the two groups (Agnew *et al.*, 1982).

Fluorocarbon propellants and hair spray

Pressurized canisters used in the administration of drugs or for example the delivery of hair lacquer contain propellants (fluorocarbons), sometimes a surface active agent (surfactant) and the active ingredient. Although fluorocarbons are said to be inert there is some evidence suggesting that they might have an adverse effect on the lungs and the heart. The acute and long-term effects of the fluorocarbon propellants, Freon 11, 12 and 114, on LMC of healthy subjects and patients with airways obstruction have been investigated by several investigators. The unanimous evidence is that these agents do not alter clearance of lung secretions (Pavia *et al.*, 1982).

The effect of a commercially available hair spray (Aqua-Net Hair Spray®) on TMV was investigated in healthy subjects. The aerosol spray, directed towards the hair, was delivered for 20 seconds. At 1 hour post exposure TMV was found to be depressed by as much as 57 per cent of baseline values despite unaltered pulmonary function tests (Friedman *et al.*, 1977a).

Effects of disease on lung mucociliary clearance (Wanner, 1977)

Chronic bronchitis

Carefully controlled studies have shown that lung mucociliary clearance (LMC) is decreased in chronic bronchitis (Pavia *et al.*, 1983a). There appears to be no relationship between impairment of lung clearance and pulmonary function indices. Some studies have claimed that clearance of lung secretions in patients with chronic bronchitis appears to be normal or even faster than that measured in healthy subjects. However, cough plays a major role in the clearance of lung secretions and can compensate for an otherwise impaired mucociliary clearance mechanism (*see* Chapter 7). Furthermore, because of the associated airways obstruction, inhaled radioaerosol tends to deposit more proximally in patients with chronic bronchitis than in healthy subjects. This central deposition, if not taken into account, gives rise to a shorter transfer path along the ciliated airways for the radioaerosol and thus may give rise to an apparent normal or even faster clearance in such patients when compared with healthy subjects.

Asthma

From autopsies carried out on asthmatics there is evidence of extensive sloughing of ciliated cells from the bronchial epithelium and often associated with mucus plugging. Such histological changes might well give rise to or result from an impaired mucociliary clearance in patients with asthma.

Marked reductions have been noted in the tracheal mucous velocities (TMV) of symptomatic asthmatics and asymptomatic, non-smoking subjects with ragweed hypersensitivity (Wanner, 1979). Studies carried out on twenty five patients with mild asthma (most on bronchodilator treatment only and a few patients on inhaled corticosteroids) demonstrated a reduced tracheobronchial mucociliary clearance compared to a healthy group matched for physical characteristics and smoking habits (Bateman *et al.*, 1983). We have also measured LMC in eight asthmatics who were in remission at the time. The pulmonary function indices of these patients were within normal limits and the patients required no therapy whatsoever for a period of 1–6 months prior to entering the study. Their lung mucociliary clearance was however found to be depressed compared to a matched control group of healthy subjects. In another study we measured LMC in a group of asthmatics who were admitted in our hospital, because of an acute exacerbation of their asthma. The measurement was carried out within 1–5 days of their admission. Their LMC was also measured at 12–16 days and at 2–4 months after admission to hospital. Our data suggested that the reduced LMC observed in these patients following their admission to hospital showed no sign of improvement 2–4 months later.

Bronchiectasis

In a carefully conducted study on bronchiectatic patients it was observed that less inhaled radioaerosol was deposited in areas with localized saccular bronchietasis. Abnormal mucociliary clearances were observed in all patients; the degree of abnormality being similar to that seen in patients with chronic bronchitis without bronchiectasis (Lourenço *et al.*, 1972).

There is some limited evidence suggesting that the abnormal mucociliary clearances seen in Polynesian bronchiectatics might be attributable to abnormalities in the ultrastructure of cilia leading to abnormal ciliary beating (Waite *et al.*, 1983).

Influenza

Influenza A virus can destroy ciliated cells in the respiratory tract. There is evidence from two laboratories that patients infected with this virus and studied within one week after the onset of symptoms had a definite retardation in clearance which was, however, reversible, with complete recovery approximately 3 months later (Camner *et al.*, 1973b).

Pneumonia

Infection with Mycoplasma pneumoniae also damages the ciliated tracheal epithelium. In patients with serologically verified infection by *M. pneumoniae*, a significant reduction in clearance was noted 10–15 days after the onset of disease, with a tendency to impairment in clearance up to one year later (Camner, 1980).

Patients with immunoglobulin deficiency

Patients with immunoglobulin deficiency, as measured in the serum, had the mucociliary clearance of their proximal airways measured. Four younger patients with symptoms of severe airway infections showed a markedly slow clearance. Older patients with less severe immunoglobulin deficiency and with a history of less severe airway infections were found to have clearances within the normal range. There was some evidence, following adequate medical treatment, that this impairment of clearance was not necessarily irreversible (Mossberg *et al.*, 1982).

Tuberculosis

There is a report (Wagner *et al.*, 1965) of clearance of particles from the tracheobronchial tree of patients with chronic pulmonary tuberculosis in various stages of activity at the time of measurement. It appears that mucociliary clearance was present, but areas were identified of alleged decreased ciliary activity resulting in local accumulation of the tracer particles.

Bronchogenic carcinoma

An early report on two patients with bronchogenic carcinoma suggested a normal tracheal and lung clearance of secretions. More recently a study on 37 patients with lung cancer claimed that mucociliary clearance from the proximal airways was reduced or absent (Matthys *et al.*, 1983).

Emphysema

In patients with emphysema, as a result of alpha$_1$-antitrypsin deficiency, but without any history of chronic bronchitis the mucociliary clearance of their proximal airways was found to be within the normal range.

Asbestosis

Asbestosis is a restrictive type of lung disease acquired following exposure to asbestos. Patients who had been certified as having the disease on the basis of clinical, radiological and pulmonary function data had no impairment of LMC.

Sjögren's syndrome

Sjögren's syndrome is characterized by deficient secretion of the lachrymal, salivary and other glands which gives rise to keratoconjunctivitis sicca, dry tongue and hoarse voice. This syndrome manifests itself mainly in postmenopausal woman and it is often associated with rheumatoid arthritis. We measured the LMC of eight female patients with this syndrome who presented with chest complaints in order to ascertain whether drying of secretions did extend into the lungs. Had this been the case a reduced clearance should have been observed. In the event no abnormality of LMC was found (Fairfax *et al.*, 1981). The pulmonary function tests of these patients indicated on average a mild restrictive defect with accompanying small airways obstruction.

Rheumatoid disease

Rheumatoid disease is a multisystem disorder which may affect the lung in several ways. Because of the increased incidence of respiratory infections and frequency of other forms of respiratory involvement we investigated the tracheobronchial mucociliary clearance in eleven patients with rheumatoid disease (Sutton *et al.*, 1982). All the patients at the time of the study were taking nonsteroidal anti-inflammatory drugs, but none were taking aspirin. The mucociliary clearance of these patients was found to be unaltered compared to that of a group of matched control subjects.

Cystic fibrosis

Lung mucociliary clearance in patients with cystic fibrosis (CF) as measured by the radioaerosol technique has on the whole shown a functioning mucociliary mechanism (Kollberg *et al.*, 1978). Direct comparison with healthy, matched groups of young children was not possible because of ethical considerations.

Tracheal mucous velocities in patients with CF have yielded rates which varied from zero to normal (Yeates *et al.*, 1976). Patients with poor oxygen tension were the ones who tended to have abnormal TMV. Nasal mucociliary clearance has been shown to be normal in CF children. Furthermore, the ultra-structure of the cilia has been reported to be normal also.

Primary ciliary dyskinesia syndrome

The primary ciliary dyskinesia syndrome—previously known as the 'immotile-cilia syndrome' (Sleigh, 1981)—is characterized by defects in the ultrastructure of cilia, male infertility and chronic infections of the lower and upper respiratory tract. This syndrome includes Kartagener's syndrome but patients lack the features of situs inversus. The ultrastructural abnormalities seen in the cilia include missing radial spokes, dynein arms and central tubules. These ultrastructural abnormalities give rise to an inefficient ciliary beat resulting in a grossly depressed LMC.

Young's syndrome

Obstructive azoospermia is a form of male infertility with absence of spermatozoa in the ejaculate. Young (1970) was the first to report a significant number of lung defects, including bronchitis and bronchiectasis, in men with obstructive azoospermia and he called this connection the Berry–Perkins–Young syndrome.

No abnormalities have been reported in the ultrastructure of cilia from the epididymis of patients with Young's syndrome. Furthermore, normal nasal ciliary beat frequency has been reported in such patients. However, the measurement of LMC in our laboratory of twenty patients with this syndrome gave clear cut evidence of a depressed clearance of lung secretions (Pavia *et al.*, 1981). It appears that this abnormality in the transportation of secretions might well be related to the properties of the secretions rather than to the cilia.

Effects of pharmacological agents on lung mucociliary clearance (Sackner, 1978)

Mucolytics and expectorants

Difficulty in expectoration is a frequent chest complaint and there is a need for effective therapeutic agents to promote bronchial clearance (Richardson and Phipps, 1978). The efficacy of mucolytic and expectorant drugs in man has hitherto been evaluated (a) subjectively, i.e. clinically or by medical questionnaire (b) by assessing the possible effects on pulmonary function indices and (c) by changes in the amount, chemical and visco-elastic properties of sputum. The measurement of lung mucociliary clearance (LMC) offers the only direct, objective, *in vivo* means of evaluating such drugs.

Bromhexine is claimed to liquefy mucus by breaking the muco-polysaccharide chains present in the mucus so facilitating its removal, by ciliary action, from the lungs. In our laboratory we administered bromhexine (16 mg tds) for 2 weeks to patients with obstructive bronchitis. A statistically significant enhancement of mucociliary clearance was observed despite the fact that the tracer radioaerosol was deposited significantly more distally after treatment. These observations are consistent with those reported from two other laboratories (Clarke *et al.*, 1980). Recently, however, the action of a single dose of intravenous bromhexine was studied in patients with chronic daily cough. This study was unable to demonstrate any acute effect of this drug, under these particular experimental conditions, on the efficiency of voluntary coughing (Camner, 1981).

Ambroxol is the eighth metabolite of bromhexine and it is claimed to have mucolytic properties. Fifteen patients, some with chronic obstructive bronchitis and others with obstructive emphysema, were given this drug at a dose of 30 mg tds for 4 days. A stimulatory effect of this drug on lung mucociliary clearance was noted in only one out of five lung regions of interest. It is worth noting that this drug caused an improvement of radioaerosol penetration within the lungs in obstructive emphysematous patients (Weiss *et al.*, 1981).

Guaiphenesin (glyceryl guaiacolate) has been used for many years as an expectorant and has been found in sputum after its oral administration to subjects. A single oral dose of 600 mg of this drug on clearance of lung secretions gave inconclusive results when studied on two separate occasions in our laboratories (Pavia *et al.*, 1983b). Another group of investigators reported that a single dose of 400 mg of guaiphenesin did not alter LMC in a group of 19 chronic bronchitics.

Compounds with free sulphydryl groups such as S-carboxymethylcysteine and acetylcysteine are believed to be able to split the disulphide bonds of the long glyco-proteins of mucus and thereby reduce its viscosity. Further, such compounds may also reduce the 'compactness' of the fibrillar structure of the mucus by replacing fucomucins by sialomucins. We studied the effect on lung clearance of 1 g qds of S-carboxymethylcysteine administered orally for 7 days in 16 patients with chronic bronchitis. The lack of an effect in our study is in agreement with that of another study which examined the action of a single dose (2 g) of this drug on TMV. More recently S-carboxymethylcysteine was shown to have no effect on either mucus properties or mucociliary transport in dogs (Pavia *et al.*, 1983b).

Lung mucociliary clearance after water aerosol administration has been shown not to differ significantly from control until some 2 hours later when there was a small but nevertheless significant acceleration.

Saline has been shown to reduce the viscosity of sputum *in vitro*, although no demonstrable advantage over a water mist has been reported. The administration of hypotonic saline (0.45 per cent) aerosol resulted in a significant enhancement of TMV in only about 30 per cent of healthy subjects studied and had no effect in patients with cystic fibrosis. We administered hypertonic saline (7.1 per cent) aerosol for 10 minutes, from an ultrasonic nebulizer to 11 chronic bronchitic patients and compared lung clearances after treatment with those in a control run. It was estimated that only a fraction of one millilitre of hypertonic saline was likely to have been deposited within the lungs. We observed that the whole lung clearance rate during the first 50 minutes was twice as fast after hypertonic saline aerosol as in the control run. Furthermore, the weight of sputum produced was also higher in the saline run and, probably, was the reason for the observed enhancement of mucus clearance as opposed to an improvement in mucociliary clearance *per se* (Pavia *et al.*, 1983b).

Aerosolized sodium 2-mercapto-ethane sulphonate administered from an ultrasonic nebulizer to 11 patients with chronic bronchitis resulted in a similar clearance curve to that following the administration of hypertonic saline but failed to reach statistical significance compared with the control baseline runs (Pavia *et al.*, 1983b).

Beta-agonists

Adrenergic drugs in addition to being effective bronchodilators might have a further role to play in the control of mucus transport in the airways in obstructive lung disease. Such drugs have attracted the interest of many investigators and their effects on ciliary beat frequency, mucus production and transport have been widely reported (Wanner, 1981).

In vitro studies on ciliated epithelium taken from animals and man have on the whole shown a stimulatory effect of beta adrenergic drugs on ciliary beat frequency and mucus production.

The subcutaneous administration of a $beta_2$ adrenergic drug, terbutaline, has given somewhat conflicting interpretations of its stimulatory effect on the clearance of tracheobronchial secretions. In one study, a marked increase in clearance was noted in healthy subjects and to a lesser extent in patients with bronchial asthma. Another investigator noted that the administration of this drug to chronic bronchitics had on average no effect on lung clearance; however there was some evidence suggesting that improvement in clearance was associated with those patients with less severe ventilatory impairment. From these studies the conclusion might be drawn that this drug promotes clearance in patients with less severely obstructed lungs. However, in other studies an enhancement of TMV was noted in patients with obstructive lung disease and cystic fibrosis patients but not in normal subjects.

The oral administration of terbutaline has been shown not to improve clearance of lung secretions in healthy subjects and in patients with chronic bronchitis. On the other hand, 20 mg of orciprenaline given to healthy subjects resulted in enhancement of TMV but had no overall effect on clearance of secretions from the lungs as a whole. This finding points to a regional effect of lung mucociliary clearance from the administration of this drug.

The effects on lung mucociliary clearance following the administration of adrenergic drugs in aerosol form is also somewhat conflicting. Epinephrine and isoprenaline administered to healthy subjects from an intermittent positive pressure breathing apparatus have shown a stimulatory effect on lung mucociliary clearance. Further, the administration of these drugs to asthmatics has resulted in an increase of their depressed clearances to levels approaching those of healthy subjects. Two to five puffs (200 μg per puff) of fenoterol administered from pressurized canisters has resulted in a two-fold increase of TMV in healthy subjects in one study; in another it had only a modest increase in normal subjects and no effect in chronic bronchitics. Conversely, a third study carried out with this drug in patients with airways obstruction has indicated that the stimulatory effect of this drug on LMC was most marked in patients with slow clearances. We have administered terbutaline from pressurized canisters at a dose of 500 μg tds for 7 days to patients with reversible airways obstruction and found that LMC was unaltered compared to control. Subsequently, a single dose of 1 mg given to asthmatics was found once again not to alter clearance. However when we doubled the dose once again (i.e. to 2 mg) we observed a significant stimulatory effect on LMC in asthmatics. These studies point to the stimulatory effect of beta adrenergic drugs on LMC being dose dependent. Salbutamol administered from pressurized canisters at a dose of 400–500 μg has been shown in two independent studies to enhance proximal tracheobronchial mucociliary clearance.

Beta antagonists (blockers)

Since the administration of beta adrenergic drugs results in an enhanced lung mucociliary clearance it is not unreasonable to expect the converse with beta antagonists (blockers). In animals the cilioexcitory effect of beta agonists has been shown to be blocked by low concentrations of propranolol (10^{-7} M). However at low concentrations propranolol in the absence of beta agonists had no effect on ciliary activity. At high concentrations (10^{-4} M) propranolol resulted in a decrease of ciliary beat frequency; this effect was attributed to the local anaesthetic properties of this drug. Intravenous administration of 3–5 mg of propranolol to dogs did not alter TMV at 15 minutes following its administration. We have investigated the acute effects of a selective (100 mg atenolol) and non-selective (160 mg propranolol) beta blocking agent on clearance of lung secretions in 12 healthy subjects. The drugs were administered 2 hours prior to the 6 hours observation periods and despite effective beta blockade with both drugs clearance was similar to that following a placebo administration (Pavia *et al.*, 1983b). Further studies are needed to ascertain the effect of beta blocking agents on lung clearance in (a) patients with airways obstruction and (b) after their long-term use by patients with cardiovascular complaints.

Methylxanthines

Theophyllines are often used for the relief of bronchospasm in patients with reversible airways obstruction. If the enhancement of mucociliary clearance following the administration of beta agonists is due to increased cyclic AMP/GMP ratio then it is not unreasonable to expect theophyllines to have a similar action. We found that the oral administration of 450 mg of aminophylline bd for 7 days in patients with airways obstruction resulted in a significant enhancement of LMC compared to the placebo run (Sutton *et al.*, 1981). In another study, aminophylline was infused at a dose of 6 mg kg^{-1} body weight in a group comprising normal and infertile males. There was a suggestion from this study that in some subjects there was enhancement of clearance of lung secretions attributable to the drug (Matthys and Kohler, 1980). The effect of aminophylline from these two human studies suggests stimulation of mucous transport in the central airways; this evidence supports earlier observations in animals. Furthermore, *in vitro* studies have shown a modest (10 per cent) increase in ciliary beat frequency as a result of aminophylline.

Corticosteroids

The precise pharmacological action of corticosteroids in asthma is not well defined. It is possible that one of the mechanisms might be the enhancement of mucociliary clearance thereby reducing the tendency to mucus plugging in small airways (Pavia *et al.*, 1983b).

We have studied the effect of a four weeks course of oral corticosteroids (prednisolone) on tracheobronchial clearance. Patients with stable asthma were studied on three occasions and their data compared with those from a healthy group with a similar age. The first assessment was carried out after a two weeks baseline period, the second after two weeks treatment with 15 mg daily of prednisolone and the third after a further two weeks at 30 mg daily. Daily (morning and night) peak expiratory flow rates were increased in the asthmatics after treatment. Alveolar deposition was significantly less in the asthmatic baseline run compared to the control group but tended to increase after treatment, reflecting the increase in airway patency. Baseline mucociliary clearance was found to be depressed in the asthmatic group, as expected, compared to the control group and despite modest but non-significant improvements after treatment did not attain control group levels. A marked decrease in frequency of coughing and expectoration was noted during the clearance measurements in the asthmatics after treatment. Our data were interpreted as giving indirect evidence of improvement in mucociliary function following treatment with corticosteroids for the following two reasons. In the baseline assessment, clearance in the asthmatics was aided significantly by productive coughing. Secondly, although after treatment the radioaerosol was deposited more distally and therefore had, on average, a longer way to travel to the trachea, clearance via the mucociliary escalator apparently was at the same rate as in the baseline run.

In vitro studies have shown modest increases in ciliary beat frequency following the topical application of prednisolone to isolated preparations of rat bronchi. Beclomethasone dipropionate is an insoluble corticosteroid used in aerosol form for the management of patients with asthma. The effect of 200 μg of this drug on TMV in conscious sheep was investigated and found not to alter it during a 1 hour observation period following its administration.

Cholinergics

Both *in vivo* and *in vitro* experiments on animals have shown a stimulatory effect of cholinergic compounds on mucociliary transport. This increase has been attributed to vagal stimulation. Using the radioaerosol technique, it has been shown that subcutaneous administration of bethanecol (dose range: 5.0–7.5 mg) to healthy, non-smoking subjects resulted in a significant enhancement of mucociliary clearance from the proximal airways (Camner *et al.*, 1974). This increase in transport may have resulted from altered or increased secretions since (a) a significant correlation was seen between salivary secretion by this drug and increases in bronchial clearance and (b) airway tone and secretion (at least from the submucosal glands) is thought to be under cholinergic control. However increase in transport can be brought about by an increase in ciliary beat frequency. Certainly cholinergic drugs such as acetylcholine and pilocarpine have been shown to increase ciliary beat frequency *in vitro*.

Anticholinergics

The bronchodilator properties of anticholinergic drugs are well known. Although several studies in asthmatic patients and chronic bronchitics have demonstrated their therapeutic value, their widespread use has not been advocated mainly because of the possibility of mucus retention in the lungs. Anticholinergic drugs have been shown to reduce sputum production and ciliary beat frequency. Both these effects could potentially inhibit the removal of lung secretions in patients with an already inefficient clearance of copious secretions and potentially cause plugging. There is one school of thought however that believes the undesirable effects to be small (Richardson and Phipps, 1978).

In our laboratory we have demonstrated that the oral administration of hyoscine (mean dose: 8 μg/kg body weight) resulted in a statistically significant retardation of lung mucociliary clearance (Pavia *et al.*, 1983b). However, the administration of methylscopolamine (0.5 mg) intramuscularly has been shown, by another group, not to alter clearance. Atropine given orally and intravenously has been shown to reduce clearance of lung secretions in man. The administration of atropine to dogs has shown conflicting results: in one study tracheal mucous transport rates were reported to have increased and in another reduced. However, a couple of studies indicate that tracheal mucus from atropinized dogs when placed on mucus-depleted frog palates was transported at normal rates. It could well be that the main effect of atropine on the mucociliary escalator is not on the physical properties of mucus. Alternative explanations are that atropine may alter (a) the rate of mucus production, (b) the periciliary fluid or (c) ciliary mechanism.

Ipratropium bromide is a synthetic anticholinergic drug which was specifically developed to relieve bronchospasm. It is claimed not to depress lung mucociliary clearance. The drug is administered topically in aerosol form. Five studies performed in three independent laboratories investigated this claim (Pavia *et al.*, 1983b). The studies were of short-term duration (up to one week), with ipratropium bromide being delivered from a jet nebulizer or pressurized inhaler to patients with chronic bronchitis or asthma and healthy subjects. The doses studied were up to five times the normal therapeutic dose (i.e. up to 5 × 0.04 mg). Three of these studies demonstrated no effect of this drug on lung mucociliary clearance whereas the remaining two gave direct or indirect evidence of a stimulatory effect on clearance. It is worth noting that relatively higher doses (0.4–0.6 mg) given to animals resulted in an increased volume of lung secretions.

Antibiotics

The increased incidence of serous otitis media observed after the introduction of penicillin for the treatment of acute otitis media led to the suspicion that penicillin might have a possible effect on the mucociliary function of the Eustachian tube.

No studies have been reported of the effects of antibiotics on lung mucociliary clearance. Epithelia of the nasal cavity, lungs and Eustachian tube are morphologically of the same type. One group studied the effect of penicillin treatment on nasal mucociliary clearance in 21 healthy subjects. Each volunteer was investigated on nine occasions: (a) three times before the administration of penicillin (b) on three consecutive days during penicillin treatment (via the mouth, 3 tablets bd, each of 10^6 IU of phenoxymethylpenicillin for 3 days) and (c) three times after treatment. No change in nasal clearance was noted as a result of the antibiotic treatment (Vintner and Elbrond, 1978).

Sodium cromoglycate

Animal experiments suggest that the release of chemical mediators may have a role to play in mucociliary dysfunction in allergic asthma.

Sodium cromoglycate is used prophylactically in asthma. Asymptomatic asthmatics with ragweed hypersensitivity demonstrated a fall in TMV to 72 per cent of baseline after challenge with ragweed. The TMV was further depressed to a level of 47 per cent that of baseline values at 1 hour after challenge. Pre-treatment with 20 mg of sodium cromoglycate however resulted in a 32 per cent increase in TMV compared to baseline with a further increase to 62 per cent after bronchial provocation with ragweed. Healthy subjects, however, treated with 20 mg of sodium cromoglycate show no alteration in their baseline TMV (Wanner, 1979).

Slow reacting substance of anaphylaxis (SRS-A) antagonist (FPL 55712)

The effect of a SRS-A antagonist (FPL 55712) on TMV has been studied in asymptomatic non-smokers with ragweed asthma. It was found that doses of ragweed resulting in a 35 per cent decrease in specific airway resistance (SG_{aw}) led to an immediate fall of TMV to 74 per cent of baseline value, returning to baseline within 2 hours. However when the patients were pre-treated with 0.5 and 1.0 per cent FPL-55712 and then challenged until the SG_{aw} fell by more than 35 per cent, this was accompanied by increases in TMV to 138 and 126 per cent respectively with return to baseline within 2 hours. The inhalation of the SRS-A antagonist following ragweed challenge resulted in preventing a fall in TMV only. These studies suggest that SRS-A liberated during airway anaphylaxis impairs mucous transport and the antigen-induced increase in TMV after pretreatment may reflect a stimulatory effect of other chemical mediators of anaphylaxis (Ahmed *et al.*, 1981). Histamine and acetylcholine administered to animals have been shown to result in an enhancement of TMV.

Aspirin

Aspirin (acetylsalicylic acid) is used for its analgesic, antipyretic and anti-inflammatory properties; it is also claimed to inhibit prostaglandin synthesis. *In vitro* studies have shown that exogenous prostaglandins increase bronchial fluid secretion whereas sodium salicylate decreases the output of serous and mucous cells of human bronchial epithelium. It is therefore possible that the administration of aspirin may give rise to an altered LMC.

Lung mucociliary clearance following the administration of aspirin has recently been tested in twelve healthy subjects. A single dose of 16 mg per kg body weight, representing the upper range of a single dose of this drug for say antipyretic purposes, was found to result in a small but nevertheless significant retardation of LMC (Gerrity *et al.*, 1983). The effect of aspirin on LMC in patients, where high doses are involved, has yet to be determined.

Oxygen therapy

A common complaint of normal human subjects breathing oxygen for prolonged periods is substernal distress; it can occur within a few hours after commencement of oxygen breathing but usually manifests itself between the 12–16th hour. The suggestion has been made that this may be the onset of acute tracheobronchitis with loss of ciliated epithelium and retention of secretions.

The possibility of this alleged pulmonary oxygen toxicity on lung mucociliary clearance has been studied by several investigators. In one study, carried out on healthy subjects, oxygen (90–95 per cent) was breathed for 6 hours. Endoscopic examination at the end of that time revealed evidence of tracheitis in all the subjects. The interesting observation made in this study was that of a depressed TMV as early as 3 hours after commencing (Sackner *et al.*, 1975). The administration of terbutaline restored depressed TMV values to control levels. In another study, healthy non-smokers inhaled either humified (95 per cent) air or oxygen (concentration: 96–100 per cent) via a facemask at 27°C for 4.5 hours and the mucous clearance measured was compared to that obtained from comparable subjects breathing air at 24 per cent relative humidity and at 25°C. Mucous clearance was observed to be reduced as a result of breathing either humified air or oxygen.

Animal experiments have shown that 100 per cent oxygen results in a marked impairment of tracheal mucous flow in cats. The adverse oxygen effects were however prevented and reversed by the administration of epinephrine compounds and adenosinetriphosphate. The observations of an inhibitory effect of oxygen on mucous clearance are not unchallenged. Administering oxygen at 100 per cent and 13 per cent to anaesthetized dogs for 10 minutes resulted in no alteration of TMV. Interestingly, the administration of 7.5 per cent of CO_2 resulted in a 31 per cent fall in TMV from baseline values.

Ethyl alcohol

The effect of acute alcohol ingestion (0.5 g/kg body weight) on LMC was investigated in a group of subjects. The average levels of alcohol at 1 hour ($68 \pm 8\,mg\,dl^{-1}$) were similar to those achieved during social drinking. Although bronchial clearance, over a 4.5 hour observation period, did not on average differ from that of the placebo run the results were interpreted by the investigator as demonstrating an effect on clearance although the direction and magnitude of the changes differed amongst individuals (Venizelos *et al.*, 1981).

Anaesthesia

Postoperative chest complications may arise from damage to the ciliated epithelium during anaesthesia causing impaired clearance and retention of secretions. As previously discussed atropine-like drugs, used in premedication, result in reduced lung mucociliary clearance; further during sleep *per se* clearance is also reduced.

The effect of analgesics, anaesthetics, humidification of anaesthetic gases and the insertion of intratracheal tubes might also delay clearance. The respiratory epithelium has been shown to be easily injured by aspiration and instrumentation.

Exposure of the respiratory mucosa to the dry gases delivered by anaesthetic systems has been shown to result in severe changes with hyperaemia, excess mucus and diminished ciliary action. However, when patients were administered gases which were properly humidified, bypass of the nasal passages by an endotracheal tube had no adverse effect on the mucosa. In the region of the inflated cuff of endotracheal tubes ciliary activity is seen to be depressed or stopped. In a similar study on 14 non-smoking females with no history of chest disease undergoing gynaecologic surgery it was observed that their mucociliary transport deteriorated with premedication, intubation, and humidification as used in routine surgical procedures (Lichtiger *et al.*, 1975).

The degree of mobilization may also have a role to play in the rate of removal of lung secretions. We have already discussed the effect of exercise on lung mucociliary clearance. A marked difference has been observed in the postoperative clearance of insufflated tantalum—a radio-opaque powder—between a group of patients undergoing orthopaedic procedures, who demonstrated a rapid clearance, and a group of patients undergoing major vascular surgery who had a delayed clearance. In the latter group segmental and lobar atelectasis developed subsequently in the regions where tantalum was unduly retained. It is worth noting that for the orthopaedic patients the duration of anaesthesia was shorter and postoperative status better with regard to depth of breathing, ability to cough and degree of immobilization (Gamsu *et al.*, 1976).

Similar mucous transport rates have been reported in the exposed trachea of dogs regardless of whether the animals were sacrificed with pentobarbital or with a blow to the head. In intact sheep 30 mg of pentobarbital or thiomylal per kg body weight was found to reduce TMV by some 35 per cent below pre-anaesthesia baseline values. Halothane has also been shown to reduce mucous flow in the trachea of dogs; this impairment was however reversible.

One report has shown that following the application of 2 per cent tetracaine there was an immediate cessation of nasal mucociliary function in human subjects which was nevertheless reversible some 45 minutes later. On the other hand, lignocaine (4 per cent) has been shown by two investigators not to adversely affect nasal mucociliary function in healthy subjects and a third report claimed that when this anaesthetic was instilled at a concentration of 2 per cent into the trachea of human subjects it had no adverse effects. Lignocaine administered *in vivo* in doses that produce local anaesthesia did not affect ciliary beat frequency when it was subsequently measured using an *in vitro* technique. Cilioinhibition has been shown to result in *in vitro* experiments but at concentrations three orders of magnitude greater than the usual therapeutic serum concentrations.

References

AHMED, T., GREENBLATT, D.W., BIRCH, S., MARCHETTE, B. and WANNER, A. (1981). Abnormal mucociliary transport in allergic patients with antigen-induced bronchospasm: role of slow reacting substance of anaphylaxis. *Am. Rev. Respir. Dis.*, **124**, 110–114

AGNEW, J.E., BATEMAN, J.R.M., PAVIA, D. and CLARKE, S.W. (1983). Mucus clearance in central and peripheral airways in asthma assessed from radionuclide images. In *Nuclear medicine and biology advances*. Edited by Raynaud, C. Oxford; Pergamon Press, pp. 2533–2536

AGNEW, J.E., LITTLE, F., PAVIA, D. and CLARKE, S.W. (1982). Mucus clearance from the airways in chronic bronchitis—smokers and ex-smokers. *Bull. Europ. Physiopath. Resp.*, **18**, 473–484

ALBERT, R.E. and ARNETT, L.C. (1955). Clearance of radioactivity dust from the lung. *Arch. Environm. Hlth.*, **12**, 99–106

BATEMAN, J.R.M., PAVIA, D., SHEAHAN, N.F., AGNEW, J.E. and CLARKE, S.W. (1983). Impaired tracheobronchial clearance in patients with mild stable asthma. *Thorax*, **38**, 463–467

CAMNER, P. (1980). Clearance of particles from the human tracheobronchial tree. *Clin. Sci.*, **59**, 79–84

CAMNER, P. (1981). Studies on the removal of inhaled particles from the lungs by voluntary coughing. *Chest*, **80** (Suppl), 824–827

CAMNER, P. and PHILIPSON, K. (1973). Urban factor and tracheobronchial clearance. *Arch. Environm. Hlth.*, **27**, 81–84

CAMNER, P. and PHILIPSON, K. (1978). Human alveolar deposition of 4 μm Teflon particles. *Arch. Environm. Hlth.*, **36**, 181–185

CAMNER, P., HELLSTROM, P-A. and PHILIPSON, K. (1973a). Carbon dust and mucociliary transport. *Arch. Environm. Hlth.*, **26**, 294–296

CAMNER, P., JARSTRAND, C. and PHILIPSON, K. (1973b). Tracheobronchial clearance in patients with influenza. *Am. Rev. Respir. Dis.*, **108**, 131–135

CAMNER, P., STRANDBERG, K. and PHILIPSON, K (1974). Increased mucociliary transport by cholinergic stimulation. *Arch. Environm. Hlth.*, **29**, 220–224

CHEN, T.M. and DULFANO, M.J. (1978). Mucus viscoelasticity and mucociliary transport rate. *J. Lab. Clin. Med.*, **91**, 423–431

CHOPRA, S.K., TAPLIN, G.V., ELAM, D., CARSON, S.W. and GOLDE, D. (1979). Measurement of tracheal mucociliary transport velocity in humans—smokers versus non-smokers (preliminary findings). *Am. Rev. Respir. Dis.*, **119** (Suppl.), 205

CLARKE, S.W., THOMSON, M.L. and PAVIA, D. (1980). Effect of mucolytic and expectorant drugs on tracheobronchial clearance in chronic bronchitis. *Eur. J. Respir. Dis.*, **61** (Suppl. 110), 179–191

FAIRFAX, A.J., HASLAM, P.L., PAVIA, D., SHEHAN, N.F., BATEMAN, J.R.M., AGNEW, J.E., CLARKE, S.W. and TURNER-WARWICK, M. (1981). Pulmonary disorders associated with Sjögren's syndrome. *Q. J. Med.*, **50**, 279–295

FAZIO, F. and LAFORTUNA, C. (1981). Effect of inhaled salbutamol on mucociliary clearance in patients with chronic bronchitis. *Chest*, **80** (Suppl.), 827–830

FRIEDMAN, M., DOUGHERTY, R., NELSON, S.R., WHITE, R.P., SACKNER, M.A. and WANNER, A. (1977a). Acute effects of an aerosol hair spray on tracheal mucociliary transport. *Am. Rev. Respir. Dis.*, **116**, 281–286

FRIEDMAN, M., STOTT, F.D., POOLE, D.O., DOUGHERTY, R., CHAPMAN, G.F., WATSON, H. and SACKNER, M.A. (1977b). A new roentgenographic method for estimating mucous velocity in airways. *Am. Rev. Respir. Dis.*, **115**, 67–72

GAMSU, G., SINGER, M.M., VINCENT, H.H., BERRY, S. and NADEL, J.A. (1976). Postoperative impairment of mucous transport in the lung. *Am. Rev. Respir. Dis.*, **114**, 673–679

GERRITY, T.R., COTROMANES, E., GARRARD, C.S., YEATES, D.B. and LOURENÇO, R.V. (1983). The effect of aspirin on lung mucociliary clearance. *New Eng. J. Med.*, **308**, 139–141

GOODMAN, R.M., YERGIN, B.M., LANDA, J.F., GOLINVAUX, M.H. and SACKNER, M.A. (1978). Relationship of smoking history and pulmonary function tests to tracheal mucous velocity in non-smokers, young smokers, ex-smokers, and patients with chronic bronchitis. *Am. Rev. Respir. Dis.*, **117**, 205–214

HILDING, A.C. (1957). Ciliary streaming in the lower respiratory tract. *Am. J. Physiol.*, **191**, 404–410

KOLLBERG, H., MOSSBERG, B., AFZELIUS, B.A., PHILIPSON, K. and CAMNER, P. (1978). Cystic fibrosis compared with the immotile-cilia syndrome. *Scand. J. Respir. Dis.*, **59**, 297–306

LICHTIGER, M., LANDA, J.F. and HIRSCH, J.A. (1975). Velocity of tracheal mucus in anaesthetized women undergoing gynaecologic surgery. *Anesthesiology*, **42**, 753–756

LIPPMANN, M., LEIKAUF, G., SPEKTOR, D., SCHLESINGER, R.B. and ALBERT, R.E. (1981). The effects of irritant aerosols on mucus clearance from large and small conductive airways. *Chest*, **80**(Suppl.), 873–877

LOURENÇO, R.V., KLIMEK, M.F. and BOROWSKI, C.J. (1971). Deposition and clearance of 2 μ particles in the tracheobronchial tree of normal subjects—smokers and non-smokers. *J. Clin. Invest.*, **50**, 1411–1420

LOURENÇO, R.V., LODDENKEMPER, R. and CARTON, R.W. (1972). Patterns of distribution and clearance of aerosols in patients with bronchiectasis. *Am. Rev. Respir. Dis.*, **106**, 857–866

MATTHYS, H. and KÖHLER, D. (1980). Effect of theophylline on mucociliary clearance in man. *Eur. J. Respir. Dis.* (Suppl. 109), 98–102

MATTHYS, H., VASTAG, E., KÖHLER, D., DAIKELER, G. and FISCHER, J. (1983). Mucociliary clearance in patients with chronic bronchitis and bronchial carcinoma. *Respiration,* **44**, 329–337

MAY, K.R. (1949). An improved spinning top homogeneous spray apparatus. *J. Appl. Phys.*, **20**, 932–938
MOSSBERG, B., BJORKANDER, J., AFZELIUS, B.A. and CAMNER, P. (1982). Mucociliary clearance in patients with immunoglobulin deficiency. *Eur. J. Respir. Dis.*, **63**, 570–578
PAVIA, D., SHORT, M.D. and THOMSON, M.L. (1970). No demonstrable long term effects of cigarette smoking on the mucociliary mechanism of the human lung. *Nature*, **226**, 1228–1231
PAVIA, D., THOMSON, M.L. and POCOCK, S.J. (1971). Evidence for temporary slowing of mucociliary clearance in the lung caused by tobacco smoking. *Nature*, **231**, 325–326
PAVIA, D., BATEMAN, J.R.M. and CLARKE, S.W. (1980a). Deposition and clearance of inhaled particles. *Bull. Europ. Physiopath. Resp.*, **16**, 335–366
PAVIA, D., BATEMAN, J.R.M., SHEAHAN, N.F., AGNEW, J.E., NEWMAN, S.P. and CLARKE, S.W. (1980b). Techniques for measuring lung mucociliary clearance. *Eur. J. Respir. Dis.*, **61** (Suppl. 110), 157–177
PAVIA, D., AGNEW, J.E., BATEMAN, J.R.M., SHEAHAN, N.F., KNIGHT, R.K., HENDRY, W.F. and CLARKE, S.W. (1981). Lung mucociliary clearance in patients with Young's syndrome. *Chest*, **80** (Suppl.), 892–895
PAVIA, D., SUTTON, P.P., AGNEW, J.E., LOPEZ-VIDRIERO, M-T., NEWMAN, S.P. and CLARKE, S.W. (1982). Lung mucociliary transport in man. In *Cellular biology of the lung*. Edited by Cumming, G. and Bonsigmore, C. New York; Plenum Publishing Corporation, pp. 205–223
PAVIA, D., SUTTON, P.P., AGNEW, J.E., LOPEZ-VIDRIERO, M.T., NEWMAN, S.P. and CLARKE, S.W. (1983a). Measurement of bronchial mucociliary clearance. *Eur. J. Respir. Dis.*, **64** (Suppl. 127), 41–56
PAVIA, D., SUTTON, P.P., LOPEZ-VIDRIERO, M.T., AGNEW, J.E. and CLARKE, S.W. (1983b). Drug effects on mucociliary function. *Eur. J. Respir. Dis.*, **64** (Suppl. 128), 304–317
PUCHELLE, E., ZAHM, J-M. and BERTRAND, A. (1979). The influence of age on bronchial mucociliary transport. *Scan. J. Respir. Dis.*, **60**, 307–313
RICHARDSON, P.S. and PHIPPS, R.J. (1978). The anatomy, physiology, pharmacology and pathology of tracheobronchial mucus secretion and the use of expectorant drugs in human subjects. *Pharmac. Ther. B.*, **3**, 441–479
SACKNER, M.A. (1978). Effect of respiratory drugs on mucociliary clearance. *Chest*, **73** (Suppl.), 958–964
SACKNER, M.A., ROSEN, M.J. and WANNER, A. (1973). Estimation of tracheal mucous velocity by bronchofiberscopy. *J. Appl. Physiol.*, **34**, 495–499
SACKNER, M.A., LANDA, J., HIRSCH, J. and ZAPATA, A. (1975). Pulmonary effects of oxygen breathing. A 6-hour study in normal man. *Ann. Intern. Med.*, **82**, 40–43
SANTA CRUZ, R., LANDA, J., HIRSCH, J. and SACKNER, M.A. (1974). Tracheal mucous velocity in normal man and patients with obstructive lung disease; effects of terbutaline. *Am. Rev. Respir. Dis.*, **109**, 458–463
SLEIGH, M.A. (1981). Primary ciliary dyskinesis. *Lancet*, **ii**, 476
SUTTON, P.P., PAVIA, D., BATEMAN, J.R.M. and CLARKE, S.W. (1981). The effect of oral aminophylline on lung mucociliary clearance in man. *Chest*, **80** (Suppl.), 889–892
SUTTON, P.P., NADIR, N., PAVIA, D., SHEAHAN, N.F. and CLARKE, S.W. (1982). Lung mucociliary clearance in rheumatoid disease. *Ann. Rheum. Dis.*, **41**, 47–51
VENIZELOS, P.C., GERRITY, T.R. and YEATES, D.B. (1981). Response of human mucociliary clearance to acute alcohol administration. *Arch. Environm. Hlth.*, **36**, 194–201
VINTHER, B. and ELBROND, O. (1978). Nasal mucociliary function during penicillin treatment. *Acta. Octolaryngol.*, **86**, 132–134
WAGNER, H.N. Jr., LOPEZ-MAJANO, V. and LANGAN, J.K. (1965). Clearance of particulate matter from tracheobronchial tree in patients with tuberculosis. *Nature*, **205**, 252–254
WAITE, D.A., WAKEFIELD, S.J., MORIARTY, K.M., LEWIS, M.E., CUTTANCE, P.C. and SCOTT, A.C. (1983). Polynesian bronchiectasis. *Eur. J. Respir. Dis.*, **64** (Suppl. 127), 31–36
WANNER, A. (1977). Clinical aspects of mucociliary transport. *Am. Rev. Respir. Dis.*, **116**, 73–125
WANNER, A. (1979). The role of mucociliary dysfunction in bronchial asthma. *Am. J. Med.*, **67**, 477–485
WANNER, A. (1981). Alteration of tracheal mucociliary transport in airway disease. Effect of pharmacologic agents. *Chest*, **80** (Suppl.), 867–870
WEISS, T., DOROW, P. and FELIX, R. (1981). Effects of a beta adrenergic drug and a secretolytic agent on regional mucociliary clearance in patients with COLD. *Chest*, **80** (Suppl.), 881–885
WOLFF, R.K., DOLOVICH, M.B., OBMINSKI, G. and NEWHOUSE, M.T. (1977). Effects of exercise and eucapnic hyperventilation on bronchial clearance in man. *J. Appl. Physiol.*, **43**, 46–50
WOLFF, R.K., DOLOVICH, M., ROSSMAN, C.M. and NEWHOUSE, M.T. (1975). Sulfur dioxide and tracheobronchial clearance in man. *Arch. Environm. Hlth.*, **30**, 521–527
YEATES, D.B., GERRITY, T.R. and GARRARD, C.S. (1982). Characteristics of tracheobronchial deposition and clearance in man. *Ann. Occup. Hyg.*, **26**, 245–257
YEATES, D.B., ASPIN, N., LEVISON, H., JONES, M.T. and BRYAN, A.C. (1975). Mucociliary tracheal transport rates in man. *J. Appl. Physiol.*, **39**, 487–495

YEATES, D.B., STURGESS, J.M., KAHN, S.R., LEVISON, H. and ASPIN, N. (1976). Mucociliary transport in trachea of patients with cystic fibrosis. *Arch. Dis. Childh.*, **51**, 28–33

YEATES, D.B., PITT, B.R., SPEKTOR, D.M., KARRON, G.A. and ALBERT, R.E. (1981a). Coordination of mucociliary transport in the human trachea and intra-pulmonary airways. *J. Appl. Physiol.: Respir., Environ. Exercise Physiol.*, **51**, 1056–1064

YEATES, D.B., GERRITY, T.R. and GARRARD, C.S. (1981b). Particle deposition and clearance in the bronchial tree. *Ann. Biomed. Eng.*, **9**, 577–592

YOUNG, D. (1970). Surgical treatment of male infertility. *J. Reprod. Fertil.*, **23**, 541–542

Chapter 7

Chest physiotherapy and cough

Philip P. Sutton

Introduction

The use of chest physiotherapy (CP) is widespread in hospital practice but at present lacks both precision in its application and objectivity in its assessment. It is used in many types of chest disorders including acute and chronic lower respiratory tract infection, bronchiectasis and cystic fibrosis, exacerbations of chronic obstructive airways disease (chronic bronchitis and emphysema) and certain stages of asthma. It may also be used prophylactically in patients thought to be at risk of developing pulmonary complications secondary to another illness (e.g. following surgery) and as treatment should complications such as infection or mucus retention become established. Also, recently physiotherapy has formed the basis of rehabilitation programmes in patients with chronic obstructive airways disease.

The aim of chest physiotherapy is to promote sputum clearance, improve airway function by reducing airways obstruction and relieve dyspnoea thereby. Ventilation and gas exchange may be improved, infection eliminated and hypoventilation, atelectasis or mucus retention corrected. On the other hand, long-term rehabilitation in patients with chronic obstructive airways disease aims to increase exercise tolerance by graduated training. As the increased level of activity occurs without alteration of pulmonary function indices, this probably involves improved respiratory muscle function.

The accepted components of CP are postural drainage (PD), percussion (PN), vibration or 'clapping', cough (or other forced expiratory manoeuvres) and breathing exercises. Postural drainage seeks to increase the drainage of tracheobronchial secretions by positioning the chest to allow gravity to exert a greater influence on various areas of the diseased lung (Gaskell and Webber, 1980). It is usually combined with cough which seems to help the final clearance of secretions from large airways. Percussion, vibration and clapping impart an energy wave transmitted through the chest wall to cause a loosening of bronchial wall mucus. Mechanical or manual percussion are both used but vibrating pads available commercially usually operate on a frequency above the natural resonant frequency of the chest. A recent development is the application directly to the airway of high-frequency ventilation but the effect of this on sputum mobilization is not yet known (although one report suggests this may inhibit mucociliary clearance (McEvoy *et al.*, 1982)). Cough and forced expiratory manoeuvres are considered in detail later but can be applied either as an adjunct to the above modes of CP or effectively alone.

This chapter will firstly look at background information useful to define those patients likely to benefit from CP (Sutton *et al.*, 1982). It will then concentrate on the recent application and objective use of the inhaled radioaerosol technique to study CP, cough and other physiotherapy manoeuvres. If sputum mobilization is the prime objective of CP then this method effectively allows the tracheobronchial secretions to be 'labelled' and their subsequent clearance, by whatever manoeuvre under investigation, visualized directly by the use of a gamma camera. Computer linked facilities will also allow regions of interest within the lung field to be defined and studied in isolation. I will not address the diagnostic or therapeutic use of (pharmaceutical) aerosols which are dealt with elsewhere and which are often used as an adjunct to CP. The advantages and limitations of radioaerosol studies will be illustrated and some recent results and recommendations affecting clinical practice which arise from them will be presented.

Background

Postural drainage

Postural drainage (PD) has been one of the components of CP most frequently studied. There is firm evidence that PD alone or when combined with other physiotherapy manoeuvres (Tecklin and Holsclaw, 1975; May and Munt, 1979; Cochrane *et al.*, 1977) will increase sputum yield above control values in patients characterized by copious tracheobronchial secretions. Alternatively, it cannot increase sputum mobilization in those patients who are termed 'poor' sputum producers (March, 1971; Newton and Stephenson, 1978). Chopra *et al.* (1977) reported an increase in tracheal mucus velocity (TMV) of 40 per cent following 15 minutes of 20 degree 'head-down' positioning in anaesthetized dogs. Wong *et al.* (1977) similarly demonstrated increased TMV after PD in patients with cystic fibrosis and in adults recovering from an acute viral infection. The latter, however, were criticized by Oldenburg *et al.* (1979) for failing to control or allow for cough and their own results using a radioaerosol technique did not find tracheobronchial clearance to be altered by PD.

Percussion, Vibration (or Clapping) and Shaking

Percussion (5 Hz) vibration (12–16 Hz), or shaking (2 Hz) have been little studied in isolation but both Denton *et al.* (1962) and Maxwell and Redmond (1979) reported percussion alone to increase sputum yield in patients with cystic fibrosis. Chopra *et al.* (1977) also found percussion alone to increase TMV by 57 per cent in animal studies. In the only study investigating mucociliary clearance and vibration, Pavia *et al.* (1976) did not find mechanical vibration to alter clearance, although the frequency chosen (40 Hz) was higher than the probable resonant frequency of the lung which is thought to be 7 to 8 Hz. Hazleman (1976) expressed the widespread clinical impression that the addition of percussion and vibration produced more sputum than PD alone but this remains unsupported by objective evidence at present.

Breathing exercises

Instructions or exercises to alter the pattern of respiration are frequently used and may transiently increase overall ventilation though they do not appear to change the underlying regional ventilation (Grimby *et al.*, 1975; Sackner *et al.*, 1974). The relationship of these breathing exercises to sputum mobilization however has not yet been explored. The value of breathing exercises during retraining of patients with chronic obstructive airways disease by altering strength or endurance of the respiratory muscles also remains a real possibility.

Changes in arterial blood gases following CP are not consistently found. One explanation advanced is that these changes would occur only following the clearance of an airway completely occluded by mucus. Frequently no significant change is demonstrated (May and Munt, 1979; Mackenzie *et al.*, 1978; Newton and Stephenson, 1978) and two studies have both reported an immediate fall in oxygen saturation in patients with little or no sputum (Connors *et al.*, 1980) and also paradoxically those with profound secretions (Huseby *et al.*, 1976). Alternatively, Morran *et al.* (1981) have demonstrated a small but significant increase in oxygen saturation following post-operative CP.

The presence of excess secretions would seem to have functional importance although this is difficult to establish firmly. The view that secretions contribute relatively little to total airway resistance may only be true in health when the main resistance to airflow occurs in large central airways and secretions are minimal, whereas small (peripheral) airway resistance dominates early in disease associated with mucus hypersecretion (Hogg *et al.*, 1968). Wanner (1979) interpreted data from McFadden and Lyons' (1968) original study to suggest that the residual airway dysfunction in patients with asthma in remission may be particularly related to the presence of excessive mucus in peripheral airways. Certainly little alteration in pulmonary function indices occurs following physiotherapy in 'poor' sputum producers (Anthonisen and Riis, 1964; March, 1971; May and Munt, 1979) whereas small but significant improvements in peak expiratory flow rates (Weller *et al.*, 1980; Tecklin and Holsclaw, 1975) specific airway conductance (Cochrane *et al.*, 1977) and maximal flow rates (Feldman *et al.*, 1979) have been found after successful sputum mobilization in patients with copious tracheobronchial secretions. The observation by Campbell *et al.* (1975) of an immediate fall in FEV_1 in patients with an exacerbation of chronic bronchitis treated by physiotherapy has not been repeated (e.g. Newton and Stephenson, 1978). However, forced expiratory manoeuvres (which may increase airway reactivity) are usually avoided in the presence of bronchospasm or deferred until this responds to inhaled bronchodilators.

Much of the above evidence illustrates an important consideration in selecting patients who may potentially benefit from CP; namely they should have excess tracheobronchial secretions and expectorate large sputum quantities (variously defined as greater than 30, 60 or 100 ml sputum daily). Murray (1979) has commented that 'if the disease is not characterized by excess respiratory secretions, chest physiotherapy has no part in its clinical management'. Sputum mobilization is central to the purpose of CP and any alterations of other parameters such as ventilation and altered gas exchange are probably secondary to this. Many of the individual results of these studies must be interpreted with caution. A common problem in the past has been in defining (and measuring) a satisfactory 'end-point' of treatment, e.g. sputum volume, forced expiratory measurements, blood gases or radiological resolution, etc. Furthermore results from early studies may have laid undue emphasis on the possible benefit from CP due to the relative lack of satisfactory medication then available. Also many investigators have failed adequately to control their study or have ignored the powerful placebo action of CP.

Cough

By passing air through tubes lined with viscoelastic fluid (representing airway secretions) Clarke *et al.* (1970) studied resistance to airflow (which was found to be greater than expected, considering the effective diameter available) and also defined four phases of flow: bubble, slug, annular and mist. They postulated that transfer of momentum, i.e. movement or shearing of secretions, could only occur during mist flow when linear velocities were of the order of 25 m s^{-1}. During forced expiration *in vivo* maximal flow rates are directly related to lung volumes (West, 1979). At any given point, if this figure is divided by airways cross-section (available from lung models—*see* Chapter 1) linear velocity is obtained. A further correction is necessary because of the dynamic compression or collapse of airways during forced expiration (*Figure 7.1*). Velocities in these regions are extremely high (around 240 m s^{-1}) and areas where this collapse occurs alters with lung volume.

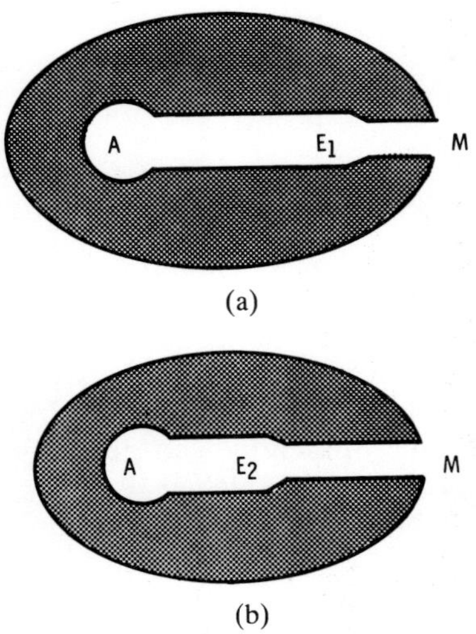

Figure 7.1 Dynamic compression of large airways during forced expiration/cough. During exhalation a pressure gradient exists between the alveoli (A) and the mouth (M). Traction preventing the conducting airways from collapsing is maximal at high lung volume (a) allowing the point of collapse to move further towards the alveoli (b) as support decreases during exhalation ($E_1 \rightarrow E_2$)

For example, at 75 per cent of vital capacity this collapse does not extend beyond the third generation, whereas at low lung volumes the airway collapse extends distally (Macklem and Wilson, 1965). By using this approach Leith (1968) established first that cough is most effective at high lung volumes and secondly that the linear velocity necessary to shear mucus is only exceeded in central airways and probably does not extend beyond the sixth or seventh (Weibel) generation. Recently, however, Scherer (1981) argued (also from theoretical considerations) that under conditions of excess mucus production the effect of cough can extend to the level of the respiratory bronchioles, i.e. the seventeenth generation. The exact mechanisms responsible for maintaining clearance of such small airways are still far from clear because just as the anatomical extent of effective cough is unknown so there is still uncertainty as to where effective mucociliary clearance begins (Agnew *et al.*, 1981). It is a well known but unexplained observation that following a forceful cough during bronchography under screening, expulsion of the radiographic medium from small airways is seen as is on occasions 'alveolarization' implying retropulsion also. It is postulated by Smalldone *et al.* (1979) that the formation of such flow-limiting segments (by dynamic collapse of the airways) during cough may locally impair mucociliary clearance.

Clearance of the tracheobronchial tree in health largely results from mucociliary transport with cough having a secondary role which only becomes important during illness. This hypothesis was supported by Puchelle *et al.* (1980) who measured the clearance of resin particles inhaled and deposited in proximal airways in 10 healthy subjects and 27 patients with chronic bronchitis. Both groups avoided coughing for 1 hour to measure their rate of mucociliary clearance and then both coughed vigorously. It was clear that mucociliary clearance was depressed in chronic bronchitis and that cough was a much more effective means of mucus clearance in these patients (*Figure 7.2*). Further information about the role of cough was

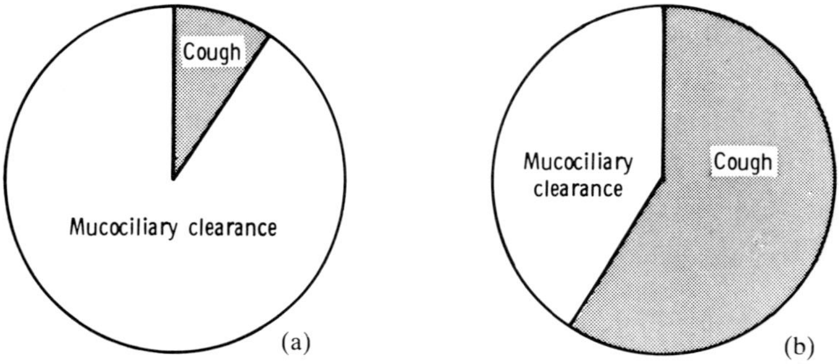

Figure 7.2 Tracheobrochial clearance in (a) health and (b) disease (adapted from Puchelle *et al.* (1980)

demonstrated by Camner *et al.* (1979). They compared tracheobronchial clearance of Teflon particles by voluntary coughing in 6 normal subjects and 8 patients with chronic obstructive airways disease. Cough did not clear particles in healthy subjects but did so only in those patients with chronic bronchitis who produced sputum (6 out of 8). Thus the presence of increased tracheobronchial secretions appeared to be an essential prerequisite for cough to be effective in tracheobronchial clearance. This point agrees well with much of the background evidence for CP and again underlines the central role of sputum mobilization in all forms of CP.

Forced expiration technique

Recently the Forced Expiration Technique (FET) has been used as an alternative to cough during CP. The FET was first described by Thompson (1973) and is currently in routine use at the Brompton Hospital, London (Gaskell and Webber, 1980). It consists of one or two forced expirations (but without closure of the glottis and the compressive phase which characterizes the start of the cough) commencing from mid-lung volume rather than total lung capacity, and continuing to residual volume (*Figure 7.3*). The transpulmonary pressure gradient is less during the FET than during cough (Langlands, 1967) and thus airway compression and closure are

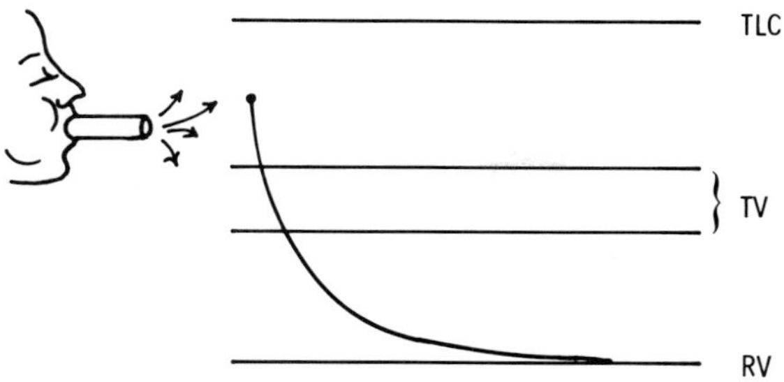

Figure 7.3 The Forced Expiration Technique (FET). The subject may practice by blowing through a cardboard tube. Note the similarity to the forced expiratory spirogram but in this instance expiration commences at *less* than total lung capacity

less and sputum clearance should be enhanced. Pryor *et al.* (1979) have demonstrated that the use of the FET with postural drainage obviates the need for an assistant (who normally provides chest percussion or vibratory shaking) in the domiciliary treatment of patients with cystic fibrosis. The efficiency of chest physiotherapy was also increased as more sputum was cleared in a shorter time. However FET was not evaluated on its own or compared to cough.

Radioaerosol studies of chest physiotherapy

Within the last decade the inhaled radioaerosol technique has been increasingly utilized by several groups of investigators to provide an objective assessment of CP, initially to study CP as a complete form of treatment and recently to evaluate its individual components. Insoluble particles labelled firmly with a gamma-emitting isotope are generated, inhaled and serve to 'tag' tracheobronchial secretions. Their subsequent clearance from the chest during CP is then monitored by external counters with suitable corrections for radioactive decay. Change in sputum expectorated should similarly parallel the clearance of radioactivity, although there are exceptions to this last point as outlined below. The design of these studies have mostly used results from past CP work and employ those patients who potentially benefit from CP, i.e. patients with large volumes of sputum production.

Thomson *et al.* (1975) employed CP during a study using the inhaled radioaerosol technique to evaluate the mucolytic, S-carboxymethylcysteine. At the end of a six-hour observation period in eight chronic bronchitics (during which there was no discernible difference in mucociliary clearance between placebo and active drug treatment) a period of CP (percussion and postural drainage) significantly increased the clearance of radioaerosol (and sputum) by approximately 22 per cent.

The efficiency of combined CP was studied slightly differently by Sackner *et al.* (1982) using aerosol deposition during rebreathing. As no change in lung mechanics occurred during CP he concluded that the alteration in deposition pattern following CP in chronic bronchitis was due to mobilization of secretions over and above that occurring during spontaneous cough.

Bateman *et al.* (1979) applied the radioaerosol method to the *in vivo* study of the efficiency of combined CP as a form of treatment. Ten patients with stable chronic bronchitis and mucus hypersecretion (mean sputum volume: 100 ml day^{-1}) underwent a 20 minute period of combined CP (postural drainage vibration, percussion and shaking—all with encouragement to cough) and a similar control period with the patients resting upright and avoiding coughing. The radiolabel was uniformly deposited throughout the tracheobronchial tree with 30 per cent of the initial burden placed in the peripheral lung regions (the outer and vertical two-fifths of the lung field as defined by an A-P orientated gamma camera). During CP clearance from the whole lung (and all regions of interest) was significantly greater than during the equivalent control period. The wet volume of sputum mobilized also increased fifteen-fold following CP. On viewing the selected lung regions clearance of the particles was increased five-fold in the central lung region, but only four-fold in the peripheral region (*Figure 7.4*).

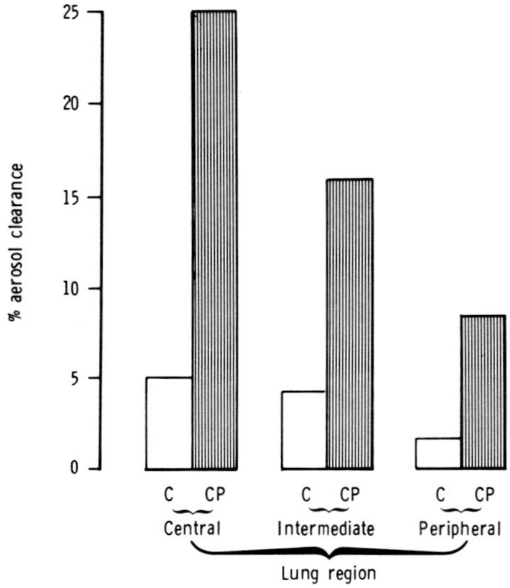

Figure 7.4 Radioaerosol clearance (in regions of interest) following control (C) or combined chest physiotherapy (CP). (After Bateman *et al.* (1979))

Although it was not stated if the difference in rates of clearance during CP from central and peripheral regions was significant, the possibility was raised that some component of CP was relatively less effective peripherally. An explanation concerned the role of cough and this possibility was addressed directly in a following study (Bateman *et al.*, 1981). Using six patients with mucus hypersecretion (160 ml day^{-1}) and a similar experimental technique, the effect of cough alone was compared to combined CP (postural drainage, vibration, shaking and percussion—all with encouragement to cough). Both treatments enhanced central lung clearance and combined CP, but *not* cough, accelerated peripheral lung clearance. Sputum volume mobilized during CP was significantly greater than during the cough study. The latter was supported by the hypothesis that the effectiveness of cough was limited peripherally and it may only be of definite value in moving secretions from large/central airways. However, it was not clear at this point as to which component of combined physiotherapy was effective either centrally or peripherally.

Oldenburg *et al.* (1979) viewed CP as an adjunct to improve the decreased mucociliary clearance present in chronic bronchitis and examined the role of the individual components of CP using the radioaerosol technique. Eight patients were studied and underwent a 20 minute period of cycling, exercises at submaximal rate, a 30 minute period of 15 degree 'head down' postural drainage and encouraged or

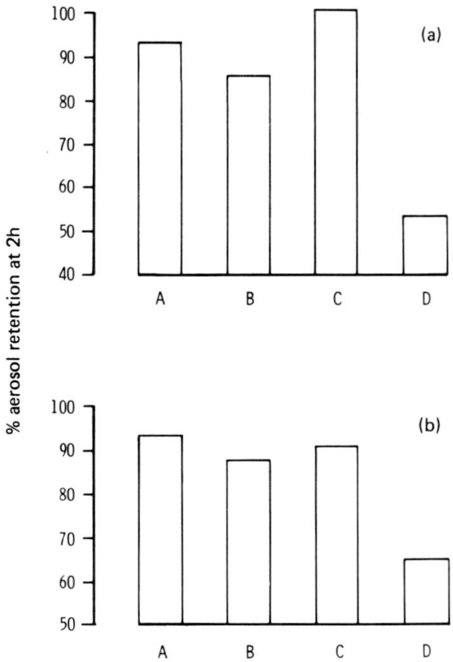

Figure 7.5 Whole lung (a) and peripheral (b) radioaerosol retention following control (A), exercise (B), postural drainage (C) and cough (D). (After Oldenburg *et al.* (1979))

directed coughing (a total of 30 minutes over the 46 minute experimental period). Postural drainage had no effect on aerosol clearance, exercise accelerated clearance somewhat, but cough proved extremely effective—both from the whole lung and peripheral regions, accelerating clearance by a factor of 7 and 6 respectively (*Figure 7.5*). These findings are at variance with others on several important points. The lack of any effect following postural drainage is contrary to the animal work of Chopra *et al.* (1977) and the results from Wong *et al.* (1977). Oldenburg and co-workers recorded the daily sputum production of their patients as quite variable ranging from 10 to 120 ml; it has been established that the beneficial action of postural drainage (at least in terms of expectoration) is only seen in those with copious sputum production. When the latter type of patient was subsequently studied (Sutton *et al.*, 1983b) enhanced particle clearance and sputum mobilization following postural drainage was clearly seen. The demonstration that cough is effective in peripheral regions of the lung differs from the implied results of Bateman *et al.* (1981) and our subsequent results.

An important technical point centres on Oldenburg's method of inhalation which deposits aerosols mainly in proximal airways and only a mean of 14 per cent of the total lung burden was deposited peripherally. (As the particles used were small and their patients lacked extreme airways obstruction, this may in part reflect the lack of a breathholding pause, which has been shown to be of critical importance in the deposition of therapeutic aerosols—Newman *et al.*, 1981.) It might be argued that firm conclusions regarding the peripheral efficacy of various manoeuvres must be guarded when only a minority of the lung activity is deposited peripherally.

The finding that exercise alone increases clearance is of interest and consistent with claims that an exercise programme is beneficial in cystic fibrosis increasing sputum yield and improving pulmonary function tests (Zach *et al.*, 1981; 1982).

However Zach's suggestion that physical exercise could replace chest physiotherapy in children with cystic fibrosis is tendentious. Certainly exercise transiently increases mucociliary clearance (Wolff *et al.*, 1977) but further study is necessary to evaluate the contribution of exercise to CP (although it clearly has an established role, albeit largely unexplained, in the long term rehabilitation of patients with chronic obstructive airways disease, e.g. Haas and Cardon (1969).

Oldenburg *et al.* (1979) gave no information about sputum mobilized during individual manoeuvres but this was presented in subsequent work from the same group. Using the same technique, Rossman *et al.* (1982) compared (a) postural drainage (b) PD + mechanical percussion (amplitude and frequency not stated) (c) combined CP (d) directed vigorous cough, and (e) a control period during which spontaneous cough was allowed. Clearance of radioaerosol from their outer and inner lung zones following each active treatment is shown in *Figure 7.6* and each

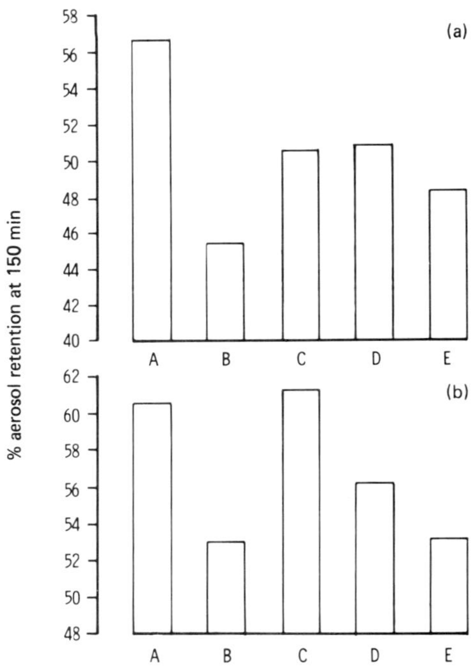

Figure 7.6 Inner zone (a) and peripheral zone (b) radioaerosol retention following control (A), cough (B), postural drainage (C), postural drainage and percussion (D) and therapist administered physiotherapy regime (E). (After Rossman *et al.* (1982))

gave increased clearance, although cough was significantly greater in both inner and outer lung zones. Sputum mobilization during cough, however, was not significantly increased over the control period, whereas this was increased following all other physiotherapy manoeuvres which were stated to be less effective. This disparity between particle clearance and sputum mobilization casts doubt on their conclusion that vigorous cough alone is as effective as other forms of physiotherapy.

A possible explanation for their demonstration of the efficacy of cough may have been due to the use of the Forced Expiratory Technique or 'huffing' in place of conventional cough. We have recently compared vigorous cough over a 30 minute period to FET and FET plus postural drainage. Ten patients with copious sputum (mean daily sputum volume: 63 ml) were studied and the superiority of FET over

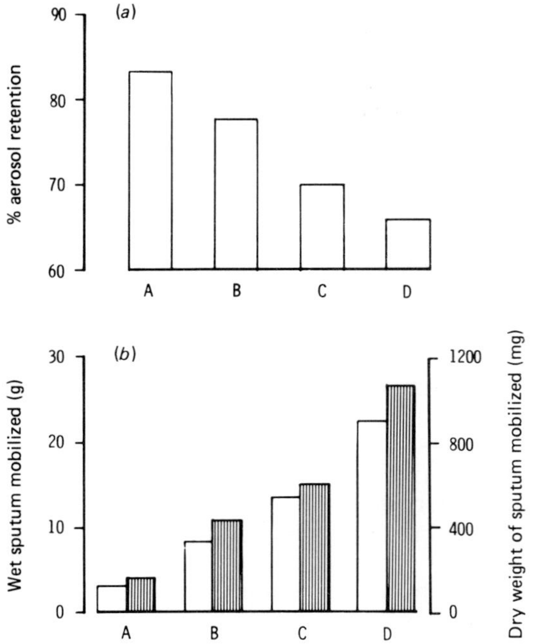

Figure 7.7 (a) Radioaerosol retention in whole lung. (b) Wet (open) and dry (shaded) weight of sputum mobilized during each treatment period. *Key*: A: control; B: cough; C: FET; D: FET plus postural drainage. (Sutton *et al*. (1983b))

cough, both in terms of aerosol clearance and sputum mobilization (*Figure 7.7*), was clearly demonstrated. This finding was further enhanced when postural drainage was included and it is suggested that both the FET and postural drainage be incorporated into standard CP.

We were able in this study to match the clearance of radioaerosol with the dry macromolecular weight of sputum mobilized during each treatment period. Recording sputum volumes directly may be misleading due to the unapparent inclusion of other material. If samples are freeze-dried then low molecular weight secretions such as saliva will contribute little and the dry macromolecular weight will represent bronchial secretions alone. Despite a carefully controlled inhalation technique designed to give uniform and widespread deposition only 10 per cent of the initial inhaled burden was deposited in the peripheral zone*. For this reason we felt constrained in any inference we could draw from our data based on peripheral zones alone. At present an accurate method of studying regional clearance from small airways has not yet been devised. Nevertheless we felt that the limited total value of cough was confirmed and the superiority of FET and PD demonstrated. In practical terms it seems unlikely that a patient who is already coughing freely can significantly increase the tracheobronchial clearance of secretions following instruction to encourage cough alone (Sutton *et al.*, 1983a).

Finally the radioaerosol technique was applied to a group of eight patients (mean daily sputum, 44 ml) to evaluate the role of percussion, vibratory-shaking and

*The term peripheral zone does not solely denote 'small airways' (diameter less than 2 mm). It is the gamma camera image of the outer 2/5th of the lung field as seen on an AP projection and almost certainly includes some large airways

TABLE 7.1. Radioaerosol clearance and sputum mobilization following (1) vibratory-shaking (with breathing exercises); (2) percussion (with breathing exercises); (3) percussion (without breathing exercises). All treatments, including control, contained postural drainage.

	Control	*1*	*2*	*3*
% radioaerosol clearance	40	43	38	44
(SE)	9	7	7	8
p		NS	NS	NS
Sputum mobilization*	157	59	50	92
(SE)	90	14	12	27
p		NS	NS	NS

*Expressed as mean specific activity ($\times 10^3$ γ counts per gramme sputum)

breathing exercises. There was no significant difference in radioaerosol clearance or sputum yield between any of these treatments (*Table 7.1*). The amount of activity cleared during each 30 minute treatment period was consistently greater than a similar group of patients studied previously and it was felt that the inclusion of postural drainage in each treatment period (including control) may have masked any additional effect of percussion, etc. Alternatively it may be argued that any value of these treatment manoeuvres is unimportant compared to simple postural drainage.

The inhaled radioaerosol technique offers also a unique approach to the evaluation of mucolytics and expectorants either alone or as adjuncts to CP and they have been reviewed by Pavia *et al.* (1980). Although mucolytic activity can often be demonstrated *in vitro* (and plausibly explained by altered sputum viscosity following the breaking of glycoprotein chains at their disulphide bonds) increased sputum clearance is not consistently demonstrated *in vivo*. For example, carboxymethylcysteine does not appear to enhance clearance whereas bromhexine and glyceryl guaiacolate does. However, despite these positive findings clinical studies have failed to demonstrate these as a useful aid to expectoration (Clarke *et al.*, 1972). Clarke and Pavia (1980) found sodium mercapto-ethane-sulphonate to enhance mucociliary clearance but only to a similar extent as hypertonic saline aerosol (although not necessarily by the same mechanism). The explanation for the increased clearance following saline was postulated as due to increased mucus production and expectoration. Saline aerosol alone seems to have no effect on tracheal mucociliary transport either in normal subjects or patients with cystic fibrosis (Wood *et al.*, 1977). Alternatively water aerosol, which also reduces sputum viscosity *in vitro* (Palmer, 1960) was found by Foster *et al.* (1976) to increase mucus clearance slightly (although this response was minimal compared to the inhaled adrenergic agents under investigation). Inhaled bronchodilators as an aid to CP have not yet been studied together with physiotherapy, although they do enhance mucociliary clearance when used alone (Foster *et al.*, 1976).

Summary

In designing studies to investigate chest physiotherapy, patient selection is important and in particular an adequate (if potential) sputum volume is critical. If the radioaerosol method is used to measure clearance during CP, then the aerosol is best monodisperse, inhaled with a standard lung volume and flow rate and with a standard breath-holding pause to achieve suitable deposition (*see* Chapters 3 and

6). This standardization is crucial when comparing results from different procedures.

Tracheobronchial clearance is a complex intervention of co-ordinated ciliary activity coupled with the overlying mucus layer of which the thickness, apparent viscosity and elasticity are important components. These factors, together with gravity, cough and other forced expiratory manoeuvres, determine mucus clearance.

There has been a need for firm evidence confirming the value of CP in certain chest disorders. Such evidence has been required (a) to ensure cost-effectiveness by refining techniques (b) to define those conditions which are most amenable to such treatment and (c) to discourage indiscriminate use.

There seems no doubt that chest physiotherapy will improve expectoration particularly in patients with copious sputum. However there is not yet unanimity about the role of the various components of CP and of coughing. In our experience of studying a total of 34 patients on 120 separate occasions, the forced expiration technique and postural drainage proved of value while that of cough alone was limited. Furthermore, manual percussion, vibratory-shaking and breathing exercises appear to add little to postural drainage. In conclusion therefore, it is suggested that FET+PD should be the mainstay of chest physiotherapy. This has the advantage of simplicity, self application and suitability for domiciliary care.

References

AGNEW, J.E., PAVIA, D. and CLARKE, S.W. (1981). Airway penetration of inhaled radioaerosol: an index to small airway function? *Eur. J. Respir. Dis.*, **62**, 239–255

ANTHONISEN, P. and RIIS, P. (1964). The value of lung physiotherapy in the treatment of acute exacerbations in chronic bronchitis. *Acta. Med. Scand.*, **175**, 715–719

BATEMAN, J.R.M., DAUNT, K.M., NEWMAN, S.P., PAVIA, D. and CLARKE, S.W. (1979). Regional lung clearance of excessive bronchial secretions during chest physiotherapy in patients with stable chronic airway obstruction. *Lancet*, **1**, 294–297

BATEMAN, J.R.M., NEWMAN, S.P., DAUNT, K.M., SHEAHAN, N.F., PAVIA, D. and CLARKE, S.W. (1981). Is cough as effective as chest physiotherapy in the removal of excessive tracheobronchial secretions. *Thorax*, **36**, 682–687

CAMNER, P., MOSSBERG, B., PHILLIPSON, K. and STRANDBERG, K. (1979). Elimination of test particles from the human tracheobronchial tree by voluntary coughing. *Scan. J. Respir. Dis.*, **60**, 56–62

CAMPBELL, A.H., O'CONNELL, J.M. and WILSON, F. (1975). The effect of chest physiotherapy upon the FEV_1, in chronic bronchitis. *Med. J. Aust.*, **1**, 33–35

CHOPRA, S.K., TAPLIN, G.V., SIMMONS, D.H., ROBINSON, G.D., ELAM, D. and COULSON, A. (1977). Effects of hydration and physical therapy on tracheal transport velocity. *Am. Rev. Respir. Dis.*, **115**, 1009–1014

CLARKE, S.W. and PAVIA, D. (1980). Lung mucus production and mucociliary clearance: methods of assessment. *Br. J. Clin. Pharmac.*, **9**, 537–546

CLARKE, S.W., CRAIG, G.M. and MAKIN, E.J.B. (1972). Clinical trial of bromhexine in severe chronic bronchitis during winter. *Thorax*, **27**, 429–432

CLARKE, S.W., JONES, J.G. and OLIVER, D.R. (1970). Resistance to two-phase gas-liquid flow in airways. *J. Appl. Physiol.*, **29**, 464–471

CLARKE, S.W., LOPEZ-VIDRIERO, M.T., PAVIA, D. and THOMSON, M.L. (1979). The effect of sodium 2-mercapto-ethane sulphonate and hypertonic saline aerosols on bronchial clearance in chronic bronchitis. *Br. J. Clin. Pharmac.*, **7**, 39–44

COCHRANE, G.M., WEBBER, B.A. and CLARKE, S.W. (1977). Effects of sputum on pulmonary function. *Br. Med. J.*, **2**, 1181–1183

CONNORS, A.E., HAMMON, W.E., MARTIN, R.J. and ROGER, R.M. (1980). Chest physical therapy; the immediate effect on oxygenation in acutely ill patients. *Chest*, **78**, 559–564

DENTON, R. (1962). Bronchial secretions in cystic fibrosis: the effects of treatment with mechanical percussion vibration. *Am. Rev. Respir. Dis.*, **86**, 41–6

FELDMAN, J., TRAVER, G.A. and TAUSSIG, L.M. (1979). Maximal expiratory flows after postural drainage. *Am. Rev. Respir. Dis.*, **119**, 239–245

FOSTER, W.M., BERGOFSKY, E.H., BOHNING, D.E., LIPPMANN, M. and ALBERT, R.E. (1976). Effect of adrenergic agents and their mode of action on mucociliary clearance in man. *J. Appl. Physiol.*, **41**, 146–152

GASKELL, D.V. and WEBBER, B.A., (Eds) (1980). *The Brompton Hospital guide to chest physiotherapy.* Oxford and London; Blackwell Scientific Publications

GRIMBY, G., OXHOJ, H. and BAKE, B. (1975). Effects of abdominal breathing on distribution of ventilation in obstructive lung disease. *Clin. Sci. Mol. Med.*, **48**, 193–199

HAAS, A. and CARDON, H. (1969). Rehabilitation in chronic obstructive pulmonary disease. *Med. Clin. North Am.*, **53**, 593–606

HAZLEMAN, B.L. (1976). Physical forms of treatment in respiratory disease. In *Respiratory disease.* Edited by Lane, D.J. London; Heinemann

HOGG, J.C., MACKLEM, P.T. and THURLBECK, W.M. (1968). Site and nature of airway obstruction in chronic obstructive lung disease. *N. Eng. J. Med.*, **278**, 1355–1360

HUSEBY, J., HUDSON, L., STARK, K. and TYLER, M. (1976). Oxygenation during chest physiotherapy. *Chest*, **70**, 430

JONES, J.G. and CLARKE, S.W. (1970). Dynamics of cough. *Brit. J. Anaesth.*, **42**, 280–285

LANGLANDS, J. (1967). The dynamics of cough in health and in chronic bronchitis. *Thorax*, **22**, 88–96

LEITH, D.E. (1968). Cough. *Phys. Ther.*, **48**, 439–447

LORIN, M.I. and DENNING, C.R. (1971). Evaluation of postural drainage by measurement of sputum volume and consistency. *Am. J. Phys. Med.*, **50**, 215–219

MACKENZIE, C.F., SKIN, B. and McASLAN, T.C. (1978). Chest physiotherapy; the effects on arterial oxygenation. *Anaesth. Analg.*, **57**, 28–30

MACKLEM, P.T. and WILSON, N.J. (1965). Measurement of intratracheal pressure in man. *J. Appl. Physiol.*, **20**, 653–666

MARCH, H. (1971). Appraisal of postural drainage for chronic obstructive pulmonary disease. *Arch. Phys. Med. Rehabil.*, **52**, 528–531

MAY, D.B. and MUNT, P.W. (1979). Physiologic effect of chest percussion and postural drainage in patients with stable chronic bronchitis. *Chest*, **75**, 29–32

MAXWELL, M. and REDMOND, A. (1979). Comparative trial of manual and mechanical percussion technique with gravity assisted bronchial drainage in patients with cystic fibrosis. *Arch. Dis. Child.*, **54**, 542–544

McEVOY, R.D., DAVIES, N.T.H., HEDENSTEIRNA, G., HARTMAN, M.T., SPRAGG, R.G. and WAGNER, P.D. (1982). Lung mucociliary transport during high-frequency ventilation. *Am. Rev. Respir. Dis.*, **126**, 452–456

McFADDEN, E.R. and LYONS, H.A. (1968). Airway resistance and uneven ventilation in bronchial asthma. *J. Appl. Physiol.*, **25**, 365–370

MORRAN, C.G., CARTER, D.C., McARDLE, C.S. and MILLS, R.J. (1981). Effect of physiotherapy on post-operative pulmonary function and complications. *Thorax*, **36**, 716

MURRAY, J.R. (1979). The ketchup bottle method. *N. Eng. J. Med.*, **300**, 1155–1157

NEWMAN, S.P. (1982). Studies of inhaled therapeutic pressurised aerosols in man; patterns of deposition and bronchodilator response. Ph.D. Thesis, University of London

NEWMAN, S.P., PAVIA, D. and CLARKE, S.W. (1981). How should a pressurized beta adrenergic bronchodilator be inhaled. *Eur. J. Respir. Dis.*, **62**, 3–22

NEWTON, D.A.G. and STEPHENSON, A. (1978). Effect of physiotherapy on pulmonary function. *Lancet*, **8**, 228–229

OLDENBURG, F.A., DOLOVICH, M.B., MONTGOMERY, J.M. and NEWHOUSE, M.T. (1979). Effect of postural drainage, exercise and cough on mucus clearance in chronic bronchitis. *Am. Rev. Respir. Dis.*, **120**, 739–745

PALMER, K.N.V. (1960). Reduction of sputum viscosity by a water aerosol in chronic bronchitis. *Lancet*, **ii**, 91

PAVIA, D., BATEMAN, J.R.M. and CLARKE, S.W. (1980). Deposition and clearance of inhaled particles. *Bull. Europ. Physiopath. Resp.*, **16**, 335–366

PAVIA, D., THOMSON, M.L. and PHILIPAKOS, D. (1976). A preliminary study of the effect of a vibrating pad on bronchial clearance. *Am. Rev. Respir. Dis.*, **113**, 92–96

PAVIA, D., THOMSON, M.L., CLARKE, S.W. and SHANNON, H.S. (1977). Effect of lung function and mode of inhalation on penetration of aerosol into the human lung. *Thorax*, **32**, 194–197

PRYOR, J.A., WEBBER, B.A., HODSON, M.E. and BATTEN, J.C. (1979). Evaluation of the forced expiration technique as an adjunct to postural drainage in the treatment of cystic fibrosis. *Br. Med. J.*, **2**, 417–418

PUCHELLE, E., ZAHM, J.M., GIRARD, F., BERTRAND, A., POLU, J-M., UNG, F. and SADOUL, P. (1980). Relationships to sputum properties in chronic bronchitis. *Eur. J. Respir. Dis.*, **61**, 254–264

ROSSMAN, C.R., WALDES, R., SAMPSON, D. and NEWHOUSE, M.T. (1982). Effect of chest physiotherapy on the removal of mucus in patients with cystic fibrosis. *Am. Rev. Respir. Dis.*, **126**, 131–135

SACKNER, M.A., SILVA, G., BANKS, J.M., WATSON, D.D. and SMOAK, W.M. (1974). Distribution of ventilation during diaphragmatic breathing in obstructive lung disease. *Am. Rev. Respir. Dis.*, **109**, 331–337

SACKNER, M.A., SHANE, D., KLAUS, V., CRITES, D., FORD, D., LEWARG, G.A. and KIM, C.S. (1982). Effect of chest physiotherapy on pulmonary secretions. *Am. Rev. Respir. Dis.*, **125**, No. 4 part 2 of 2 parts, 137

SCHERER, P.W. (1981). Mucus transport by cough. *Chest*, **80**, 830–833

SMALLDONE, G.C., HON, H., SWIFT, D.K. and WAGNER, H.N. (1979). Effect of flow-limiting segments and cough on particle deposition and mucociliary clearance in the lung. *Am. Rev. Respir. Dis.*, **120**, 747–758

SUTTON, P.P., PAVIA, D., BATEMAN, J.R.M. and CLARKE, S.W. (1982). Chest physiotherapy: a review. *Eur. J. Respir. Dis.*, **63**, 188–201

SUTTON, P.P., LOPEZ-VIDRIERO, M.T., PAVIA, D., NEWMAN, S.P. and CLARKE, S.W. (1983a). Effect of chest physiotherapy on the removal of mucus in patients with cystic fibrosis. *Am. Rev. Respir. Dis.*, **127**, 390–391

SUTTON, P.P., PARKER, R.A., WEBBER, B.A., NEWMAN, S.P., GARLAND, N., LOPEZ-VIDRIERO, M.T., PAVIA, D. and CLARKE, S.W. (1983b). Assessment of the forced expiration technique, postural drainage and directed coughing in chest physiotherapy. *Eur. J. Respir. Dis.*, **64**, 62–68

TECKLIN, J.S. and HOLSCLAW, D.S. (1975). Evaluation of bronchial drainage in patients with cystic fibrosis. *Phys. Ther.*, **55**, 1081–1084

THOMPSON, B.J. (1973). The physiotherapist's role in the rehabilitation of the asthmatic. *N.Z. J. Physiotherapy*, **4**, 11–16

THOMSON, M.L., PAVIA, D., JONES, C.J. and McQUISTON, T.A.C. (1975). No demonstrable effect of S-Carboxymethylcysteine on clearance of secretions from the human lung. *Thorax*, **30**, 669–673

WANNER, A. (1979). The role of mucociliary dysfunction in bronchial asthma. *Am. J. Med.*, **67**, 477–485

WELLER, P.H., BUSH,E., PREECE, M.D. and MATHEW, D.J. (1980). Short term effect of chest physiotherapy on pulmonary function with cystic fibrosis. *Respiration*, **40**, 53–56

WEST, J.B. (1979). *Respiratory physiology—the essentials.* Baltimore; Williams and Wilkins, 2nd edn

WOLFF, R.F., DOLOVICH, M.B., OBMINSKI, G. and NEWHOUSE, M.T. (1977). The effects of exercise and eucapnic hyperventilation on bronchial clearance in man. *J. Appl. Physiol.*, **43**, 46–50

WONG, J.W., KEENS, T.G., WANNAMAKER, E.M., CROZIER, D.N., LEVISON, H. and ASPIN, N. (1977). Effects of gravity on tracheal mucus transport rates in normal subjects and patients with cystic fibrosis. *Paediatrics*, **60**, 146–152

WOOD, R.E., HOROWITZ, J.G. and MANCINI, N. (1977). Effect of saline aerosol on tracheal mucociliary transport in normal subjects and patients with cystic fibrosis. *Am. Rev. Resp. Dis.*, **115**, 295

ZACH, M., OBERWALDER, B. and HASLER, F. (1982). Cystic fibrosis; physical exercise versus chest physiotherapy. *Arch. Dis. Child.*, **57**, 587–589

ZACH, M.S., PURREY, B. and OBEWALDER, B. (1981). Effect of swimming on forced expiration and sputum clearance in cystic fibrosis. *Lancet*, **2**, 1201–3

Chapter 8

Clearance of inhaled particles from the alveoli

J. Gareth Jones

Introduction

This chapter is concerned with the complex mechanisms for clearing inhaled particles from the alveoli. Although these mechanisms tend to minimize the deleterious effects of inhaled particles on lung structure and function the clearance process itself may, in some circumstances, be the cause of lung damage. Part of the chapter is, in consequence, concerned with recent developments in the techniques for studying the effects of these particles on the lung in terms of changes in the solute permeability of the alveolar capillary interface.

It is well known that the structure of the lung maximizes the area of the gas exchanging interface exposed to the external environment. This vast exposed area not only facilitates the rapid transfer of respiratory gases across that interface but is itself exposed to toxic gases or particles which are entrained in the inspired gas. These may dissolve in or deposit upon the epithelial lining layer which covers both the conducting airways and the gas exchanging interface. In the case of toxic gases or vapours the site of damage to the epithelium depends upon the solubility of the gas. Toxic *soluble* gases may damage the large conducting airways and *insoluble* gases predominantly damage the terminal, alveolated airways.

Toxic particulate material damages different parts of the lung depending upon its site of deposition, composition and clearance. As pointed out earlier in this volume, particles more than 5 μm in diameter tend to impact against the walls of large airways whereas particles smaller than 5 μm may reach the alveolated region and deposit by sedimentation (0.2–5 μm) or by Brownian movement (~0.1 μm) (Newhouse *et al.*, 1976). A remarkable exception is asbestos where particles up to 300 μm in length and about 1 μm in diameter have been found in the alveoli. It is believed that these fibres which are entrained in the inspired gas are orientated parallel to the laminar airstream and in this way may be carried to the terminal airways. Particles ranging between 0.1 and 0.5 μm in diameter show least tendency to be retained in the lung (less than 20 per cent retention) which is a negligible amount compared to the retention of particles larger and smaller than this range.

Inhaled particles may consist of aqueous aerosols containing micro-organisms, toxic vapours, radioactive substances or organic and inorganic dusts. Provided that these aerosols have low lipid solubility, the walls of the conducting airway and alveoli provide an effective barrier to rapid absorption. Consequently, particles which are deposited in the *conducting airways* are removed by mucociliary clearance whereas those that deposit in the *terminal airway units* are cleared by two main processes:

1. *Non-absorptive*, where particles are transported from the alveoli to the ciliated region where they are removed by the mucociliary clearance mechanism.
2. *Absorptive* which is of two main subtypes:
   (a) Direct penetration into the epithelial cells with subsequent cell death and muco-ciliary clearance of cell debris *or* penetration right through the epithelium into the interstitial space and either deposition or clearance by lymph or vascular drainage.
   (b) Phagocytosis and destruction within the phagocytic system or transport to lymphatics.

The non-absorptive mechanism will be mentioned only briefly, the subject having being discussed in detail in an earlier part of this volume. The major emphasis in this chapter is on the absorptive mechanisms of alveolar clearance.

This absorptive mechanism implies (a) a unique and selective permeability function for the respiratory epithelium and (b) a complex cell mediated clearance system which will be discussed in detail. Inhaled toxic particles may exert a deleterious effect on lung function which may be direct or indirect. However, it is a remarkable paradox that despite the vast onslaught of potentially harmful particles on the alveolar epithelial surface there has been an extraordinary lack of interest on the part of investigators in developing clinically applicable methods of studying the deleterious effects of inhaled particles on alveolar epithelial *function*. While considerable attention has been paid to the effects on the patency of conducting airways the functional changes in the alveolar epithelium have been almost ignored, deleterious effects being inferred from the structural rather than the functional approach. Recent developments using small hydrophilic probe molecules (Jones *et al.*, 1982a) have opened the way for detailed, minimally invasive, studies to be made of the harmful effects of inhaled particles and vapours on the permeability function of the alveolar epithelium in both animals and man.

Bearing in mind the different pathways for the clearance of particles deposited in the alveoli the chapter will be subdivided into:

1. The structure and newer aspects of function of the constituent parts of the alveolar-capillary interface.
2. Alveolar clearance mechanisms for specific particles.

Structure and function of the alveolar capillary interface

The alveolar wall consists of an epithelial cell layer in close proximity to the vascular endothelial layer. In some parts these two cell layers are separated by an interstitial space which contains connective tissue and the origins of the pulmonary lymphatic system. The alveolar epithelium is coated with a thin layer of liquid which may be secreted by the alveolar epithelium. In this liquid lies the crucially important humoral and cellular defence mechanism of the lung.

The lining layer of liquid

Secretion and surface properties

This layer contains the phospholipids dipalmitoyl lecithin and dipalmitoyl phosphatidyl ethanolamine whose fundamental property is to reduce the tension of the alveolar surface. The surface tension lowering material or surfactant is found predominantly in the alveoli, negligible amounts occurring in the liquid lining the conducting airways.

Secretion of surface active material has been difficult to study because broncho-alveolar lavage itself may interfere with the production of the material. Increased secretion of surfactant in intact lungs occurs with hyperventilation and with β adrenergic and cholinergic stimulation (Oyartzun and Clements, 1977; 1978). The secretion of saturated phosphatidylcholine by isolated alveolar type II cells is also stimulated by β adrenergic agonists, cholera toxin and the calcium ionophore A23187 (Mason *et al.*, 1982).

Regulation of the thickness of the alveolar liquid is important to minimize the diffusion distance between alveolar gas and blood. However, the concept of a finite layer of liquid lining the alveoli has been challenged by Hills (1982). He suggests that the cationic surfactants found on the alveolar walls act also as water repellants. He predicts that the properties of these surfactants result in an essentially dry alveolar surface, any alveolar liquid being confined to the corners of the alveoli. At this point it is worth noting that the alveoli, like numerous soap bubbles in contact, have many faceted plane surfaces with sharp corners at the junctions of surfaces rather than the popular conception of multiple small spheres. The events occurring in these corners have been the subject of recent intense discussion and controversy. There is further controversy about the magnitude of the passive forces that govern fluid movement across the alveolar epithelium (Guyton and Moffat, 1981; Wilson, 1981). The force resulting from surface tension may draw fluid into the alveolar lumen and this force may be very large at the corners of alveoli where the radius of curvature, 0.5 μm, is minute (Gil *et al.*, 1979). There are three possible implications of these large corner forces (a) re-absorption of fluid from the alveolar space can occur only if the interstitial pressure is subatmospheric (b) there may be an active transport mechanism. This has been confirmed by Mason *et al.* (1982) who showed that alveolar type II cells grown in culture produce a polarized epithelium which actively transports fluid and electrolyte from the alveolar subphase to the interstitium. (c) Hills (1982) presents persuasive evidence that the surface properties of the fluid in the alveolar corners can itself act as very effective 'corner pumps' which function as a self regulating mechanism in the resolution of pulmonary oedema. This implies that there is no necessity for a low interstitial space pressure to maintain a 'dry' alveolus.

Non-specific factors mediating bacterial resistance

There are a number of important nonspecific soluble factors in the lining liquid which affect the resistance to infection and represent the first line of defence against toxic particles depositing on the alveolar wall. The distribution of these factors vis-a-vis the alveolar surface and the surface of the bronchial wall is not known with complete certainty. One of these factors is α_1 antitrypsin, deficiency of which leads to severe lung damage owing to the lack of ability to remove a variety of proteolytic enzymes that reach the alveolar surface following infection or inflammation. The enzyme *lysozyme* is bactericidal and is found in large amounts in the secretions on mucous surfaces. *Interferon* is probably produced by lymphocytes in the alveolar liquid and is an important agent eliminating virus infection. *Lactoferrin* is secreted by polymorphonuclear leucocytes (PMN) and is an important bacteriostatic mechanism. Only trace amounts of C_3, C_4 and C_6 of the *complement system* are present in broncho-alveolar washings. Whether these are truly representative of undisturbed alveolar liquid is unknown. *Factor B* of the properdin pathway is only about 6 per cent of the concentration found in serum. It seems likely, however, that an increase in permeability of the alveolar wall caused by inflammation will result in a rapid diffusion into the alveolar space of large molecular weight serum components.

The opsonic protein, *fibronectin*, mediates the binding of gelatin coated particles to monocytes. Fibronectin has been demonstrated in human bronchoalveolar fluid in higher concentration in smokers than non-smokers (Villiger *et al.*, 1982). The likely source of fibronectin is the alveolar macrophage and the combined action of the macrophage and fibronectin acts as a specific endogenous opsonic mediator for the uptake of deuterated collagen, fibrin or staphylococci in the lower respiratory tract.

All mucosal surfaces tend to have a secretory *IgA antibody* as a primary defence mechanism (Newhouse *et al.*, 1976). Relatively small numbers of cells secreting *IgE, IgG and Ig M* have been found in the upper respiratory tract but the IgE secreting cells are more numerous in the upper airway than in peripheral lymphoid tissue. The role of IgA in the respiratory tract secretions is obscure. Patients deficient in IgA do not necessarily have an increased prevalence of respiratory tract infection but the response to infection is to increase IgA, IgM and, in the lower respiratory tract, IgG (Kaltreider *et al.*, 1974). The ratio of IgG to IgA in bronchoalveolar washings resemble that found in the serum.

Alveolar epithelium

The lung is lined by a continuous layer of epithelial cells which extends from the ciliated columnar cells of the conducting airway via an abrupt transition to the flattened cells of the alveolar region. Two main cell types make up the alveolar epithelial layer, these are the squamous type I and granular type II pneumocytes. Type II cells make up more than half of the alveolar epithelial cells but because of their cuboidal shape they cover less than 5 per cent of the surface area. Type II cells differentiate into type I cells and repair the epithelial surface after injury. They are also responsible for the production of surface active material. In contrast to the type II cell the type I cell, 0.2 μm in thickness, may cover an area equivalent to a disc 50 μm in diameter.

The type I and II cells are held together by very tight junctions called Zonulae occludentes. The characteristic feature of this type of junction bestows on the epithelium a ten-fold greater resistance to the permeation by hydrophilic probe molecules than that of the pulmonary vascular endothelium. The permeability of the epithelium and endothelium can be compared using the dimensions of the pore radii between the cells. The equivalent pore radius of the paracellular channels between epithelial cells is about 1 nm which is a quarter of the pore radius found between the adjacent endothelial cells. This implies that the epithelium represents an almost complete barrier to the passage of macromolecules such as horseradish peroxidase (MW 40 000 daltons, molecular radius >3 nm) or ferritin (MW 500 000 daltons). The structural basis for this difference in permeability has been elucidated using freeze fracture electron microscopy. The epithelial tight junction is characterized by a network of sealing strands made up of a row of protein molecules on each of the adjacent cell walls and these molecules interdigitate like a zip (Staehelin and Hull, 1977). The greater the number of strands the more impermeable is the junction and the higher is the transepithelial electrical resistance. This very low permeability implies that *active transport* of salt and water across the epithelial layer is important for the normal functional integrity of this barrier. The general arrangement of these strands suggests that the tightness of the junction can be varied according to the physiological needs of the tissue. In this way it can be hypothesized that the intercellular strands can reversibly unzip to permit lymphocytes, macrophages and polymorphonuclear leucocytes to enter or leave the air space without creating a large leak of solute and water.

The ad-epithelial *basement membrane* is made up of thin collagen fibres (Kefalides, 1966) and the similarities in structure and antigenic properties of the alveolar and the glomerular basement membranes (Pasternak *et al.*, 1965) may underlie the Goodpasture syndrome. Functionally, however, the alveolar basement membrane, unlike that of the glomerular basement membrane does not appear to be a barrier to macromolecules such as horseradish peroxidase or Ferritin (Gonzalez-Crussi and Boston, 1972; Laweryns and Baert, 1977).

The impermeability of the normal epithelial junctions to penetration by macromolecules implies that the main mechanism of transport of large particles across the normal epithelium is either by endocytosis through the substance of the epithelial cell itself or by phagocytosis and subsequent penetration of the epithelium. Transcellular transport will be discussed under Alveolar Clearance Mechanisms and is an active process compared to the passive diffusion of paracellular transport.

The vascular endothelium

The capillary endothelium is made up of highly metabolically active cells which are also held together by tight junctions. These, however, have fewer sealing strands than the epithelium and the equivalent pore radius of the paracellular channels between these cells is about 4 nm (Schneeberger-Keeley and Karnofsky, 1968). Unlike the epithelium the endothelium is freely permeable to horse-radish peroxidase but not to Ferritin. Albumin (MW 65 000 daltons molecular radius 3.6 nm) can diffuse through this layer, the concentration of albumin in pulmonary lymph being about 50 per cent that of plasma (Staub, 1974).

Lymphatic system

The pulmonary lymphatic system (Lauweryns and Baert, 1977) is a network which is subdivided into a pleural plexus and a peribronchial plexus which anastomose at the hilar lymph nodes. Within the lung the lymphatics are very thin-walled structures which are never seen as far distally as the alveolar walls or in the interalveolar septa (Lauweryns and Baert, 1977). They are divided into (a) collecting channels and (b) lymphatic capillaries. The collecting channels are made up of endothelial cells with relatively tight junctions and have a more substantial wall structure containing smooth muscle and conical monocuspid valves. The lymphatic capillaries are made up of endothelial cells with loose junctions and frequent large intercellular gaps. Consequently, the basement membrane of these capillaries is of the interrupted type which contrasts with the well-developed basement membrane of the pulmonary capillaries. This type of loose structure is consistent with the very high permeability of the walls of the lymphatics to macromolecules which is of fundamental importance in a clearance system. There is, however, a long diffusion distance from the interalveolar space to the juxta alveolar lymphatic endings. Furthermore the average lymph flow is 400 times slower than the pulmonary blood flow (Meyer *et al.*, 1969). Despite these apparent disadvantages the very leaky nature of the terminal ends of the lymphatic capillaries compared to the vascular endothelium has been shown to result in a highly efficient lymphatic clearance of macromolecules introduced into the alveoli. Following instillation of albumin into the alveoli the amount of albumin cleared by the lymphatics was 37 times greater than that cleared by the capillaries (Meyer *et al.*, 1969).

The pathway of albumin through the normal alveolar epithelium in this type of experiment is probably not via the paracellular route because the equivalent pores are too small (1 nm). The more likely path is via pinocytosis through the cell wall itself.

The alveolar macrophage

Morphology

In contrast to the conducting airways where the major clearance mechanism is the mucociliary transport system, the alveolar macrophage is mainly responsible for clearing particles deposited in the alveoli. The role of the alveolar macrophage has been reviewed by Newhouse *et al.* (1976) and by Hocking and Golde (1979) and is the subject of rapidly expanding interest in pulmonary research. Alveolar macrophages vary in diameter from 15 to 50 μm, lie in contact with the surfactant lining of the alveoli (Weibel and Gil, 1968) and have a striking number of cytoplasmic inclusions which differ in smokers and non-smokers. In the former group, these inclusions are needle-like crystals of the aluminium silicate, kaolinite, which is present in cigarette smoke and is engulfed by the macrophages. The alveolar macrophages are readily obtained in animals and man by lung lavage. Several studies have shown that 1×10^5 cells are recovered per millilitre of lavage fluid in normal subjects (Reynolds and Newball, 1974; Weinberger *et al.*, 1978). Of these 86 per cent are macrophages, 10 per cent lymphocytes and 4 per cent neutrophils. In cigarette smokers the total number of cells recovered increases by a factor of two with a particular increase in the number of alveolar macrophages. In contrast, following inhalation of dust such as asbestos, there is a considerable increase in neutrophils similar to that seen in cryptogenic fibrosing alveolitis (Turner-Warwick *et al.*, 1981).

Origins of alveolar macrophages

Alveolar macrophages, like other monocytes, are ultimately derived from the bone marrow (Van Furth and Cohn, 1968). The alveolar macrophage has two developmental lines (Bowden and Adamson, 1982). Under normal circumstances the majority of cells originate directly from blood monocytes. Other alveolar macrophages may be derived from cells located in the interstitial space which may be marrow-derived colony-forming units. These may represent an important source of alveolar macrophages when the circulating monocyte supply to the lung is diminished as in some leukaemia patients (Golde *et al.*, 1974) or in animals following whole body irradiation (Bowden and Adamson, 1982).

Regulation of activity of alveolar macrophages

Antigens and lymphocyte dependent phagocytosis. Many of the inhaled particles which deposit in the alveolar region of the lung behave as antigens and initiate an immune response that involves cooperation between lung lymphocytes and alveolar macrophages. This response is two-fold: (a) antibody formation and (b) cellular reactions (Unanue, 1980). The B and T lymphocytes, derived from the bone marow and thymus respectively, are the specific antigen recognition cells. The B cells have antigen specific receptor proteins in their plasma membranes and form antibodies to specific antigens. The T cells exert a regulatory role having *helper* (TH), *suppressor* (TS) or *cytolytic* (TC) function. The alveolar macrophages, polymorphonuclear neutrophils and mast cells are the effectors whose role it is to remove bacterial, viral, toxic or inert particles that reach the alveoli.

The B cell recognition of antigen protein is controlled by the genetic code within the major histocompatibility complex (MHC). However, it should be remembered that immunity does not result simply from interactions between antigens and B lymphocytes but occurs only after prior contact between the antigen and the alveolar macrophage. As pointed out by Unanue (1980), macrophages (having non-specific function) and lymphocytes (having specific function) are interdependent, *one cannot function without the other*, the interrelationship being determined genetically by the immune response (Ir) genes which are located in the genetic segment labelled I in the MHC. In man, this location is termed HLA-D in contrast to the classic transplantation locations HLA-A, B, and C. The Ir genes control the degree of response (high or low) to proteins, the Ia antigens being surface proteins also coded in the I region. The Ia molecules of the macrophage control the recognition of antigen by the T cell. Not all macrophages bear the Ia molecule, only those that do can cooperate with the T cell. Thus the macrophage is not only a scavenger of antigen, but the antigen stimulates the alveolar macrophage to secrete biologically active molecules which regulate the function of the T cells. Stimulation of B lymphocytes requires not only antigen but a signal from the activated T lymphocyte (*Figure 8.1*).

The activated T cell stimulates the macrophage by secreting several powerful mediators called *lymphokines*. These lymphokines include chemotactic factor (CF), macrophage migration inhibition factor (MIF) and macrophage activating factor (MAF). Once the macrophages are activated by these lymphokines they operate independently of any lymphocyte control and mop up the antigens that initiated the original reaction.

Macrophages and neutrophils have surface membrane receptors for the Fc fragment of IgG and for C_3 which are both important opsonins in initiating particle attachment and phagocytosis (Rowlands and Daniels, 1975). The number and

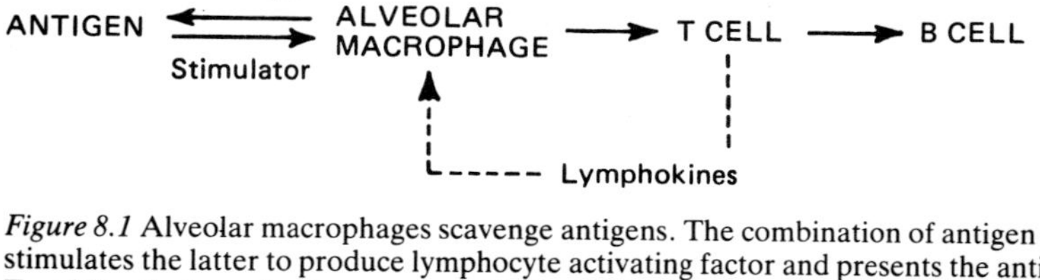

Figure 8.1 Alveolar macrophages scavenge antigens. The combination of antigen and macrophage stimulates the latter to produce lymphocyte activating factor and presents the antigen to the receptors on T and B cells. Lymphokines produced by lymphocytes regulate, in turn, the function of the macrophage

affinity of these receptors is increased by immunization with Bacillus Calmette-Guerin (Montarroso *et al.*, 1978). Specific antibody, administered either by intramuscular or aerosol route, will also enhance bacterial binding and phagocytosis.

Opsonin independent phagocytosis. In addition to antigen stimulation and activation by the opsonins IgG and complement, an opsonin independent system has recently been discovered which mediates phagocytosis of particulate activators by alveolar macrophages (Czop *et al.*, 1982). It has been shown that alveolar macrophages are effective phagocytes of some infectious particles in the absence of antibody. It was presumed that avid phagocytosis occurred as a result of direct interaction between the macrophage, plasma membrane and foreign particles. It has now been demonstrated that the alveolar macrophage, like the polymorphonuclear leukocyte (Roos *et al.*, 1981) and peripheral monocytes (Czop *et al.*, 1981), possesses a recognition unit on its plasma membrane that is specific for particles (such as zymosan) that activate the alternative pathway of complement. This implies that inhaled aerosols of infectious agents and toxins (e.g., endotoxin) which are capable of initiating the alternative complement pathway also initiate a phagocytic response as part of the alveolar clearance mechanism. Furthermore, it was found that the activity of this recognition unit was selectively augmented by the protein fibronectin (MW 440 000 daltons). Alveolar macrophages normally secrete fibronectin (Villiger *et al.*, 1982) which suggests a self-enhancing mechanism for the alveolar macrophage to augment its own phagocytic activity.

Alveolar macrophage function

Besides their *phagocytic* and *killing* activity alveolar macrophages have other important effector functions. These include the *secretion* of a vast number of mediators which are of fundamental importance in the cellular and humoral components of the inflammatory and immunological processes in the lung. Other effector functions not discussed here are their role in combating tumour growth, the remodelling of tissues and in healing of lung injury.

Phagocytic and killing function. Considerable attention is being directed to the killing mechanisms of alveolar macrophages and polymorphonuclear neutrophils (Hocking and Golde, 1979; Weissman *et al.*, 1980; Badwey *et al.*, 1979). The process of phagocytosis by alveolar macrophages and neutrophils has been divided into seven stages (Stossel, 1976) (*Table 8.1*).

Stossel and Hartwig (1975; 1976) showed that contact and recognition of particles by the cell membrane of the macrophage activated a system of contractile proteins in regions of pseudopod formation in the macrophage wall which were responsible for pseudopod movement and engulfment of the particle. Once engulfed, a

TABLE 8.1. Sequence in phagocytosis by alveolar macrophages and neutrophils

1. Particle recognition
2. Reception of message to initiate phagocytosis
3. Transmission of message from receptor to effector
4. Adhesion of cell membrane to particle
5. Assembly of pseudopodia
6. Particles engulfed by pseudopodia
7. Fusion of pseudopodia

bacterial particle may be subject to a poorly understood microbicidal mechanism. Non-bacterial particles may also react with the macrophage depending on the physicochemical properties of the particle. The main microbicidal mechanisms within the alveolar macrophage and neutrophil include:

1. Generation of hydrogen peroxide
2. Catalase transfer from the granular fraction of the cytoplasm
3. Lysosomal enzymes and lysosomal cationic proteins
4. The superoxide anion

Impairment of both phagocytosis and killing by alveolar macrophages may occur following virus infections (Jackab and Green, 1972; Warshauer *et al.*, 1977), ethanol, irradiation, cytotoxic and other drugs, metabolic acidosis, uraemia or hypoxia (Hocking and Golde, 1979).

Secretory functions of alveolar macrophages. Macrophages may also react with neutrophils, platelets and with the complement, kinin and coagulation cascades (Nathan *et al.*, 1980). All of these reactions may stimulate the secretory function of the alveolar macrophages. Among the most important secretory products which may affect both the adjacent inhaled particle and the integrity of nearby pulmonary tissue are *lysozymes* and *proteases* such as plasminogen activator, collagenase and elastase. Following activation of macrophages, the secretion of proteases by the macrophage is influenced in at least four ways (Nathan *et al.*, 1980).

1. By endotoxin, foreign proteins, bacteria or other inhaled particles.
2. By immune complexes which may augment or suppress the release of proteases.
3. By lymphokines which promote secretion not only of proteases but also prostaglandins. Newly formed prostaglandin reacts with endotoxin to stimulate macrophage secretion of collagenase.
4. By corticosteroid or indomethacin which suppress the secretion of certain proteases whereas phorbol esters and colchicine enhance it.

Alveolar macrophages not only interact with complement but also synthesize complement components. As pointed out by Nathan *et al.* (1980) the anaphytalox-ins C_3a and C_5a stimulate macrophage migration but a product of the alternative complement pathway,B_b, inhibits migration and promotes cell spreading over the alveolar surface.

Inhalation of acidic fumes or of acidic gastric contents stimulates the release of lysosomal acid hydrolases which were formerly regarded solely as intracellular digestive enzymes. Damage to surrounding lung cells may follow enzymatic degradation of collagen and basement membranes.

Not only are the hydrolases secreted into the external environment of the macrophage but so also are the same potent oxidizing mediators that are normally involved in *intracellular* killing. These potent oxidants are potentially very damaging to surrounding structures such as the alveolar epithelial wall. Until recently, however, it has not been possible to detect the functional consequences of this damage at an early stage in man. The new technique developed specifically to make such measurements (Jones *et al.*, 1982) will be discussed in the next section.

Stimulated macrophages also secrete endogenous pyrogen and are thought to be the only source of this small protein hormone (Nathan *et al.*, 1980). In addition to causing fever, endogenous pyrogen may be synonymous with 'lymphocyte activating factor' discussed under regulation of alveolar macrophages.

Alveolar clearance mechanisms

This will be discussed in four parts:

1. Absorption through epithelium
2. Phagocytosis of particles by macrophages
3. Transport pathways
4. Clearance kinetics

Absorption through the epithelial wall

We have emphasized that the alveolar epithelial wall presents a much greater barrier to the passage of lipid insoluble particles than does the endothelial wall. The two routes that may be taken by particles crossing the epithelial wall are *transcellular* and *paracellular*.

The transcellular path

Lauweryns and Baert (1977) have reviewed some aspects of macromolecular transport across the pulmonary epithelial cell and showed that particles of different size and chemical composition are handled in different ways by the alveolar epithelium. They compared the transepithelial transport of ferritin and carbon particles from the lung and showed that, whereas both particles were endocytosed by the alveolar type I cells, ferritin was transported across the epithelium much more readily than carbon. They noticed that carbon was endocytosed only when there was a relative excess of carbon particles in the alveoli compared to ferritin. Not all the ferritin was subsequently released into the interstitial space, a large number of these particles being digested by dense secondary lysosomes within the epithelial cells. Carbon, on the other hand, is released into the interstitial space, little appearing within epithelial lysosomes. Retention of carbon in the epithelial cell is associated with desquamation of these cells which are shed into the alveolar lumen. This desquamation is related not only to the load of inhaled dust but to the toxic physico-chemical properties of the particles. Cell death is most likely after absorption of toxic materials such as plutonium (Sanders and Adee, 1970) and asbestos (Suzuki *et al.*, 1972).

One of the dramatic differences in the distribution of ferritin and carbon in the lung is the appearance of the alveolar macrophages which absorb very much larger amounts of carbon than ferritin.

The paracellular path

Hydrophilic substances which are not transported through the cell can pass through the epithelium by passive diffusion through the junction: the paracellular pathway. The permeability of the alveolar epithelium is ten times smaller than the pulmonary vascular endothelium for hydrophilic solutes ranging in molecular weight from 50 to 100 000 daltons (Staub, 1974). As pointed out above this difference in permeability is a function of the tightness of the intercellular junctions of these two layers, the effective pore radius of the alveolar epithelium being about 1 nm and of the endothelium about 4–8 nm. It is known that the permeability of the *epithelial barrier* may increase considerably in a number of disease processes summarized in

TABLE 8.2. Factors associated with increased alveolar barrier permeability

Inhalation
Gastric contents
Fire smoke
Oxygen (prolonged high FIO_2)
Nitrogen dioxide
Ozone
Acrolein
Infections
Viral
Gram-negative bacteria
Pneumocystis Carinii
Legionella
Emboli
Fat
Air
Amniotic fluid
Drugs/Poisons
Aspirin
Bleomycin
Busulphan
Nitrofurantoin
Heroin
Alloxan
Paraquat
Ethchlorvynol
Miscellaneous
Uraemia
Neurogenic
Pancreatitis
Post-cardiopulmonary Bypass
Trauma

Table 8.2. The evidence for this increase in permeability is derived from measurements of an increase in the albumin concentration in pulmonary oedema fluid appearing in many of these conditions (Fein *et al*., 1980). This clearly implies that a severe abnormality of epithelial function may occur whereby albumin, with a molecular radius approximately 4 nm, can leak through the epithelial layer into the alveolar space. It is now known that lesser degrees of permeability defect can occur in the human alveolar epithelium (Jones *et al*., 1982) without there being pulmonary oedema or any other signs or symptoms. This has been demonstrated only recently using low molecular weight solutes as probes of epithelial permeability (Jones *et al*., 1980; Rinderknecht *et al*., 1980). This technique will be outlined below.

Measurement of permeability of the paracellular pathway in man. Method: We have used ^{99m}Tc diethylenetriamine pentacetic acid (^{99m}Tc DTPA) MW 492 daltons, approximate molecular radius 0.57 nm (Jones *et al*., 1980) as a probe molecule to derive an index of permeability of the paracellular pathway in the human lung. This probe molecule is one of a family of stable chelates that are chemically inert, electrically neutral and easily labelled with γ-emitting tracer molecules. Because of the small molecular radius compared to that of albumin an increased paracellular transport of this probe molecule is a more sensitive guide to increased epithelial permeability than that obtained using the protein. The probe molecule is introduced into the lung by inhalation and its rate of transfer from the alveoli to blood is measured either with the gamma camera or with a pair of scintillation detectors. Because the alveolar epithelium accounts for more than 90 per cent of the resistance to paracellular transport of hydrophilic molecules the technique is most sensitive to changes in epithelial permeability, large changes in endothelial permeability having only a small effect on the result (Jones *et al.*, 1982).

The γ-labelled probe molecule is deposited in the alveoli using an aqueous aerosol. This was generated using a standard Acorn jet nebulizer which produced particles up to 8 μm in diameter. To achieve a clinically useful mass of particles in the range 0.5–1 μm the output of the nebulizer was modified either by passing the aerosol through a horizontal plate elutriator or through a short (5 cm) column filled with 3 mm ball bearings (Jones *et al.*, 1983). This gives an aerosol with 90 per cent of particles <2 μm. The regional distribution of this aerosol in the lung in normal and abnormal subjects was very similar to the scintigrams produced with ^{81m}Kr. The alveolar deposition of small particles in abnormal lungs may be further enhanced if the carrier gas composition is 80 per cent helium and 20 per cent oxygen (Swift *et al.*, 1982).

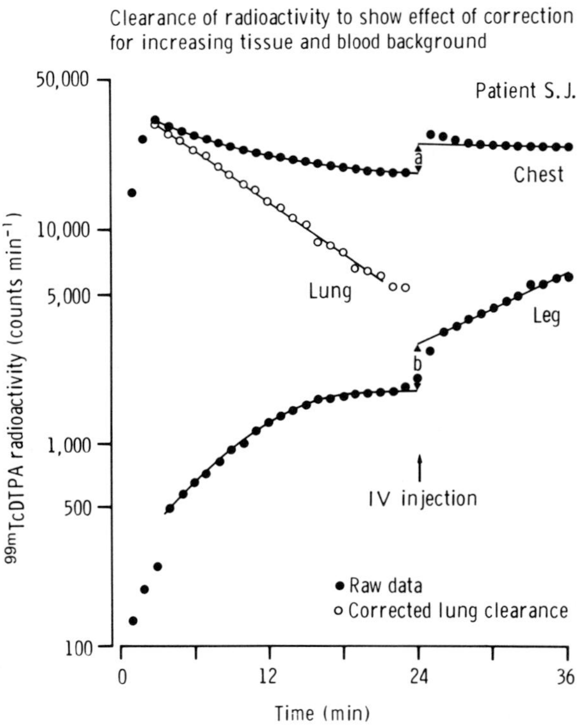

Figure 8.2 Shows the change in radioactivity (^{99m}Tc DTPA) measured with scintillation detectors over the chest (lung and pulmonary vascular tissue) and leg (vascular tissue). To derive a correction factor to eliminate the effect of radioactivity in pulmonary vascular tissue a small dose of ^{99m}Tc DTPA is injected intravenously. The quotient a/b is derived and used to multiply each value of leg activity which is then subtracted from the chest activity to give the lung clearance curve. The slope of this curve is expressed as the $T_{1/2}$LB which is the clearance rate from lung to blood. (From Jones *et al.* (1983) with permission of authors and publisher)

Subjects breathed the modified aerosol at a slow respiratory rate for 3 minutes then the rate of disappearance of the probe molecules from the lung was plotted and the transfer rate from lung to blood was calculated as previously described (Jones *et al.*, 1980). Particular emphasis is placed on corrections being applied for the contribution of radioactivity in vascular tissue within the field of the lung detector (Jones *et al.*, 1980). These corrections are omitted from the technique described by Rinderknecht *et al.* (1980), and this may result in large errors in deriving the index of permeability but also precludes the measurement of multi-exponential clearance curves, an important finding in cases of severe lung damage (Jones *et al.*, 1983; Royston *et al.*, 1983a). The index of pulmonary epithelial permeability is expressed as the half-time clearance rate of ^{99m}Tc DTPA from lung into blood ($T_{1/2}$LB).

Results; Cigarette smokers: Using this technique we have found that the epithelium of the normal lung presents a high degree of resistance to the trans epithelial transfer of these chelates, the mean $T_{1/2}$LB being 59 ± 5 min (sem). However, we have shown that symptomless cigarette smokers have a much greater epithelial permeability, the $T_{1/2}$LB being 17 ± 3 min (sem) (Jones *et al.*, 1980). This finding is consistent with the observation of Simani *et al.* (1974) that exposure of experimental animals to cigarette smoke leads to an increase in permeability of the intercellular epithelial junctions to the electron-dense tracer molecule, horse-radish peroxidase (MW 40 000 daltons). This is a considerably larger molecule (approximate molecular radius 2.5 nm) than ^{99m}Tc DTPA and implies that smoke may induce an increased permeability of the pulmonary epithelium to quite large molecules without causing epithelial damage of sufficient severity to induce oedema. In fact the changes in permeability of the junctions are probably

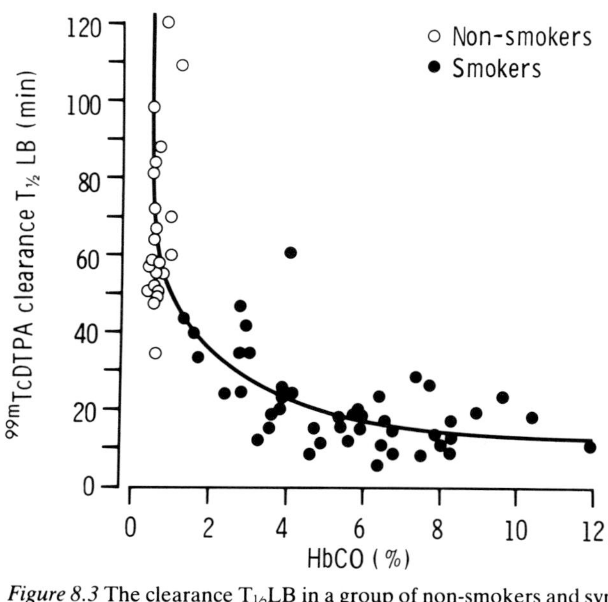

Figure 8.3 The clearance $T_{1/2}$LB in a group of non-smokers and symptomless cigarette smokers is plotted against the carboxyhaemoglobin (HbCO). A highly significant ($p < 0.001$) hyperbolic relationship exists between HbCO and $T_{1/2}$LB. This establishes a dose response relationship between cigarette smoke exposure and alveolar epithelial permeability. It does not necessarily imply that carbon monoxide itself is the causal agent of this abnormality. (From Jones *et al.* (1983) with permission of authors and publisher)

non-uniform, the transfer rate of hydrophilic solute through the epithelium being a function not only of the size but also the distribution of these functional pores.

The degree of increase in permeability ($T_{1/2}LB$) is related hyperbolically to cigarette smoke exposure represented by the carboxyhaemoglobin level in venous blood (*Figure 8.3*) (Jones *et al.*, 1983). This is not to say that epithelial damage is caused by carbon monoxide alone although we have shown that carbon monoxide exposure induces an increase in permeability in experimental animals (Fein *et al.*, 1979). With cessation of smoking there is a decrease in permeability both to ^{99m}Tc DTPA and to HRP (Minty *et al.*, 1981; Hulbert *et al.*, 1981). Although this occurred rapidly in animal experiments, in our human studies there was a significant improvement after one day without cigarettes, but even after three weeks the group had still not returned to the normal non-smoking range. The most rapid recovery was observed in subjects with the least increase in permeability.

The mechanisms of increased permeability in cigarette smokers and the significance of this change for the alveolar clearance of inhaled particles from the lung has yet to be determined. Cigarette smoke contains a vast number of toxic constituents that are capable of damaging epithelial surfaces directly. Alternatively, cigarette smoke exposure is a well known cause of proliferation of alveolar macrophages (Damarest *et al.*, 1979) and it has been postulated that these abnormal macrophages may release a number of elastolytic and proteolytic enzymes that are capable of damaging lung tissues (Hocking and Golde, 1979). Whether or not this chronic effect in loosening epithelial junctions is related to the subsequent development of emphysema is unknown.

There is still considerable conflict about the effect of cigarette smoking on transepithelial clearance of macromolecules and dusts. Although there may be an increased solute permeability of the epithelium, other adverse effects of cigarette smoke may impair the active cellular transport mechanisms which normally remove inhaled particles from the alveoli.

Other causes of an increased alveolar epithelial permeability: Inhaled toxic materials such as NO_2, SO_2, O_3, cadmium and asbestos are all capable of inducing epithelial damage either to the intercellular junctions or to the cell membranes themselves. Detailed studies of lung permeability after this type of exposure have not yet been reported in either animals or man. The technique using labelled chelates was originally developed to study alveolar epithelial permeability in animals (Jones *et al.*, 1978; 1982a). In these animal studies, changes were reported in epithelial permeability which were severe enough to lead to pulmonary oedema after inhalation of either hydrochloric acid or hypotonic saline (Jones *et al.*, 1978) and after fat embolism (Jones *et al.*, 1982b).

In a recent study in man we have shown that there is an increase in alveolar epithelial permeability after cardiopulmonary bypass (Royston *et al.*, 1983b). The latter observation is of particular interest in relationship to the aetiology of permeability type pulmonary oedema and the adult respiratory distress syndrome. There is a considerable body of evidence which suggests that damage to the alveolar/capillary interface may be caused by complement activation either by the classical or the alternative pathways (Jacob *et al.*, 1980; Hammerschmidt *et al.*, 1980; Craddock *et al.*, 1977). This leads to the production of C_3a and C_5a which are chemotactic for polymorphonuclear leucocytes causing them to aggregate on the vascular endothelium particularly in the lung. The activated polymorphs, together with further complement components up to C_9, may act as potent cell-wall damaging agents which are thought to increase the permeability not only of the endothelium but, because of its close proximity, the alveolar epithelium. Recent studies, however, showed that complement activation with cobra venom factor, zymosan activated plasma, or direct administration of C_5a (Webster *et al.*, 1982) or following intravenous endotoxin (Jones and Berry, 1983) produced a pulmonary aggregation of polymorphs, but caused no change in epithelial permeability. This implies that complement activation as an isolated event may be an insufficient insult to produce lung injury.

From these early experiments we conclude that the pulmonary epithelium, although normally a formidable barrier, can have its permeability altered very significantly by a number of physiological, chemical and immunological mediators that may be highly relevant to particle clearance through the alveolar epithelium. This change in the permeability of the epithelium may lead to increased absorption and clearance of some toxic materials into the lymphatics and capillaries and can be measured using a simple aerosol technique which can be applied to both animals and to man. The permeability technique is clearly of considerable but yet unexplored value in determining the degree of alveolar epithelial damage following inhalation of industrial dusts and other toxic aerosols. The relationship between increased alveolar epithelial permeability in cigarette smokers and the alveolar clearance of inhaled particles has not, so far, been clearly established.

One of the therapeutic implications of increased alveolar epithelial permeability is as follows. It has been shown that inhaling an aerosol of DTPA is of value in removing the transportable fraction of accidentally inhaled $^{238}PuO_2$ (Stather, personal communcation and Stather *et al.*, 1982). It was suggested that because of the longer retention time in the lung of inhaled DTPA compared to DTPA administered intravenously, the aerosol form of DTPA was much more effective in clearing $^{238}PuO_2$. The clearance half time of inhaled DTPA from the lung was about 75 minutes in the two subjects studied. This compares reasonably well with our non-smoking subjects but is almost an order of magnitude greater than some of our cigarette smokers. This implies that in smokers the method may not have such a great advantage over the intravenous administration and may have to be used more frequently in smokers than non-smokers to achieve the same clearance efficiency.

Phagocytosis of particles by macrophage

Effect of size and composition of particles on alveolar macrophage uptake

The majority of particles deposited in the alveoli are taken up by the alveolar macrophages which may be transported from the alveolar region to the ciliated airways where they are eliminated by mucociliary clearance. Alternatively, the macrophage, having phagocytosed the particles, may migrate through the epithelial wall into the interstitial space and either deposit the particles for distribution in the lymphatics or re-enter the airway in the ciliated zone (Lauweryns and Baert, 1977). The size of the particles determines not only the likelihood of deposition in the alveolar region but the probability of their being taken up by the alveolar macrophage (Hahn *et al.*, 1977). Following inhalation of particles in the aerodynamic diameter range 0.5–3.4 μm it was shown that the number of ingested particles (of either fused aluminosilicate or $^{239}PuO_2$) was proportional to the size of the particle. The optimum particle size for phagocytosis may be about 2–3 μm, polystyrene particles 6 μm in diameter being phagocytosed to a much smaller extent than 3 μm particles (Holma, 1967) and particles smaller in diameter than 0.26 μm being only minimally taken up by the macrophages. Other studies (Weisman and Korn, 1967) have shown that the rate of phagocytosis of polystyrene beads is a function of the mass of beads administered. This suggested that there was an accumulation of beads at specific sites on the cell surface until an optimum mass was reached at which time the beads were ingested.

Although small particles can be absorbed by alveolar macrophages in larger numbers they also exert a greater effect on the macrophage compared to the *same total mass* of large particles in the macrophage (Aranyi *et al.*, 1977). They compared particles of fly ash ranging from 2–8 μm which were either uncoated or coated with PbO, MnO_2 or NiO. It was evident that the smaller the particles, regardless of the coating, the greater was the impairment of viability of the macrophage per unit mass of particles. This is probably due to the larger total surface area of the small particles which results in greater interaction with the lysosomal membrane within the macrophage. This result differs somewhat from that reported by Sandusky *et al.* (1977), who showed that alveolar macrophages exposed to 5.7 μm polystyrene divinyl benzene beads released much more elastase and acid phosphatase than macrophages exposed to polystyrene latex beads 1.1 μm in diameter. Both sized particles were phagocytosed to the same degree by alveolar macrophages although the differences in chemical composition of the particles may have had important effects on the results.

The effect of the chemical composition of particles on phagocytosis by macrophages has been further studied by Camner and Lundborg (1977). They coated Teflon particles 4–5 μm in diameter with either carbon, manganese, aluminium, uranium, chromium or beryllium. Particles were exposed to alveolar macrophages either with or without added serum. The serum opsonins coat the particles and considerably increase phagocytosis. Carbon-coated particles were phagocytosed faster than any other type of particle in this study. The rates of phagocytosis were in the order carbon > aluminium and chromium > silver, manganese and uranium. Alveolar macrophages from animals previously exposed to nickel dust showed an enhanced ability to phagocytose both nickel- and silver-coated particles compared to non-exposed macrophages. It has also been noted (Johnson *et al.*, 1975) that macrophages from rabbits previously infected with bacteria cleared both the original bacteria and unrelated organisms to a greater extent than uninfected animals.

Effect of particle phagocytosis on chemotaxis of alveolar macrophages and neutrophils

The administration of different insoluble materials into the lung such as barium sulphate, carbon, coal dust and iron oxide results in an increased recovery of both alveolar macrophages and neutrophil cells in bronchoalveolar lavage (Brain, 1971). The response is maximal 24 hours after exposure and, for particles such as iron oxide, the alveolar leucocytes return to normal after 3 days (Kavet *et al.*, 1978). Following a single inhalation of 0.2 mg of quartz however, there is an interesting difference in the response of neutrophils and macrophages and there is a persistent increase in the number of alveolar leucocytes for at least 90 days (Morgan *et al.*, 1980). The rapid rise in neutrophils peaks after one day whereas the macrophage response peaks after 4 days (*Figure 8.4*). The number of neutrophils recovered is considerably greater than the number of alveolar macrophages, the peak response showing an 18-fold increase in neutrophils but only a 2-fold increase in macrophages.

One of the problems in evaluating the response of alveolar macrophages to these stimuli is equating the change in cell population in lavage fluid with the change in actual cell population in the lung. For example, if the function of the macrophage changed so that they could be more easily washed from the alveolar

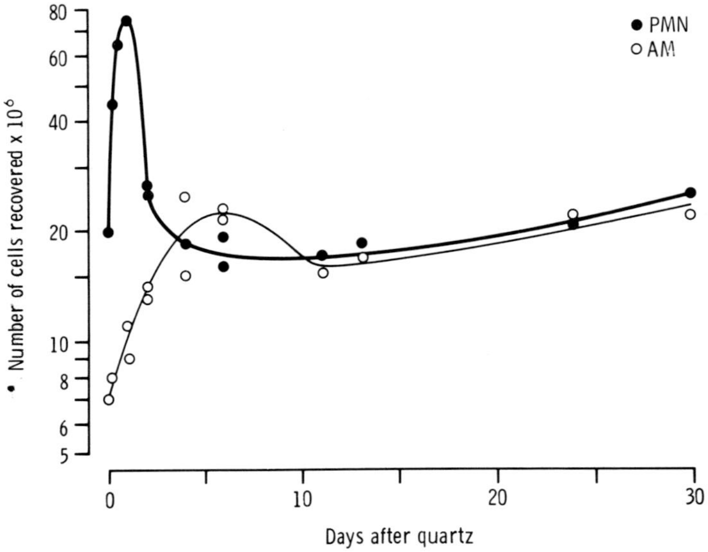

Figure 8.4 Following a single inhalation of quartz there is a difference in the time course and degree of response of the alveolar macrophages and the polymorphonuclear leucocytes. The persistently raised cell count is thought to be associated with chronic inflammation caused by quartz. Inert dusts produce a transient rise in cell count which falls within a day or so to control values

walls, there may be an increase in macrophages in lavage fluid without any real increase in macrophages in the lung. Morgan *et al.* (1980) have addressed this problem by quantitating not only the macrophages in the lavage fluid but also the macrophages in the lung by exposing the animals to an aersol of either ^{141}Ce-labelled cerium oxide or ^{233}Pu-labelled thorium oxide. In this way the total number of free alveolar macrophages in the lung could be estimated knowing the lung burden of radioactive dust and the average dust content per macrophage. This method confirmed that there was in fact a real increase in alveolar macrophages 4 days after quartz exposure. The increase in neutrophils was attributed to a brisk response to the chemotaxins released from injured macrophages which are damaged during particle phagocytosis. The initial release of neutrophil chemotactic factors from macrophages is unrelated to the cytotoxicity of the phagocytosed particles and occurs rapidly (<24 hours) after exposure to a particle load. The chronic elevation of neutrophils and macrophages may be an index of cytotoxicity (Morgan *et al.*, 1980).

Release of a neutrophil chemotactic factor from macrophages after phagocytosis of heat-killed staphylococcus aureus has been demonstrated by Hunninghake *et al.* (1978). This factor (MW 5000 daltons) is generated *in vivo* or *in vitro*. Release of macrophage factors chemotactic for macrophages themselves has been demonstrated by Miller *et al.* (1980). They showed that exposure of the lungs to quartz dust resulted in the release of specific chemotactic factors which may be the mechanism which directs macrophages to migrate into the alveolar spaces.

The effect of inhaled toxic material on alveolar macrophage function

Gases and vapours. Hocking and Golde (1979) have reviewed some of the toxic effects on alveolar macrophages. Relatively insoluble gases such as ozone and nitrogen dioxide pass into the alveolated part of the lung where they exert damaging effects on the alveolar macrophages. Both nitrogen dioxide and ozone reduce the phagocytic and bactericidal activity of alveolar macrophages and increase the susceptibility to bacterial infection. Alveolar macrophages are very sensitive to the effects of NO_2. Thirty minutes exposure of macrophages to 0.1–2 ppm resulted in a considerable decrease in both bactericidal activity and a reduced content of adenosine triphosphate (Dawson and Schenker, 1979).

In animals continuously exposed to different concentrations of NO_2 then challenged with an aerosol of streptococcus pyogenes, there was a distinct relationship between concentration of NO_2 and mortality (Gardner and Graham, 1977) (*Figure 8.5*). Mice were the most sensitive, hamsters had intermediate sensitivity and squirrel monkeys the least sensitivity to this effect of NO_2. The current United States ambient air quality standard for NO_2 is 0.05 ppm annual arithmetic mean of 24-hour values. The biological effect threshold is 0.5 ppm and the World Health Organisation recommends that 0.15 ppm should not be exceeded more than once per month.

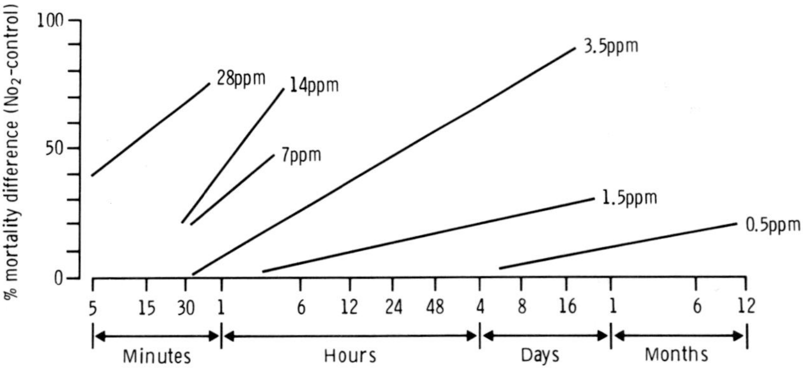

Figure 8.5 Groups of mice are exposed continuously to different concentrations of NO_2 then challenged by an inhalation of streptococci. The mortality was compared with that in non-challenged mice. (Redrawn from Gardner and Graham (1977), with permission of authors and publisher)

Exposure to 0.2 ppm ozone for 3 h also increases the mortality following challenge with streptococcus pyogenes (Coffin and Gardner, 1972). Nitrogen dioxide inhibits virus-induced production of interferon whereas ozone has no such effect. Prolonged exposure to high concentrations of oxygen can produce severe lung damage which may be related to release of free radicals from either macrophages or neutrophils (Deneke and Fanburg, 1982).

Non-gaseous toxins. Macrophages are also damaged by exposure to aerosols of nickel, cadmium, lead, manganese, chromium and vanadium (Hocking and Golde, 1979). The emphysema which develops in man after exposure to cadmium may be partly related to the damaged alveolar macrophages releasing lysosomal enzymes and proteases over long periods of time. The dust particles themselves are cytotoxic (Miller *et al.*, 1980) and the damaging effects of inhalation of these dusts may be due both to a direct effect on the epithelial walls and to an indirect effect from release of cytotoxic enzymes and free radicals from the alveolar macrophages. There are two consequences of this damage (1) the lung is less able to defend itself against exposure to further dust or bacteriologic loads and (2) enzymes are released by the macrophages which lead to damage to adjacent lung tissues (Hocking and Golde, 1979).

This suggests that following inhalation of such well-known toxic dusts as silica and asbestos lung injury may be initiated either by direct cytotoxic effect or by the proteolytic enzymes released after phagocytosis of these particles by the alveolar macrophages. An alternative mechanism for asbestos induced lung injury has recently been proposed by Schoenberger *et al.* (1982). They proposed that chrysotile asbestos, when introduced into the lung, induced a release of neutrophil chemotactic factor from the alveolar macrophage, particularly in the presence of serum which opsonizes the cells and enhances the release of chemotactic factor. This, together with asbestos induced complement activation was thought to enhance the cell damaging effect which was completed by the release of collagenase from neutrophils stimulated by macrophage derived neutrophil chemotactic factor.

Smoke inhalation. We have pointed out above that there are differences in the ultrastructure of macrophages in smokers and non-smokers. Inhalation of cigarette smoke may have divergent effects on the function of the alveolar macrophage (Demarest *et al.*, 1979). Acute and high levels of smoke exposure inhibit chemotactic response of the macrophage whereas low levels of exposure stimulate macrophage function (Holt and Keast, 1977). It is well known that cigarette smoking increases the yield of macrophages in alveolar lavage fluid by a factor of 4 (Demarest *et al.*, 1979). It is not known which cigarette smoke constituent is responsible for this effect but the latter authors suggest that the highly irritant aldehyde, acrolein, may be responsible. This may be the cause of the increased alveolar epithelial permeability that we have previously documented in man (Jones *et al.*, 1980) and in experiments on animals we have shown that 500 ppm of acrolein produces a severe permeability type pulmonary oedema (Beeley *et al.*, 1982). It also seems likely that the epithelial damage in cigarette smokers may be due to a macrophage mediated effect.

Fire smoke inhalation in man results in a rapid influx of neutrophils into the lung. It was suggested that this impaired the chemotaxis of macrophages possibly because of the release of enzymes from neutrophils such as proteases, elastase and cathepsin G, all of which inactivate complement derived chemotactic factors (Demarest *et al.*, 1979). Using our ^{99m}Tc DTPA technique for measuring alveolar epithelial permeability we have recently shown that a group of Naval fire-fighting instructors who were exposed daily to fire smoke had a significant increase in epithelial permeability. None of these subjects smoked cigarettes.

Transport pathways from the alveolar spaces

The nature of the barrier through which particles must pass from the alveolar space has been described and the various mechanisms that are responsible for removing particles deposited in the alveolar lumen have been reviewed. It has been pointed out that the two routes of clearance of phagocytosed particles are either to the ciliated region or into the lymphatic system (Lippmann *et al.*, 1980).

Having phagocytosed particles the macrophages may be transported from the alveolar walls to the ciliated region. This may occur because of the differences in surface tension between the two regions, the lower surface tension surfactant spreading into the higher surface tension in bronchial fluid carrying the macrophages with it. The gradient of interfacial tension along the walls of the conducting airways and alveoli is accentuated during each inspiration and this may enhance macrophage transport from the alveolar region.

The other route from alveolus to the bronchial tree is the interstitial path. This has been proposed and discussed at length by Brundelet (1965), Green (1973) and Lauweryns and Baert (1977), who showed that particle-laden macrophages pass through the epithelial wall into the lymphatic spaces. In these spaces, alveolar liquid, cells and uningested particles flow between alveoli in two possible directions (1) centripetally, in lymphatics that begin at the centre of the secondary lobule (centrilobular) as blind pouches which then run towards the hilum as periarteriolar periarterial lymphatics. (2) Centrifugally, to lymphatics that lie in the perivenous position (perilobular) around the margins of the lobules in subpleural or peribronchial positions. These, ultimately, also drain to the hilar lymph nodes.

At the level of the alveolar-bronchiolar junction there are small collections of lymphatic tissue which Macklin (1955) called the lymphatic sumps. These have been extensively studied by Brundelet (1965) and Green (1973), who showed that dust-laden macrophages which had passed through the alveolar wall into the lymphatics then re-entered the broncho-alveolar lumen at the sites of these lymph sumps.

The effect of particle load on the clearance mechanism was studied by Ferin (1977), using inhaled titanium oxide. At low concentrations the main clearance pathway was the mucociliary route involving macrophage phagocytosis of TiO_2. With an increasing load of TiO_2 there was an increased translocation into the lymphatic system. At lung loads greater than 1 mg per lung there was an abrupt increase in the TiO_2 in the hilar lymph nodes, the translocation to the lymph nodes being faster than total clearance from the lung (*Figure 8.6*).

They suggested that if alveolar macrophages can phagocytose only a small fraction of a large number of deposited particles, then non-phagocytosed particles may be translocated into lymphatics. Even at very low lung loads some particles will be found in the lymphocytes which have escaped the phagocytic action of the

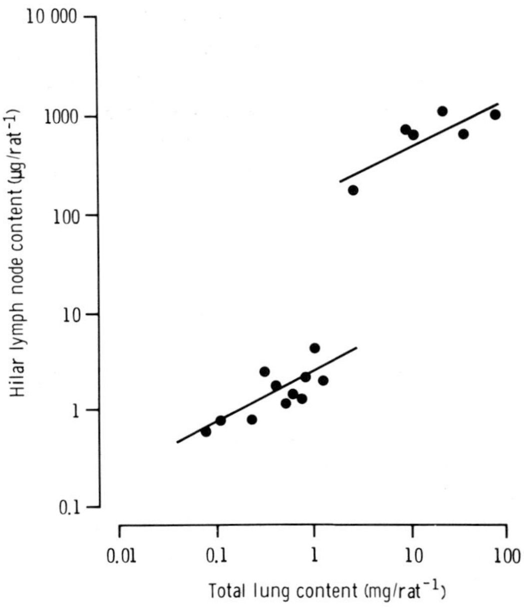

Figure 8.6 Plot of total lung content of titanium oxide on the first day following a single exposure against the amount transferred to the hilar lymph nodes 25 days post exposure. At 25 days with low exposure (<1 mg per rat) the alveoli still contain TiO_2 particles most of which lie within the alveolar macrophages. The hilar nodes are almost free of particles. At loads > 1 mg per rat there is an abrupt spill-over into the hilar nodes. (Redrawn from Ferin (1977) with permission of the author and publisher)

macrophage. The initial uptake of particles by macrophages is rapid and is increased with increasing numbers of macrophages by prior instillation of carbon (La Belle and Brieger, 1960) although the clearance rate from the lung itself is not affected.

In the case of asbestos, Morgan *et al.* (1977) found that whereas the initial deposition of dust in the lung was uniform, within a few months there was evidence of subpleural focal collections. They showed that following inhalation of asbestos, the uptake by macrophages was complete in 24 hours and that fibres longer than the diameter of the macrophage (12 μm) were found embedded in the alveolar wall. Shorter fibres are ingested by macrophages and transported to hilar nodes. Asbestos can also be phagocytosed by bronchial epithelium and can be transported intracellularly both free in the cytoplasm and in phagolysosomes (Craighead and Mossman, 1982).

In Heppleston's (1953) experiments with coal dust he found that most of it is rapidly taken up by alveolar macrophages. Initially scattered in the alveoli, coal dust later appeared in proximal alveoli in focal collections around the terminal bronchioles. The appearance of foci of atmospheric dust in the peribronchiolar and subpleural regions is also a well-known pathological feature of the lungs of town dwellers. Particles eliminated from the lung by mucociliary clearance are ultimately either expectorated or swallowed and eliminated from the gastrointestinal tract. This may be relevant to asbestos which is implicated in causing cancer of the alimentary tract and kidney although the carcinogenic potential of this dust in the gastrointestinal tract is low (Craighead and Mossman, 1982).

Alveolar clearance kinetics

It has been pointed out by Bohning *et al.* (1982) that there is little quantitative data on the alveolar clearance kinetics of insoluble particles in man. Because the potential hazard of inhaled particles is likely to increase in proportion to their residence time it is important to relate the clearance mechanisms to the clearance rate. There is an increasing concern about the health hazards of inhaled particles. Although the accumulation of certain types of dust is directly related to the development of lung disease, there is little data on the clearance rates of these dusts because of the health hazard in volunteer studies. Animal studies have been undertaken but the results are not easy to extrapolate to man. There is, however, a fairly characteristic pattern of clearance after deposition deep in the lung. Particles deposited in the conducting airways are removed in a day or so by mucociliary clearance. Particles deposited in the alveoli are cleared by a much slower process with a half-time ranging in man from 60 to several hundred days (Bailey *et al.*, 1982).

As indicated elsewhere in this book mucociliary transport rates show very wide variation between subjects but are reproducible within individuals, increasing with increasing airway size. The clearance time for large airways is 0.75 h, for intermediate airways about 3 h and for the small conducting airways about 24 h.

Clearance from the alveoli is represented by a multi-exponential curve which is thought to correspond to the different mechanisms of clearance. The fastest exponential with a half-time measured in days or weeks may correspond to clearance by alveolar macrophages. A slower phase with a half-time which may be hundreds of days is associated with the slow penetration through the alveolar epithelium of large insoluble particles. For example, haematite dust introduced into the lungs of cats, rats or hamsters has an initial fast clearance phase with a $T_{1/2}$ of about 10 days which precedes a second slower phase with a $T_{1/2} > 100$ days. The slow phase permeability of the epithelium to these particles is inversely related to molecular weight and particle size.

Most of the clearance data published in the literature is based on animal studies. *Table 8.3* summarizes the slow phase $T_{1/2}$ of a number of some compounds that have been used to study alveolar clearance in these experiments. In the majority of these studies this slow phase was preceded by a faster phase with a half time of about 10 days (Morrow *et al.*, 1966). Studies of the alveolar clearance kinetics in man are fairly limited. As pointed out by Lippmann *et al.* (1980) human studies have to be confined to non-toxic particles. These particles can be either radiolabelled or, if ferrimagnetic, detected with external electromagnetic coils.

TABLE 8.3. Half-time clearances from the alveoli of the slow phase of various particles in animals

	$T_{1/2}$ slow component days
$^{131}BaSO_4$	8
^{203}HgO	33
$^{54}MnO_2$	34
$^{59}Fe_2O_3$	58
UO_2	>200
Coal dust	>700

Studies by Bohning *et al.* (1982) using 3.6 μm (MMAD) diameter polystyrene particles labelled with ^{85}Sr showed that clearance occurred in at least two phases with half-times of about 30 and 296 days, the fast component clearing about 27 per cent of the inhaled particles. They argued, as pointed out above, that the fast component was probably explained by macrophage clearance and the slow component by passive penetration of the alveolar epithelium. They found that cigarette smokers not only lost the fast clearance phase but had evidence suggestive of an accelerated clearance in the slow phase in the early years of smoking and a prolongation of the slow phase in later years. The abolition of fast phase clearance in smokers was attributed to the toxic effects of cigarette smoke on alveolar macrophages.

In a similar study in man Bailey *et al.* (1982) examined the clearance rate of 1.2 μm and 3.9 μm diameter fused aluminosilicate particles labelled ^{85}Sr and ^{88}Y respectively. Three phase exponential clearance curves were found with half-times of about 1 day, 20 days and >300 days. The data suggested that the fastest component corresponded to mucociliary clearance of particles deposited in conducting airways. The fraction of lung associated with the intermediate phase was greater for the 3.9 μm particles. There was however a wide individual variation in long-term clearance which was thought to be more important than that of particle size from the point of an occupational health standpoint. The latter workers also tabulated the available clearance data in man for 14 other studies of the clearance of labelled iron oxide and polystyrene. The published curves in limited numbers of smokers and non-smokers showed a very wide distribution of half-times which ranged from 33 to 750 days. There appeared to be no consistent difference in clearance between these two groups.

The other approach to measuring dust retention and clearance from the alveoli is magnetopneumography. This is a non-invasive technique for estimating the amount of magnetizable dusts in the lung (Kalliomaki, 1977). Cohen (1973) was the first to observe that weak magnetic fields could be detected over the chest of subjects who had inhaled ferrimagnetic particles. The apparatus used has been described by Cohen (1973) and Freedman *et al.* (1981). It consists of a pair of large electromagnetic coils for magnetization of the intrapulmonary particles and a separate magnetometer called a superconducting quantum interference device (SQUID) for measuring remnant magnetic moment (RMM) induced by the coils. Using the latter device as little as 0.02 mg of Fe_3O_4 can be detected in the lungs. They found that after inhaling 2.8 μm (MMAD) particles of Fe_3O_4 non-smoking subjects had multiexponential curves with an average half-time of about 70 days. In the three cigarette smokers studied the half-time was >300 days. These are very small numbers of smokers but the authors were confident that they were representable results. In a different study Freedman *et al.* (1982) examined the retention of ferrimagnetic dust in the lung of several different occupational groups. These included steel arc welders, machinists, coal miners, former asbestos insulators and controls. As expected the welders had very much greater lung metal content than the other group. This correlated well with the numbers of years of exposure and radiographic abnormality but not with cigarette smoking history. This evidence seems to conflict with the apparent delayed clearance of magnetic particles in smokers reported by Cohen *et al.* (1979).

Further studies are indicated to establish a clearer relationship between alveolar clearance mechanisms and the different phases of the alveolar clearance curves and elucidate the effects of smoking on particle retention in the lung. If smoking does retard toxic particle elimination from the alveoli then there is an increased risk of lung damage. This may be the basis of the increased susceptibility to lung cancer in asbestos workers who smoke cigarettes. Our studies (Jones *et al.*, 1982) and those of Inoue *et al.* (1976) clearly show an increased alveolar permeability to low molecular weight water soluble particles in man and animals exposed to cigarette smoke. This increase in permeability may not be relevant to the direct clearance through the epithelial wall of larger molecular weight particles. Nevertheless it is a clear indicator of damage to the alveolar epithelium. The delay in clearance of the early phase of clearance has been attributable to effects of toxic dusts on the macrophage phase of clearance. This effect does not appear at first sight to explain the delay in the slow phase of clearance although Ogden (1982) suggests that the double exponential clearance curve is not necessarily representative of two clearance mechanisms. His suggestion is that if two clearance mechanisms were working simultaneously on a dust load, the clearance curve would not appear as two exponentials but as one, whose delay constant would be the sum of the constants of two constituent exponentials. Thus if the epithelial permeability were increased by, say, a factor of 3, but the macrophage transport reduced by a much greater factor, there could well be a delay in the summed clearance curve.

On the basis of our study of the functional effects on the alveolar epithelium of inhaled particles, such as cigarette smoke, it is certainly technically easier and quicker to measure the effects of inhaled particles on alveolar wall function. Using this technique one can evaluate the effects of different toxic aerosols on alveolar permeability and relate these functional changes both to aerosol composition and concentration and to the detailed responses of the alveolar macrophage and neutrophil population.

Acknowledgement

The author acknowledges the contributions of his colleagues: B. Minty, D. Royston and N. Veall.

References

ARANYI, C., ANDRES, S., EHRLICH, R., FENTERS, J.D., GARDNER, D.E. and WATERS, M.D. (1977). Cytotoxicity to alveolar macrophages of metal oxides adsorbed on fly ash. In *Pulmonary macrophage and epithelial cells*. Edited by Sanders, C.L., Schneider, R.P., Dagle, G.E., and Ragan, H.A. Virginia; Technical Information Center, Energy Research & Development Administration

BADWEY, J.A., CURNUTTE, J.T. and KARNOVSKY, M.L. (1979). The enzyme of granulocytes that produces superoxide and peroxide. *New Eng. J. Med.*, **300**, 1157–1160

BAILEY, M.R., FRY, F.A. and JAMES, A.C. (1982). The long-term clearance kinetics of insoluble particles from the human lung. *Ann. Occup. Hyg.*, **26**, 273–290

BEELEY, J.M., CROW, J., JONES, J.G., LYNCH, R.D., MINTY, B. and PRYCE, P. (1982). Treatment of inhalation damage to the lungs with corticosteroids. *Am. Rev. Resp. Dis.*, **125**, 156

BOHNING, D.E., ATKINS, H.L. and COHN, S.H. (1982). Long-term particle clearance in man; normal and impaired. *Ann. Occup. Hyg.*, **26**, 259–271

BOWDEN, D.H. and ADAMSON, I.Y.R. (1982). Alveolar macrophage response to carbon in monocyte-depleted mice. *Am. Rev. Resp. Dis.*, **126**, 708–711

BRAIN, J.D. (1971). The effects of increased particles on the number of alveolar macrophages. In *Inhaled particles III,* Proceedings of a BOHS Symposium, London, Sept. 1970. pp. 200–233. London; Unwin Brothers Ltd.

BRUNDELET, P.J. (1965). Experimental study of the dust clearance mechanism of the lung. *Acta. Pathol. Microbiol. Scand.*, **175**, 1–141

CAMNER, P. and LUNDBORG, M. (1977). Alveolar macrophages and Teflon particles coated with carbon and metals. In *Pulmonary macrophage and epithelial cells*. Edited by Sanders, C.L., Schneider, R.P., Dagle, G.E. and Ragan, H.A. Virginia; Technical information center. Energy Research and Development Administration, pp. 405–413

COFFIN, D.L. and GARDNER, D.E. (1972). Interaction of biological agents and chemical air pollutants. *Ann. Occup. Hyg.*, **15**, 219–234

COHEN, D. (1973). Ferromagnetic contamination in the lungs and in other organs of the human body. *Science*, **180**, 745–748

COHEN, D., ARAI, S.F. and BRAIN, J.D. (1979). Smoking impairs long-term dust clearance from the lung. *Science*, **204**, 514–517

CRADDOCK, P.R., FEHR, J., DALMASSO, A.P., BRIGHAM, K.L. and JACOB, H.S. (1977). Hemodialysis leukopenia. Pulmonary vascular leukostasis resulting from complement activation by dialysis cellophane membranes. *J. Clin. Invest.*, **59**, 879–888

CRAIGHEAD, J.E. and MOSSMAN, B.T. (1982). The pathogenesis of asbestos-associated diseases. *New. Eng. J. Med.*, **306**, 1446–1455

CZOP, J.K. McGOWAN, S.E. and CENTER, D.M. (1982). Opsonin-independent phagocytosis by human alveolar macrophages: Augmentation by human plasma fibronectin. *Am. Rev. Resp. Dis.*, **125**, 607–609

DAWSON, S.V. and SCHENKER, M.B. (1979). Health effects of inhalation of ambient concentrations of nitrogen dioxide. *Am. Rev. Resp. Dis.*, **120**, 281–292

DEMAREST, G.B., HUDSON, L.D. and ALTMAN, L.C. (1979). Impaired alveolar macrophage chemotaxis in patients with acute smoke inhalation. *Am. Rev. Resp. Dis.*, **119**, 279–286

DENEKE, S.M. and FANBURG, B.L. (1982). Oxygen toxicity of the lung: an update. *Br. J. Anaesth.*, **54**, 737–750

FEIN, A., GROSSMAN, R.F., JONES, J.G., HOEFFEL, J. and McKAY, D. (1980). Carbon monoxide effect on alveolar epithelial permeability. *Chest*, **78**, 726–731

FEIN, A., GROSSMAN, R.F., JONES, J.G., OVERLAND, E., PITTS, L., MURRAY, J.F. and STAUB, N.C. (1979). The value of edema fluid protein measurement in patients with pulmonary edema. *Am. J. Med.*, **67**, 32–38

FERIN, J. (1977). Effect of particle content of lung on clearance pathways. In *Pulmonary macrophage and epithelial cells*. Edited by Sanders, C.L., Schneider, R.P., Dagle, G.E. and Ragan, H.A. Virginia; Technical Information Center, Energy Research & Development Administration, pp. 414–423

FREEDMAN, A.P., ROBINSON, S.E. and GREEN, F.H.Y. (1982). Magnetopneumography as a tool for the study of dust retention in the lung. *Ann. Occup. Hyg.*, **26**, 319–335

FREEDMAN, A.P., ROBINSON, S.E., O'LEARY, K., GOODMAN, L. and STELLMAN, J.M. (1981). Non-invasive magnetopneumographic determination of lung dust loads in steel arc welders. *Br. J. Ind. Med.*, **38**, 384–388

GARDNER, D.E. and GRAHAM, J.A. (1977). Increased pulmonary disease mediated through altered bacterial defenses. In *Pulmonary macrophage and epithelial cells.* Edited by Sanders, C.L., Schneider, R.P., Dagle, G.E. and Ragan, H.A. Virginia; Technical Information Center, Energy Research & Development Administration, pp. 1–21

GIL, J., BACHOFEN, H., GEHR, P. and WEIBEL, E.R. (1979). Alveolar volume-surface area relation in air—and saline-filled lungs fixed by vascular perfusion. *J. Appl. Physiol.*, **47**, 990–1001

GOLDE, D.W., FINLEY, T.N. and CLINE, M.J. (1974). The pulmonary macrophage in acute leukaemia. *N. Engl. J. Med.*, **290**, 875–878

GONZALEZ-CRUSSI, F. and BOSTON, R.W. (1972). The absorptive function of the neonatal lung. Ultrastructural study of horseradish peroxidase uptake at the onset of ventilation. *Lab. Invest.*, **26**, 114–121

GREEN, G.M. (1973). Alveolobronchial transport mechanisms. *Arch. Intern. Med.*, **131**, 109–114

GUYTON, A.C. and MOFFAT, D.S. (1981). Role of surface tension and surfactant in the transepithelial movement of fluid and in the development of pulmonary edema. *Prog. Resp. Res.*, **15**, 62–75

HAHN, F.F., NEWTON, G.J. and BRYANT, P.L. (1977). *In vitro* phagocytosis of respirable-sized monodispersed particles by alveolar macrophages. In *Pulmonary macrophages and epithelial cells.* Edited by Sanders, C.L., Schneider, R.P., Dagle, G.E. and Ragan, H.A. Virginia; Technical Information Center, Energy Research & Development Administration, pp. 424–435

HAMMERSCHMIDT, D.E., WEARER, L.J., HUDSON, L.D., CRADDOCK, P.R. and JACOB, H.S. (1980). Association of complement activation and elevated plasma CSa with adult respiratory distress syndrome. *Lancet*, **1**, 947

HEPPLESTON, A.G. (1953). Pathological anatomy of simple pneumoconiosis in coal workers. *J. Path. Bacter.*, **66**, 235–246

HILLS, B.A. (1982). What forces keep the air spaces of the lung dry. *Thorax*, **37**, 713–717

HOCKING, W.G. and GOLDE, D.W. (1979). The pulmonary alveolar macrophage. *New Eng. J. Med.*, **301**, 580–587, 639–645

HOIDAL, J.R. and NIEWOEHNER, D.E. (1982). Lung phagocyte recruitment and metabolic alterations induced by cigarette smoke in humans and hamsters. *Am. Rev. Resp. Dis.*, **126**, 548–552

HOLMA, B. (1967). Lung clearance of mono- & di-disperse aerosols determined by profile scanning and whole body counting: A study on normal and SO_2 exposed rabbits. *Acta. Med. Scand.* (Suppl.), **473**, 1–102

HOLT, P.G. and KEAST, D. (1977). Environmentally induced changes in immunological function. Acute and chronic effects of inhalation of tobacco smoke and other atmospheric contaminants in man and experimental animals. *Bacteriol. Rev.*, **41**, 205–216

HULBERT, W.C., WALKER, D.C., JACKSON, A. and HOGG, J.C. (1981). Airway permeability to horseradish peroxidase in guinea pigs: the repair phase after injury by cigarette smoke. *Am. Rev. Resp. Dis.*, **123**, 320–326

HUNNINGHAKE, G.W., GALLIN, J.I. and FAUCI, A.S. (1978). Immunologic reactivity of the lung. The *in vivo* and *in vitro* generation of a neutrophil chemotactic factor by alveolar macrophages. *Am. Rev. Resp. Dis.*, **117**, 15–23

INOUE, S., MICHEL, R.P. and HOGG, J.C. (1976). Zonulae occludentes in alveolar epithelium and capillary endothelium of dog lungs studied with the freeze fracture technique. *J. Ultrastruct. Res.*, **56**, 215–225

JACKAB, G.J. and GREEN, G.M. (1972). The effect of Sendai virus infection on bactericidal and transport mechanisms of the microme lung. *J. Clin. Invest.*, **51**, 1989–1998

JACOB, H.S., CRADDOCK, P.R., HAMMERSCHMIDT, D.E. and MOLDOW, C.F. (1980). Complement-induced granulocyte aggregation. An unsuspected mechanism of disease. *New Eng. J. Med.*, **302**, 789–794

JOHNSON, J.D., HAND, W.L., KING, N.L. and HUGHES, C.G. (1975). Activation of alveolar macrophages after lower respiratory tract infection. *J. Immunol.*, **115**, 80–84

JONES, J.G. and BERRY, M. (1983). Pulmonary function following intravenous E. coli 0111:B4 endotoxin. *Br. J. Anaesth.*, **55**, 245–246P

JONES, J.G., MINTY, B.D. and ROYSTON, P. (1982a). The physiology of leaky lungs. *Br. J. Anaesth.*, **54**, 705–721

JONES, J.G., ROYSTON, D. and MINTY, B.D. (1983). Changes in alveolar-capillary barrier function. *Am. Rev. Resp. Dis.*, **127**, S51–S59

JONES, J.G., BERRY, M., HULANDS, G.H. and CRAWLEY, J.C.W. (1978). The time course and degree of change in alveolar-capillary membrane permeability induced by aspiration of hydrochloric acid and hypotonic saline. *Am. Rev. Respir. Dis.*, **118**, 1007–1013

JONES, J.G., MINTY, B.D., ROYSTON, D. and ROYSTON, P. (1983). Carboxyhaemoglobin and pulmonary epithelial permeability. *Thorax.*, **38**, 129–133

JONES, J.G., MINTY, B.D., LAWLER, P., HULANDS, G., CRAWLEY, J.C.W. and VEALL, N. (1980). Increased alveolar epithelial permeability in cigarette smokers. *Lancet*, **1**, 66–68

JONES, J.G., MINTY, B.D., BEELEY, J.M., ROYSTON, D., CROW, J. and GROSSMAN, R.F. (1982b). Pulmonary epithelial permeability is immediately increased after embolisation with oleic acid but not with fat. *Thorax*, **37**, 169–174

KALLIOMAKI, P.L., KARP, P.J., KATILA, T., MAKIPAA, P. and TOS-SAVAINEN, A. (1976). Magnetic measurements of pulmonary contamination. *Scand. J. Work Environ. Health*, **4**, 232–239

KALTREIDER, H.B., KYSELKA, L. and SALMON, S.E. (1974). Immunology of the lower respiratory tract II. The plaque-forming response of canine lymphoid tissues to sheep erythrocytes after intrapulmonary air intravenous immunization. *J. Clin. Invest.*, **54**, 262–270

KAVET, R.I., BRAIN, J.D. and LEVENS, D.J. (1978). Characteristics of pulmonary macrophages lavaged from hamsters exposed to iron oxide aerosols. *Lab. Invest.*, **38**, 312–319

KEFALIDES, N.A. (1966). A collagen of unusual composition and a glycoprotein isolated from canine glomerular basement membrane. *Biochem. Biophys. Res. Commun.*, **22**, 26–32

La BELLE, C.W. and BRIEGER, H. (1960). The fate of inhaled particles in the early post exposure period. II. The role of pulmonary phagocytosis. *Arch. Environ. Health*, **1**, 423–427

LAUWERYNS, J.M. and BAERT, J.H. (1977). Alveolar clearance and the role of the pulmonary lymphatics. *Am. Rev. Resp. Dis.*, **115**, 625–683

LIPPMANN, M., YEATES, D.B. and ALBERT, R.E. (1980). Deposition, retention, and clearance of inhaled particles. *Br. J. Ind. Med.*, **37**, 337–362

MACKLIN, C.C. (1955). Pulmonary sumps, dust accumulations, alveolar fluid and lymph vessels. *Acta. Anat. (Basel)*, **23**, 1–21

MASON, R.J., WILLIAMS, M.C. and WIDDICOMBE, J.H. (1982). Secretion of fluid transport by alveolar type II epithelial cells. *Chest*, **5**, 615–635

MEYER, E.C., DOMINGUEZ, E.A. and BENSCH, K.G. (1969). Pulmonary lymphatic and blood absorption of albumin from alveoli. A quantitative comparison. *Lab. Invest.*, **20**, 1–8

MILLER, K., CALVERSLEY, A. and KAGAN, E. (1980). Evidence of a quartz-induced chemotactic factor for guinea pig alveolar macrophages. *Environ. Res.*, **22**, 31–39

MINTY, B.D., JORDAN, C. and JONES, J.G. (1981). Rapid improvement in abnormal pulmonary epithelial permeability after stopping cigarettes. *Br. Med. J.*, **282**, 1183–1186

MONTARROSO, A.M. and MYRUICK, Q.N. (1978). Effect of BCG vaccination on the IgG and complement receptors on rabbit alveolar macrophages. *J. Reticuloendothelial Soc.*, **24**, 93–99

MORGAN, A., HOLMES, A. and TALBOT, R.J. (1977). The fate of inhaled asbestos fibres deposited in the rat lung: A quantitative approach. In *Pulmonary macrophage and epithelial cells*. Edited by Sanders, C.L., Schneider, R.P., Dagle, G.E. and Ragan, H.A. Virginia; Technical Information Center, Energy Research & Development Administration

MORGAN, A., MOORES, S.R., HOLMES, A., EVANS, J.C., EVANS, N.H. and BLACK, A. (1980). The effect of quartz, administered by intratracheal instillation, on the rat lung. 1. The cellular response. *Environ. Res.*, **22**, 1–12

MORROW, P.E., GIBB, F.R. and GAZIOGLU, K. (1966). The clearance of dust from the lower respiratory tract of man: An experimental study. In *Inhaled particles and vapours II*. Edited by Davies, C.N. Oxford; Pergamon Press, 351–358

NATHAN, C.F., MURRAY, H.W. and COHN, Z.A. (1980). Current Concepts: The macrophage as an effector cell. *N. Eng. J. Med.*, **303**, 622–625

NEWHOUSE, M., SANCHIS, J. and BIENENSTOCK, J. (1976). Lung defense mechanisms. *New Eng. J. Med.*, **295**, 1045–1052

OGDEN, T.L. (1982). Discussion. *Ann. Occup. Hyg.*, **26**, 290

OYARZUN, M.J. and CLEMENTS, J.A. (1977). Ventilatory and cholinergic control of pulmonary surfactant in the rabbit. *J. Appl. Physiol.*, **43**, 39–45

OYARZUN, M.J. and CLEMENTS, J.A. (1978). Control of lung surfactant by ventilation, adrenergic mediators and prostaglandins in the rabbit. *Am. Rev. Resp. Dis.*, **117**, 879–891

PASTERNACK, A., LINDER, E. and KUHLBACK, B. (1965). Glomerulonephritis with initial pulmonary haemorrhage. *Acta. Med. Scand.*, **177**, 601–605

REYNOLDS, H.Y. and NEWBALL, H.H. (1974). Fluid and cellular milieu of the human respiratory tract. *J. Lab. Clin. Med.*, **84**, 559–573

RINDERKNECHT, J., SHAPIRO, L., KRAUTHAMMER, M., TAPLIN, G., WASSERMAN, K., USZLER, J.M. and EFFROS, R.M. (1980). Accelerated clearance of small solutes from the lungs in interstitial lung disease. *Am. Rev. Respir. Dis.*, **121**, 105–117

ROOS, D., BOT, A.A.M., van SCHAIK, M.L.J., de BOER, M. and DAHA, M.R. (1981). Interaction between human neutrophils and zymosan particles: The role of opsonin & divalent cations. *J. Immunol.*, **126**, 433–440

ROWLANDS, D.T. and DANIELE, R.P. (1975). Surface receptors in the immune response. *N. Eng. J. Med.*, **293**, 26–32

ROYSTON, D., MINTY, B., LOCKWOOD, G. and JONES, J.G. (1983a). An Index of the permeability factor (Kep) and pulmonary oedema in man. *Br. J. Anaesth.*, **5**, 246

ROYSTON, D., MINTY, B., JONES, J.G., WALLWORK, J. and HIGENBOTTAM, T. (1983b). Alveolar-capillary barrier permeability to ^{99m}Tc-DTPA following cardiopulmonary bypass. *Thorax*, **38**, 236

SANDERS, C.L. and ADEE, R.R. (1970). Ultrastructural localization of inhaled 239 PuO_2 particles in the alveolar epithelium and in macrophages. *Health Phys.*, **18**, 293–295

SANDUSKY, C.B., COWDEN, M.W. and SCHWARTZ, S.L. (1977). Effect of particle size on regurgitative exocytosis by rabbit alveolar macrophages. In *Pulmonary macrophage and epithelial cells*. Edited by Sanders, C.L., Schneider, R.P., Dagle, G.E. and Ragan, H.A. Virginia; Technical Information Center, Energy Research and Development Administration, pp. 85–105

SCHNEEBERGER-KEELEY, E.E. and KARNOVSKY, M.J. (1968). The ultrastructural basis of alveolar-capillary membrane permeability to peroxidase used as a tracer. *J. Cell. Biol.*, **37**, 781–793

SCHOENBERGER, C.I., HUNNINGHAKE, G.W., KAWANAMI, O., FERRANS, V.J. and CRYSTAL, R.G. (1982). Role of alveolar macrophages in asbestosis: modulation of neutrophil migration to the lung after acute asbestos exposure. *Thorax*, **37**, 803–809

SIMANI, A.S., INOUE, S. and HOGG, J.C. (1974). Penetration of the respiratory epithelium of guinea pigs following exposure to cigarette smoke. *Lab. Invest.*, **31**, 75–81

STAEHELIN, L.A. and HULL, B.E. (1978). Junctions between living cells. *Sci. Am.*, **238**, 140–152

STATHER, J.W., STRADLING, G.N., SMITH, H., PAYNE, S., JAMES, A.C., STRONG, J.C., HAM, S., SUMNER, S.,BULMAN, R.A., HODGSON, A., TOWNDROW, C. and ELLENDER, M. (1982). Decorporation of $^{238}PuO_2$ from the hamster by inhalation of chelating agents. *Health Physics*, **42**, 520–525

STAUB, N.C. (1974). Pulmonary edema. *Physiol. Rev.*, **54**, 678–811

STAUB, N.C. (1978). Pulmonary edema due to increased microvascular permeability to fluid and protein. *Circ. Res.*, **43**, 143–151

STAUB, N.C. (1981). Pulmonary edema due to increased microvascular permeability. *Ann. Rev. Med.*, **32**, 291–312

STOSSEL, T.P. (1976). The mechanism of phagocytosis. *J. Reticuloendothel. Soc.*, **19**, 237–245

STOSSEL, T.P. and HARTWIG, J.H. (1975). Interactions between actin, myosin and an actin binding protein from rabbit alveolar macrophages: alveolar macrophage myosin MG_{2+}-adenosine triphosphatase requires a cofactor for activation by actin. *J. Biol. Chem.*, **250**, 5706–5712

STOSSEL, T.P. and HARTWIG, J.H. (1976). Interactions of actin, myosin and a new actin binding protein of rabbit pulmonary macrophages II. Role in cytoplasmic movement and phagocytosis. *J. Cell Biol.*, **68**, 602–619

SUZUKI, Y., CHURG, J. and ONO, T. (1972). Phagocytotic activity of the alveolar epithelial cells in pulmonary asbestosis. *Am. J. Pathol.*, **69**, 373–388

SWIFT, D.L., CARPIN, J.C. and MITZNER, W. (1982). Pulmonary penetration and deposition of aerosols in different gases: fluid flow effects. *Ann. Occup. Hyg.*, **26**, 109–117

TURNER-WARWICK, M., HASLAM, P.L., LUKOSZEK, A., TOWNSEND, P., ALLAN, F., DuBOIS, R.M., TURTON, C.W.G. and COLLINS, J.V. (1981). Cells, enzymes and interstitial lung disease. *J. Roy. Coll. Phys. Lond.*, **15**, 5–16

UNANUE, E.R. (1980). Cooperative between mononuclear phagocytes and lymphocytes in immunity. *New. Eng. J. Med.*, **303**, 977–985

VAN FURTH, R. and COHN, Z. (1968). The origin and kinetics of mononuclear phagocytes. *J. Exp. Med.*, **128**, 415–433

VILLIGER, G., HEYMACH, G.J., BROEKELMANN, T.J., KELLEY, D.G., KUHN, C. and McDONALD, J.A. (1982). Human bronchoalveolar fibronectin. Quantification of an opsonic protein and its synthesis by alveolar macrophages. *Chest*, **81**, 455–475

WARSHAUER,D., GOLDSTEIN, E. and AKER, S. (1977). Effect of influenza viral infection on the ingestion and killing of bacteria by alveolar macrophages. *Am. Rev. Resp. Dis.*, **115**, 269–277

WEBSTER, R.O., LARSEN, G.L., MITCHELL, B.C., GOINS, A.J. and HENSON, P.M. (1982). Absence of inflammatory lung injury in rabbits challenged intravascularly with complement derived chemotactic factors. *Am. Rev. Res. Dis.*, **125**, 335–340

WEIBEL, E.R. and GIL, J. (1968). Electron microscopic demonstration of an extracellular duplex lining layer of alveoli. *Respir. Physiol.*, **4**, 42–57

WEINBERGER, S.E., KELMAN, J.A., ELSON, N.A., YOUNG, R.C., REYNOLDS, H.Y., FULMER, J.D. and CRYSTAL, J.D. (1978). Bronchoalveolar lavage in interstitial lung disease. *Ann. Intern. Med.*, **89**, 459–466

WEISMAN, R.A. and KORN, E.D. (1967). Phagocytosis of latex beads by acanthaemoeba I. Biochemical Properties. *Biochemistry*, **6**, 485–497

WEISSMANN, G., SMOLEN, J.E. and KORCHAK, H.M. (1980). Release of inflammatory mediators from stimulated neutrophils. *N. Eng. J. Med.*, **303**, 27–34

WILSON, T.A. (1981). Effect of alveolar wall shape on alveolar water stability. *J. Appl. Physiol.*, **50**, 222–224

Chapter 9

Therapeutic aerosols

Stephen P. Newman

The inhaled route for respiratory drugs

Therapy of respiratory disorders by inhalation has been practised for thousands of years, with records dating back to ancient civilizations in several parts of the world. These involved primarily the inhalation either of hot aromatic vapours or of smokes derived from burning various types of plant leaf. Until the isolation of beta adrenoreceptor stimulants during the first half of this century, the most effective drugs for the treatment of asthma were atropine-like compounds such as Atropa Belladona and Datura Strammonium. Indeed, the asthma cigarette, comprising trace quantities of the latter compound, proved to be an effective bronchodilator. The development of both modern technology and medical research has led to tremendous strides not only in the types of drug available for treating respiratory disorders, but also in the range of devices for delivering these drugs as aerosols to the respiratory tract.

The inhaled route has several well-recognized advantages over other routes for administration of drugs to the respiratory tract. Since the drug is delivered directly to its required site of action, only a small quantity is required for an adequate therapeutic response, and there is consequently a low incidence of systemic side-effects compared to oral or intravenous administration. Furthermore, the onset of action of inhaled drugs is generally more rapid than that achieved by oral delivery. At least one bronchodilator drug is claimed to yield a significant improvement in lung function within 30 seconds of being inhaled.

Several problems or disadvantages have been proposed for inhaled therapeutic agents, but many of these can be dismissed on closer examination (Clark, 1979; 1982). It has been suggested, for instance, that therapeutic aerosols do not reach the lung periphery in patients with obstructive airway disease, and that effectiveness might be reduced in the presence of mucus hypersecretion. However, studies of bronchodilator response have shown enhancement of tests thought to reflect primarily 'small' airway obstruction, and excess mucus does not seem to be a problem unless the airways are actually plugged. Although it has been suggested that patients maintained for long periods on bronchodilators might develop tolerance to the acute effects of these drugs, tolerance does not occur in asthmatic subjects for the dose levels normally administered (Paterson *et al.*, 1979; Tattersfield, 1982). Fears about the safety of bronchodilator drugs delivered by chlorofluorocarbon propellants from metered dose inhalers have proved largely unfounded. Propellants may cause heart palpitations if used in sufficient quantity, but metered dose aerosols are believed to be safe if used in the recommended dose (*Lancet*, 1975).

The real problems of aerosol therapy stem from the simple fact that it is much harder to inhale an aerosol than to swallow a tablet. The lungs have evolved in such a way that it is quite difficult for inhaled particles to penetrate deeply into the respiratory tract unless they are of an ideal size and are inhaled in the correct manner. There is great potential for misuse of inhalation devices and patients are often instructed inadequately about the limitations of aerosol therapy. Physicians must ensure that patients receive adequate tuition in the use of inhalation devices and should check regularly that no faults have developed in patient technique (Crompton, 1982). Although many patients may have difficulty using particular inhalation devices (notably the metered dose inhaler), these problems can be overcome by use of an alternative type of delivery system. In addition to using inhalation devices correctly patients must know the circumstances under which to use the various types of drug, and that medical advice should be sought if the inhaled treatment ceases to be effective. At the same time, the pharmaceutical companies and the manufacturers of nebulizers must ensure that the aerosols being administered to patients are in fact suitable for inhalation. It may be little use to administer a drug by the inhaled route if the drug particles are too large to pass into the lungs or if the inhaler or nebulizer is used in such a way that delivery to the lungs is very low.

There is no doubt that a variety of drugs delivered as aerosols are very effective in the treatment of a range of respiratory disorders, and this has been demonstrated in many clinical trials. By contrast, little emphasis has been placed upon the scientific background of aerosol therapy, and little attention paid to the aerodynamic behaviour of therapeutic aerosols. This problem was highlighted by Brain (1980), reporting on the proceedings of the second 'Sugarloaf' Symposium on the scientific basis of respiratory therapy. The major recommendation for research on aerosol and humidity therapy was for studies of the 'distribution of retained clinical aerosols and its relation to response'. More specifically it was stated that the 'effects of particle size, breathing patterns, lung volume, pulmonary disease and airway caliber on the spatial distribution of aerosols within the respiratory tract should be determined'. A number of other deficiencies in our knowledge were pointed out, in particular the inadequate characterization of therapeutic aerosols, the need to quantify the smallest drug dose which will give an optimal therapeutic effect, and the importance of correlating the site of drug deposition with the location of receptor sites.

In trying to solve some of these problems, the physical scientist can play an important role. In particular, he can help to ensure that the various inhalers and nebulizers are designed in such a way that they produce aerosols of the right size, and furthermore that the devices are used so as to optimize bioavailability of the drug. This chapter will discuss recent work involving aerosolized drugs which has gone some way to fulfilling the needs outlined above. The types of inhalation device and respiratory drug and the features that we require of therapeutic aerosols and their delivery systems will be outlined. Recent research and development aimed at improving the efficiency of aerosol therapy will then be discussed for each type of inhalation device in turn.

Preliminary considerations

Choice of inhalation device

There are essentially three types of delivery system for therapeutic aerosols—the nebulizer, the pressurized metered dose inhaler (MDI), and the dry powder inhaler—all of which were illustrated and described in detail in Chapter 4. Nebulizers convert a liquid into a fine mist, either by means of compressed gas (jet nebulizer), or by high frequency sound waves (ultrasonic nebulizer). The MDI consists of the drug either suspended or dissolved in chlorofluorocarbon propellants at a high pressure. Each time the inhaler is actuated, a metered quantity of drug is released in the form of a spray. In the dry powder inhaler, the drug is present as a finely-milled powder in a gelatin capsule, mounted in a special breath-actuated device. The patient's inspiratory effort produces a turbulent airstream which serves to empty the contents of the capsule.

Each type of device has a role to play. MDIs are very popular, particularly for bronchodilator therapy, because of their compactness, unobtrusiveness, portability and apparent simplicity of use. Dry powder inhalers though less convenient could directly replace MDIs should the use of chlorofluorocarbon propellants be proscribed at some future date, but at present dry powder inhalers are reserved chiefly for those patients who have difficulty mastering the technique of using MDIs. Nebulizers are the least portable type of inhalation device, since the jet nebulizer generally requires either an electrically-driven compressor, an air or oxygen cylinder, or even a foot-pump to drive it. Hand-held squeeze-bulb nebulizers exist, but these are rarely used for oral inhalation now. The ultrasonic nebulizer requires access to a mains electricity supply, and as in the case of jet nebulizers, portability is limited. However, nebulizer therapy is particularly useful in hospitals or in the home under a variety of circumstances, for instance when the patient does not respond to therapy administered from an MDI, or when emergency treatment is required. Furthermore, there is greater flexibility in the range of drug solution that may be nebulized compared to MDIs and to dry powder inhalers. Since a range of inhalation devices exists, patients finding difficulty with a particular device can be given treatment with an alternative type, so that the benefits of the inhaled route can be made available to most patients. There is probably little clinical difference between the results of treatment with the various devices, providing that the patient's condition is stable and the devices are used correctly (Lourenço and Cotromanes, 1982a).

Types of aerosolized drugs

Bronchodilators are the most widely used form of therapeutic aerosol. They can act rapidly to reverse bronchospasm in asthmatic subjects, but in addition when given regularly they may exert a prophylactic effect in asthmatics and bronchitics alike. There are three types of bronchodilator—sympathomimetic (beta-adrenergic agonist), anticholinergic and methyl xanthine (Paterson, 1977; Paterson *et al.*, 1979). Sympathomimetic agents stimulate adrenergic receptors on smooth muscle cells in the airway walls, causing relaxation of smooth muscle fibres and subsequent bronchodilatation. Adrenaline and isoprenaline (*Figure 9.1*) were used for this purpose in the first half of this century, but these compounds also produce unwanted cardiovascular side-effects since isoprenaline stimulates beta receptors in the heart while adrenaline stimulates both alpha and beta receptors causing

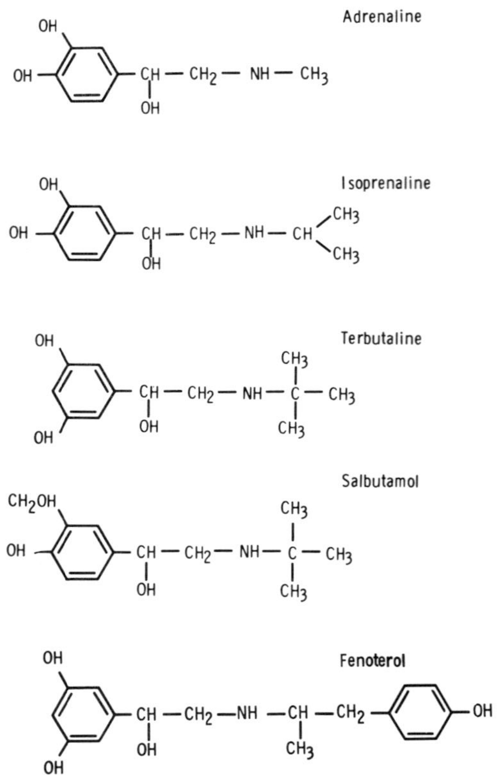

Figure 9.1 Chemical structures of 5 beta-adrenergic stimulants. Although their formulae are basically similar to those of adrenaline and isoprenaline, greater beta-2 selectivity in terbutaline, salbutamol and fenoterol have been achieved by alterations in the substituent group at the amine end of the molecules. Alterations in the hydroxyl groups on the benzene ring prevent the action of catechol-*O*-methyl transferase on terbutaline, salbutamol and fenoterol, and this may explain their relatively long durations of action

tachycardia and hypertension. During the last 15 years, a group of compounds have been introduced which act selectively on the beta-2 receptors in the bronchial tree in doses of only a few hundred micrograms, whilst having little effect on cardiac beta-1 receptors or on alpha receptors (Leifer and Wittig, 1975). Terbutaline, salbutamol and fenoterol (*Figure 9.1*) are three of the best known selective beta-2 stimulants. Differences in their chemical structures compared to those of adrenaline and isoprenaline give not only greater selectivity, but also generally ensure a longer duration of action than non-selective beta-stimulants. Although anticholinergic substances have long been known as bronchodilators, their use has been restricted owing to fears that they may dry lung secretions and cause mucus plugging. However, the synthetic anticholinergic agent, ipratropium bromide, appears not to possess this undesirable side-effect, and in the normal therapeutic dose has no adverse effect on the rate of mucus clearance from the lung. Ipratropium bromide has a slower onset of action compared to the selective beta-2 stimulants, but its duration of action is similar, and it is effective when as little as 40 μg is administered from an MDI. Methyl xanthines such as theophylline and aminophylline are effective oral bronchodilators, but clinical trials with these compounds in aerosol form have been limited. A minimum serum level of this type of drug following systemic absorption may be required for effective bronchodilatation.

Sodium cromoglycate (SCG) is not a bronchodilator, in that it is not effective once bronchoconstriction has occurred, but is very useful as a prophylactic agent in preventing the onset of asthmatic attacks (Cox, 1969). It is believed to inhibit the release of chemical mediators from mast cells in bronchial smooth muscle, hence preventing the onset of bronchoconstriction. Although this substance is available in an MDI, or as a nebulizer solution, it is best known as a dry powder in gelatin capsules delivered from the breath-actuated 'Spinhaler' device.

Corticosteroids (Williams, 1974) are frequently used for treatment of asthma or bronchitis in those patients whose symptoms cannot be controlled adequately by bronchodilators or sodium cromoglycate. Although their mechanism of action is poorly understood, it is probable that they decrease airway resistance by an anti-inflammatory effect. However, oral corticosteroids have drawbacks, since regular treatment with large doses may give rise to a number of undesirable systemic side-effects, notably suppression of the hypothalamic-pituitary-adrenal axis and the development of Cushingoid features. These problems appear to have been partially solved by several new aerosolized corticosteroids, of which beclomethasone dipropionate, betamethasone valerate and budesonide are the best known. Since these drugs are effective when delivered from an MDI in doses of only a few hundred micrograms, systemic side-effects do not normally occur, although local side-effects (oropharyngeal candidiasis and dysphonia) are observed in a small proportion of patients.

Nebulizers may be used to produce aerosols of several other types of compound, including 'bland' aerosols of distilled water or saline intended to produce humidification (Miller, 1973). The value of antibiotic therapy has been questioned in the past (Williams, 1974), but recently a combination of two nebulized antibiotics (carbenicillin and gentamicin) were found to be an effective form of treatment for respiratory tract infection in patients with cystic fibrosis (Hodson *et al.*, 1981). Other less common therapeutic aerosols have included mucolytics such as 2-mercapto-ethane-sulphonate and *n*-acetylcysteine, prophylactic agents such as ketotifen and clemastine, prostaglandins, local anaesthetics, surfactants, and even vaccines for the prevention of influenza and tuberculosis (Lourenço and Cotromanes, 1982b).

Site of action

Despite their widespread use, the site to which even the most commonly used therapeutic aerosols should be delivered is still very imprecisely understood. Most investigations into this question have involved sympathomimetic or anticholinergic bronchodilators since their rapid effect can be closely monitored. The available evidence points to a topical action, since maximal response to a beta-agonist occurs within minutes of inhalation, when plasma levels of drug are very low. Many bronchodilators are effective by the oral route in doses approximately ten times those required by aerosol, and it is possible that a proportion of the therapeutic effect from a bronchodilator aerosol arises from drug deposited in the oropharynx and then absorbed either via the buccal mucosa or from the gastrointestinal tract. However, the swallowed fraction is largely metabolized in the gut wall or liver and only a small proportion enters the circulation in an active form. Several studies in which a few hundred micrograms of beta-agonist have been placed deliberately in the buccal cavity of subjects with reversible airways obstruction, and therefore not inhaled, have found that this mode of administration is ineffective (Newman *et al.*, 1981a).

It is safe to say that the majority of the therapeutic effect attained from an inhaled beta-agonist is derived from the fraction of the dose deposited in the lungs (Paterson *et al.*, 1979), and that the first requirement of this type of compound as well as that of most other aerosolized drugs, is to deliver an adequate amount to the lungs. Beta-agonists probably act primarily by a direct effect on bronchial smooth muscle, although absorption of the drugs via the airways and subsequent redistribution to the lungs via the systemic circulation may also play a role. However, this will depend upon the degree to which the drug is metabolized within the body, and this will in turn depend upon the site from which absorption takes place. The large airways are drained by the bronchial veins, and drugs absorbed from this site will be recirculated and will reach the lungs as if by intravenous injection. The blood supply to the smaller airways drains directly into the pulmonary veins and absorbed drugs will pass into the left ventricle and could undergo 'first-pass' metabolism in the liver before reaching the lungs again. The cardiac stimulating effects of inhaled beta-agonists are thought to be derived chiefly from the fraction of the dose deposited in the lungs and absorbed via the airways (Paterson *et al.*, 1979), although the incidence of these side-effects is low.

While the necessity for delivering respiratory drugs to the lungs is well established, the exact locations of the receptor sites within the bronchial tree are poorly understood. Many studies have compared the effects of beta-agonists and anticholinergic agents on tests of lung function thought to reflect either 'small' or 'large' airway calibre, and although on balance the results suggest that beta-agonists act primarily on small airways while anticholinergic agents act primarily on the larger airways (Ingram *et al.*, 1977; Hensley *et al.*, 1978), the studies have not been in agreement (Douglas *et al.*, 1979; Tashkin *et al.*, 1980). Direct identification of the location of receptor sites by light microscopic autoradiography (Barnes *et al.*, 1982) may be more helpful. These have indicated that in the ferret lung, the highest concentrations of beta-receptors are in the small conducting airways with lower concentrations in the larger airways. There are also good numbers of receptors in alveolated zones. These findings suggest that beta-agonists should be directed towards the peripheral airways, although probably for the time being, the safest policy is to aim to distribute the particles throughout the large airways, small airways and alveolated zones.

Requirements of delivery systems

From the above considerations, it is possible to list the criteria for an 'ideal' delivery system. Such a system should permit the drug particles to reach the lungs, and there should be only minimal losses in the oropharynx, on the inhalation apparatus and in the exhaled air. Drug efficacy should be reproducible, and there should be neither systemic nor local side-effects. The inhalation device should be simple to use, portable, unobtrusive and cost-effective. The devices currently available do not meet these requirements well. In particular, only about 10 per cent of the available dose reaches the lungs from metered dose inhalers, nebulizers and dry powder inhalers. The MDI is portable and unobtrusive, but many patients find it difficult to use. Nebulizers on the other hand, are easier to use, but are more bulky and less portable than MDIs. Practical necessities and limitations are a major reason why inhalation devices are less than ideal in their characteristics, and it is unlikely that a perfect inhaler will ever be devised. However, there is no doubt that existing systems can produce aerosols more suitable for inhalation, and can be used more satisfactorily by patients if the limitations of the inhalation devices are better understood and if proper account is taken of the laws governing aerosol behaviour.

Factors affecting drug deposition

As previously described in Chapter 3, several processes account for the deposition of aerosols within the respiratory tract, or on the inhalation apparatus itself. For therapeutic aerosols, losses of drug by inertial impaction within the upper airways or within the inhalation device predominate. As will be described, only a small proportion of the dose reaches the bronchial tree, and here deposition will take place by a combination of impaction (in the large central airways) and gravitational sedimentation (in the smaller peripheral airways and in alveolated zones).

Many factors affect aerosol deposition (Chapter 3) but essentially these can be simplified into (a) particle aerodynamic diameter (the product of diameter and the square root of particle density), (b) inhalation mode and (c) the physical characteristics of the subject who inhales the aerosol. Within certain limitations, it is possible to alter particle size and mode of inhalation to deliver aerosol to the lungs of patients with a wide range of airway obstruction. In order to improve drug delivery, it is necessary to reduce impaction losses which take place before the aerosol has a chance to get to the bronchial tree.

Aerosol size is probably the most important factor determining the site of deposition. Typical deposition patterns for monodisperse aerosols of various sizes inhaled by normal subjects during steady breathing are shown in *Figure 9.2*. Submicronic particles will either be exhaled or delivered entirely to the alveolated zones, while at the other end of the scale, particles >8 μm aerodynamic diameter may be deposited primarily in the oropharynx and cannot reach the lungs. Oropharyngeal deposition rises to about 100 per cent for particles of aerodynamic

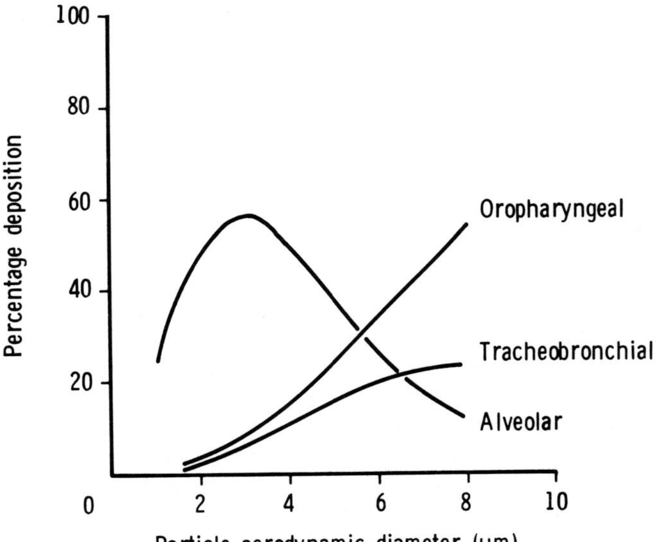

Figure 9.2 Schematic deposition patterns for stable particles in the size range 1 to 8 μm inhaled during steady breathing conditions by normal subjects. Below 1 μm aerodynamic diameter, few particles deposit on the conducting airways, while the majority of the aerosol is deposited in the oropharynx if particle size exceeds 8 μm

diameter 15 μm. It is difficult to specify an 'ideal' size for a therapeutic aerosol, partly because it is not certain where the aerosol should be deposited within the lungs, and partly because of the difficulty of predicting the aerodynamic behaviour of therapeutic aerosols. These aerosols are heterodisperse and are inhaled during very artificial breathing manoeuvres by patients with abnormal airways. Deposition patterns are further complicated by a number of factors including evaporation, hygroscopic growth and particle agglomeration. However, some general conclusions can be drawn from what we know about stable aerosols. Particles in the 1 to 5 μm size band are likely to be delivered to all parts of the lung—that is, to large airways, small airways and alveoli—with only small oropharyngeal losses. Providing the size distribution is not too wide (geometric standard deviation, GSD $\lesssim$2.0), the mass median aerodynamic diameter (MMAD) is a good index of the effective aerosol size (Task Group on Lung Dynamics, 1966), and this suggests that the manufacturers of respiratory drugs and inhalation devices should aim to deliver an aerosol with an MMAD below 5 μm, and with a GSD not exceeding 2.0. Further evidence is required, however, to support the use of aerosols confined entirely to the submicronic range.

In addition to changes in particle aerodynamic diameter, drug delivery may also be altered substantially by changes in the inhalation mode. Slow, deep inhalation is likely to deliver an aerosol to peripheral parts of the lung, and a subsequent period of breath-holding enables particles to sediment under gravity at their furthest point of penetration. By contrast, rapid inhalation enhances deposition in the oropharynx and in large central airways.

As the severity of airway obstruction increases, the probability of impaction in central airways rises, and aerosols are less able to reach the lung periphery. This suggests that smaller aerosols should be used to treat severely obstructed patients, and perhaps also for treating children. However, it is unclear how practical such an approach would be, and it would certainly add to the complexity of aerosol therapy. Over and above any effects of airway obstruction on aerosol deposition, there is also a wide inter-subject variability in aerosol deposition, so that an apparently optimal inhalation manoeuvre may result in low lung deposition in some patients.

Nebulizers

Fundamentals

While it is possible to estimate on a theoretical basis the 'ideal' size of a therapeutic aerosol, it is by no means clear that nebulizers are either designed or used in such a way that aerosols of this size are produced. The details of particle size given by the manufacturers of nebulizers is often very sparse and very misleading. For instance, it is common to quote the distribution of particles by number, and information is often limited to a statement that no more than a certain fraction of particles exceeds a given size. However, while the number distribution is of interest, it is much less important than the mass distribution. Therapeutic aerosols are generally heterodisperse (GSD > 1.22, Chapter 3), and under these circumstances, the number distribution and the mass distribution of aerosols may be very different (*Figure 9.3*). The majority of the mass of a heterodisperse aerosol may be contained in few, relatively large, particles, since the mass of a particle is proportional to the cube of its diameter. Particle size information restricted to the number distribution only can

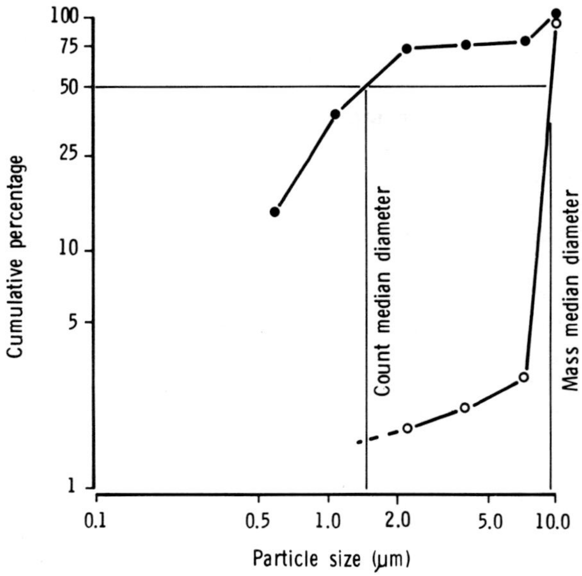

Figure 9.3 Comparison of number and mass distributions for a commercially available jet nebulizer (Hudson 'Up-draft'). The manufacturer's data sheet states that 77 per cent of the particles are <10 µm diameter, and the cumulative number distribution (closed circles) indicates a count median diameter between 1 and 2 µm. This would suggest that the aerosol is ideal for inhalation. However, the cumulative mass distribution (open circles), calculated from the number distribution, is totally different since more than 95 per cent of total mass comprises droplets outside the respirable range. The mass median diameter is close to 10 µm (this is an underestimate since it has been assumed in this calculation that the largest particles in the distribution are no more than 10 µm in diameter)

give a very false impression of the true aerosol characteristics. Proper sizing measurements, quoting MMAD and GSD, are of vital importance if a nebulizer is to be assessed for its ability to provide an aerosol within the respirable range.

The size distributions of aerosols released from jet and ultrasonic nebulizers have been reviewed by Mercer (1981). The mass median diameters (MMDs) of aerosols from jet nebulizers ranged between 1.2 and 6.9 µm (GSDs 1.7–2.2), and the MMDs from ultrasonic nebulizers were 3.7 to 10.5 µm (GSDs 1.4–2.0). At first sight, these size distributions seem suitable for inhalation, with the possible exception of aerosols released from some types of ultrasonic nebulizer. However, it must be borne in mind that these sizes were measured as the aerosols left the nebulizers, in other words after the larger droplets had impacted on baffles and other structures within the devices themselves and had been returned to the nebulizer reservoirs. The internal design of the nebulizer will play a major part in determining the size of particles released. The baffles within the nebulizer must be designed in such a way as to trap large particles, but to permit as many particles as possible within the respirable range to leave the device. The operating characteristics of the nebulizers have an important influence on the sizes of the aerosols released. The MMD of aerosols released from jet nebulizers is inversely proportional to the flow rate of compressed gas through the device (Clay *et al.*, 1983a), and hence it is important to state not only the characteristics of the aerosol produced, but also the precise conditions under which this aerosol is generated. Aerosol size may lie outside the 'ideal' size band if jet nebulizers are operated at only 4 ℓ min^{-1}, and flow rates of 6 or 8 ℓ min^{-1} may be required for optimal aerosol characteristics. The size of aerosols released from ultrasonic nebulizers is inversely proportional to the operating frequency, but it is often not possible for the user to alter this.

It is also of fundamental importance to know both the rate of aerosol output, and the total amount of drug released from nebulizers. If a jet nebulizer is weighed intermittently as nebulization proceeds, then it is possible to assess both the mass of aerosol released per unit time, and ultimately the total amount of solution released. Output rate is proportional to the rate of gas flow through the nebulizer. When the nebulizer ceases to emit aerosol, it is important to note that it is not empty. As much as half the solution initially placed in the reservoir remains in the nebulizer as a 'dead volume', being trapped as droplets on baffles and other internal structures. The greater the volume of nebulizer solution placed initially in the reservoir, the smaller the percentage dead volume (Clay *et al.*, 1983a). 4–6 ml of solution is required for more efficient emptying of the reservoir, in contrast with the drug companies' data compendium sheets, which often recommend a volume fill of only 2 ml.

During the first few minutes of nebulization, there is a small initial drop in nebulizer output rate, probably related to the marked temperature drop (~10 deg C) which occurs in the reservoir soon after nebulization commences. This in turn may affect the physical characteristics of the nebulizer solution. The temperature drop also means that patients inhale a cold aerosol, which could induce bronchoconstriction. By contrast, aerosols released from ultrasonic nebulizers are relatively warm, since they are electrically generated. It should also be borne in mind that owing to solvent evaporation, the drug solution becomes steadily more concentrated within the reservoir, and the volume of drug released may be less than the volume of liquid leaving the reservoir.

In conclusion, high aerosol output rate and small particle size occur when the flow of compressed gas through the device is relatively high (approximately 8 ℓ min^{-1} is often ideal). A high output rate would offset the fact that a relatively large volume of fluid (4–6 ml) is required for more efficient emptying of the reservoir, and in practice, treatment times can be restricted to about 10 minutes. The rate of output, volume released and particle size vary somewhat according to the brand of nebulizer, and some brands are definitely more suitable than others in terms of the delivery of adequate amounts of suitably sized aerosol. Whatever type of nebulizer is used, it is vital to ensure that bacterial contamination does not occur, and regular cleaning is essential.

Deposition and clinical efficacy

Deposition studies using jet or ultrasonic nebulizers are relatively easy to perform. A radioactive solution is placed in the nebulizer reservoir, and it is assumed that the droplets released have similar aerodynamic properties to droplets of drug solution. The radionuclide ^{99m}Tc is used most frequently, since it has a short half-life, and is available in a variety of chemical forms (Chapter 4). Aerosol present in the lungs is measured by one of several types of detector, the most usual of which is the gamma camera. Counts emanating from the chest may be compared with those obtained from a known amount of radioaerosol in order to ascertain the percentage of the dose reaching the lungs. A popular technique involves the use of a 'phantom', which is a container filled with radioactive solution and designed in such a way that

TABLE 9.1. Lung deposition of aerosols released from nebulizers

Type of nebulizer	*Aerosol*	*Percentage of dose reaching lungs*	*Authors*
Ultrasonic	$^{99m}TcO_4$	1% (mean)	Asmundsson *et al.* (1973)
Jet	$^{99m}TcO_4$	2% (mean)	Asmundsson *et al.* (1973)
Ultrasonic	^{111}In and ^{99m}Tc labelled colloids	7–32%	Lin *et al.* (1974)
Ultrasonic	^{99m}Tc labelled phytate	3–23%	Wasnich *et al.* (1976)
Ultrasonic	^{99m}Tc labelled albumin	2–11%	Ruffin *et al.* (1978a)
Jet	^{99m}Tc labelled albumin microspheres	12% (mean)	Lewis *et al.* (1981)

it resembles radionuclide distributed in the lungs. A typical lung phantom consists of a low density substance such as urethane foam with a slab of tissue equivalent material to represent the chest wall and a layer of radioactive material to simulate radioaerosol located in the mid-thorax (Asmundsson *et al.*, 1973). A gamma camera linked to a computer also lends itself to measurement of radioaerosol in specific lung zones, since computer-generated 'regions of interest' may be selected, for instance in central and peripheral lung, or at the bases and apices.

The percentage of the aerosol dose reaching the lungs from jet and ultrasonic nebulizers has been assessed in many studies (*Table 9.1*). Although there are wide variations between the results of the various studies, owing to differences in the type of nebulizer, volume of solution used, nebulization time, breathing pattern and radionuclide counting procedures, the data are in agreement that the greater part of the aerosol dose is unavailable to the lungs. As a rule of thumb, about 10 per

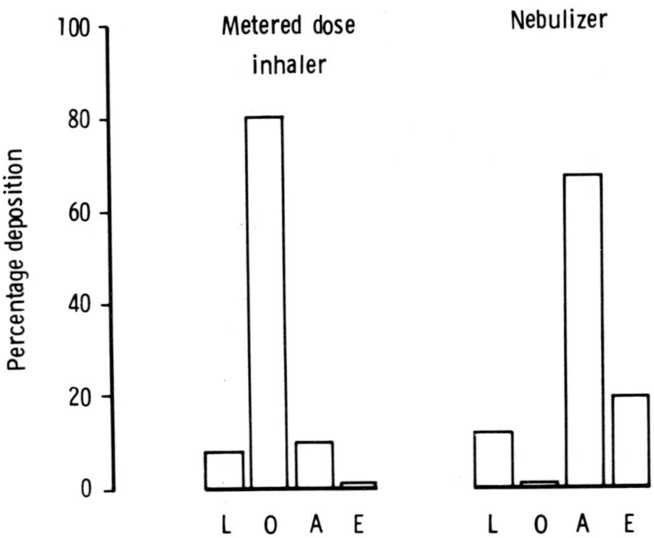

Figure 9.4 Deposition patterns for therapeutic aerosols released from an MDI (Newman *et al.*, 1981b) and from a jet nebulizer (Lewis *et al.*, 1981). Only about 10 per cent of the dose reaches the lungs (L) from each device, but the division of the remainder of the dose between oropharynx (O), inhalation apparatus (A) and exhaled air (E) is totally different

cent of the dose reaches the lungs. A typical deposition pattern for nebulized aerosol is shown in *Figure 9.4*, the data being taken from Lewis *et al.* (1981). About two-thirds of the aerosol dose remained within the apparatus itself (within the nebulizer and on the mouthpiece) and only 12 per cent of the dose reached the lungs on average. Oropharyngeal losses were very low, but one-fifth of the dose was exhaled.

The so-called 'soup' technique (Chapter 4), involving the nebulization of a solution which comprises both radiolabelled compound and drug, has permitted a number of very interesting studies to be performed. Ruffin *et al.* (1978b) mixed the beta-agonist fenoterol and $^{99m}TcO_4$ in the reservoir of an ultrasonic nebulizer, and were able to quantify the mass of drug delivered to the lungs. Maximal bronchodilatation occurred when only about 30 μg of drug was deposited in the lungs, and further deposition of drug did not enhance the therapeutic effect. This technique is also useful for performing 'selective' deposition studies, in other words altering the deposition pattern deliberately by means of changes in both particle size and inhalation mode. The effects of a histamine/$^{99m}TcO_4$ aerosol deposited centrally or diffusely within the lung were compared by this means (Ruffin *et al.*, 1978c). A small dose of centrally deposited histamine was as effective as a large dose of diffusely deposited histamine in causing bronchoconstriction, and it was inferred that the receptor sites for histamine lie chiefly in central airways. Although a broadly similar study was performed with a fenoterol/$^{99m}TcO_4$ aerosol, no definite conclusion was reached regarding the location of the receptor sites for beta-agonists (Ruffin *et al.*, 1981).

Surprisingly little attention has been given to the effects of changes in the inhalation mode on the deposition of aerosols released from nebulizers. Ryan *et al.* (1981) found that fast vital capacity inhalations resulted in a lower lung dose and a more central deposition pattern than slow vital capacity inhalations. The distributions of the dose within the lung produced by tidal breathing and by slow vital capacity breaths were not significantly different. Gottschalk *et al.* (1978) found that compared to tidal breathing, deposition of aerosol from an ultrasonic nebulizer could be enhanced by deep inhalation with breath-holding. Although intermittent positive pressure breathing (IPPB) is often used to assist nebulizer therapy, this technique gives a similar deposition pattern to that attained by quiet breathing (Dolovich *et al.*, 1977). The clinical value of IPPB attachments to nebulizers is questionable (Lourenço and Cotromanes, 1982b).

There have been few studies comparing the efficacies of particles of different sizes inhaled from nebulizers, although those studies which have been performed suggest that within or close to the 'ideal' size band (<5 μm), small changes in particle size might not be of major importance. Similar bronchodilator effects have been noted for fenoterol aerosols with MMADs 0.55 and 2.4 μm (Dolovich *et al.*, 1981a). A change in particle size from 1.3 to 3.6 μm did not alter the quantity of methacholine aerosol required to produce a given degree of bronchoconstriction (Ryan *et al.*, 1981).

Metered dose inhalers

Fundamentals

The size distributions of aerosols released from MDIs are at present inadequately characterized. The MMADs of metered dose aerosols have been measured by a laser particle sizing technique (Hiller *et al.*, 1978), and lie between 2.8 and 4.3 μm

(GSDs 1.5–2.1). Similar data were obtained by Sackner *et al.* (1981) using a cascade impactor (MMADs 3.3–5.5 μm, GSDs 2.0–2.2). As in the case of nebulizers, these measurements indicate aerosols of sizes suitable for inhalation, but these data are misleading since the measurements have been carried out after most or all of the propellants have evaporated. The aerosols released from MDIs consist of the drug particles with a coating of propellants which does not evaporate for some time and distance after actuation. At the actuator orifice, the MMD of the propellant droplets may exceed 30 μm (Morén, 1981). Propellant evaporation takes place but contrary to popular belief, this is not immediate. Even at a distance of 25 cm from the canister, the MMD may be as high as 10 μm. The evaporation process results in a sudden cooling of the aerosol spray (Sanders, 1970). Since evaporation of the aerosol constituents is taking place while the drug is being inhaled, the effective aerosol size is constantly changing, and it is difficult to predict the site of deposition within the lungs.

The velocity of the propellant droplet spray as it leaves the canister is very rapid. Published data for hair spray aerosols have indicated velocities >30 ms^{-1} (67 miles per hour) at the actuator orifice (Rance, 1974), and the droplets may not decelerate to a speed less than that of the inhaled air until they have travelled more than 20 cm from the canister. Propellant droplet velocity is approximately proportional to vapour pressure. The high initial droplet size and high velocity of the spray as it leaves the canister make deposition in the oropharynx very likely, and few droplets are able to get beyond the back of the throat and penetrate into the lungs. Further research is necessary to find propellants with small yet slowly moving droplets, but it is difficult to find suitable alternatives to the chlorofluorocarbons. Furthermore, it would be necessary for the pharmaceutical companies to conduct wide-ranging trials to demonstrate the safety of new delivery systems.

Changes in propellant droplet size and velocity can be produced by altering the propellant mixture. The various chlorofluorocarbon propellants have different boiling points, and influence the aerosol characteristics in different ways. A low boiling point propellant (such as propellant 12) will contribute more to the initial droplet velocity, but will result in smaller droplet size and more rapid evaporation (Morén, 1981). Propellants with higher boiling points (such as propellant 11) will remain in the liquid phase for a longer period of time and will make the drug particles seem larger than they really are. The numbering system used to denote the various propellants defines the number of carbon, chlorine and fluorine atoms present in the propellant molecules. Propellant vapour pressure varies not only with the propellant mixture, but also according to the ambient temperature, and a given aerosol spray would have different characteristics in hot and in cold weather.

Alterations in the metering volume (that is, the volume of propellant released in each actuation) may also change the effective aerosol size. Since propellant evaporation depends upon the acquisition of heat from the surrounding atmosphere, it is likely that propellant droplets derived from a 50 or 100 μl metered volume will evaporate more slowly than droplets from a 25 μl metered volume, and will be effectively larger on arrival at the patient's lungs (Morén, 1981). It is interesting to note that the formulations of metered dose aerosols commercially available in the UK vary somewhat according to brand. Most metered dose aerosols employ a 1:2:1 ratio of chlorofluorocarbons 11:12:114, giving a propellant vapour pressure of 374 kPa at 20°C. The metering volume is usually 25 or 50 μl (400 or 200 doses per canister). The most widely used bronchodilator aerosol (salbutamol) and corticosteroid aerosol (beclomethasone dipropionate) are unusual in that

TABLE 9.2. Contents of typical 'suspension' and 'solution' metered dose aerosols used for delivery of the bronchodilator isoprenaline

Type of aerosol	*Product*	*Metered volume* (μl)	*Weight of drug per dose* (μg)	*Propellant mixture*	*Other ingredients*	*MMAD** (μm)	*GSD**
Suspension	'Medihaler-ISO' (Riker)	25	80	Chlorofluorocarbons 11:12:114 in ratio 1:2:1	Sorbitan trioleate surfactant	2.8	1.8
Solution	'Isuprel mistometer'	50	130	Chlorofluorocarbons 12:114 in ratio 1:4	Ethanol cosolvent Ascorbic acid preservative	4.3	2.1

*After complete evaporation of propellants, from Hiller *et al.* (1978)

their metering volume is 63 μl, and there is a high concentration of chlorofluorocarbon 12, giving a particularly high vapour pressure and a more forceful spray. Either glass or metal canisters are available with MDIS, but the latter permit higher vapour pressures to be attained.

A reduction in actuator orifice diameter will reduce the propellant droplet size, but care must be taken to minimize valve clogging and particle agglomeration which could adversely affect the uniformity of drug delivery. Moisture content must be minimized in order to reduce hygroscopic effects (Gorman and Hall, 1973), although the change in particle size within the respiratory tract as a result of hygroscopic growth is smaller than that predicted on theoretical grounds (Hiller *et al.*, 1981), possibly because the presence of propellants and other constituents exerts a protective effect against hygroscopic growth. The use of MDIs has been restricted largely to the delivery of bronchodilators and corticosteroids. These drugs may be formulated as suspensions of crystals or as solutions. Suspension aerosols also contain surface active agents such as oleic acid, sorbitan trioleate or lecithin to reduce particle agglomeration and to lubricate the valve mechanism, while solution aerosols, in which the drug is mixed uniformly with the propellant, contain not only ethanol or glycol in high concentrations as a cosolvent, but may also contain trace quantities of a range of preservatives and flavouring agents (Gorman and Hall, 1973). The influence of these compounds on effective aerosol size is largely unknown, although it is likely that the presence of slowly evaporating ethanol in solution aerosols retards the rate of droplet shrinkage. The contents of typical suspension and solution aerosols are shown in *Table 9.2*.

In addition to their large droplet size and velocity, metered dose aerosols differ in another important respect from nebulized aerosols, in that they are introduced into the inhaled air stream as a bolus, rather than continuously throughout the breath. Although there is no evidence that this in itself reduces drug efficacy, the patient must learn the technique of coordinating inhalation with firing the aerosol if the drug is to be carried into the lungs. Failure to coordinate is probably the major form of misuse of metered dose aerosols, and may be observed in a significant fraction of patients who use the devices (Crompton, 1982). The apparent simplicity of MDIs is therefore very misleading.

Deposition studies

The first indirect estimates of metered dose aerosol deposition come from pharmacokinetic studies using bronchodilators labelled with the beta-emitting

TABLE 9.3. Lung deposition of aerosols released from metered dose inhalers

Technique used	*Percentage of dose reaching lungs*	*Authors*
^{3}H labelled bronchodilators (pharmacokinetics)	<10%	Davies (1975)
^{77}Br labelled ipratropium bromide	13–29% (mean 16%)	Short *et al.* (1981)
^{99m}Tc labelled solution aerosol	13.6%*	Dolovich *et al.* (1981b)
^{99m}Tc labelled Teflon particles	7–17% (mean 8.8%)	Newman *et al.* (1981b)
^{99m}Tc labelled Teflon particles	7–25% (mean 14.1%**)	Newman *et al.* (1982a)
^{3}H labelled bronchodilators (with activated charcoal)	0.8–10.1% (mean 2.9%)	Davies (1982)

*Maximum dose to right lung multiplied by a factor of 2
**Using 'optimal' inhalation technique

isotope ^{3}H. Levels of the drugs and their metabolites in plasma and urine, measured by liquid scintillation counting, are similar after inhalation and after oral administration (Davies, 1975). It was thus concluded that the majority of the dose ($\gtrsim$90 per cent) is deposited in the oropharynx and is subsequently swallowed, and that $<$10 per cent of the dose reaches the lungs (*Table 9.3*). These findings were largely confirmed by measuring the quantity of drug recovered in mouthwashings, although this process is inevitably inefficient, and some of the drug is always swallowed. However, comparison of drug losses in mouthwashings between various inhalation manoeuvres or with different aerosol formulations enables a qualitative estimate to be made of the relative amounts of drug available to the lungs (Morén, 1981).

As described in Chapter 4, studies with gamma-labelled bronchodilator drugs have been limited by the lack of suitable radionuclides, although such measurements would constitute a 'gold standard' for metered dose aerosol deposition measurements. Although there have been no published studies with gamma-labelled beta-agonists, the anticholinergic agent ipratropium bromide has been labelled with the gamma-emitting isotope ^{77}Br (Short *et al.*, 1981), and its deposition in the lung measured (*Table 9.3*). On average, 16 per cent of the dose reached the lungs, and about 80 per cent was deposited in the oropharynx, in close agreement with the findings of earlier pharmacokinetic studies.

As an alternative to labelling the drug itself, a system of inert 'replacement' particles may be used—these may be solid particles or liquid droplets, simulating formulations in which the drug is present as a suspension or as a solution respectively. The radionuclide ^{99m}Tc is probably the most suitable material for this purpose, although the choice of radionuclides and test aerosols was discussed more fully in Chapter 4. Direct measurement of a pressurized suspension aerosol has been performed by making particles of Teflon, firmly labelled with ^{99m}Tc, using a spinning disc generator (Newman *et al.*, 1981b). These particles had an MMAD (3.2 μm) similar to that of commercially available metered dose aerosols after complete evaporation of propellants, but a smaller GSD (1.2), indicating a narrower spread of particle size. Deposition was assessed from profile scanning along the length of the body using a whole body counter. As for jet nebulizers, only about 10 per cent of the dose reached the lungs (*Table 9.3*), but compared to the nebulizer, the fate of the remainder of the dose was quite different (*Figure 9.4*). More than 80 per cent of the dose was lost by impaction in the oropharynx and about 10 per cent of the dose was deposited on the actuator. Since the Teflon particles are insoluble, it is possible to assess alveolar deposition by measuring the percentage of aerosol retained in the lungs after 24 hours, and in this respect the method has a marked advantage over direct labelling of the drug. About one-third of the aerosol deposited in the lungs penetrated to the alveolated zones and about two-thirds was on the conducting airways. Deposition of a pressurized solution aerosol was studied by Dolovich *et al.* (1981b) who incorporated $^{99m}TcO_4$, ethanol cosolvent and propellants into an MDI. After propellant evaporation, the droplets released had an MMAD of 2.15 μm and a GSD 2.44. The maximum quantity of aerosol reaching the right lung of healthy subjects was 6.8 per cent of the dose (*Table 9.3*). A modification of the pharmacokinetic technique also enables a direct estimate to be made of lung deposition. If activated charcoal is used to block the absorption of drug which has been deposited in the oropharynx and swallowed, then the entire swallowed fraction is excreted in the faeces. Drug appearing in the urine must have arrived there following its deposition in the lung and subsequent absorption through airway surfaces. By this technique, it was shown that on average <10 per cent of the dose reached the lungs, the data being in broad agreement with those obtained by other techniques (Davies, 1982).

Effect of inhalation mode

The effects of changes in inhalation manoeuvre on lung deposition and/or clinical efficacy of metered dose aerosols have been studied by several groups of workers. Bronchodilators are generally employed for studies of drug efficacy, owing to the rapid and easily measurable response that they elicit. There is agreement that the aerosol should be inhaled slowly (approximately 30 $\ell\ \text{min}^{-1}$) if maximal deposition in the lung (Newman *et al.*, 1982a; Dolovich *et al.*, 1981b) and maximal therapeutic effect (Newman *et al.*, 1981a) are to be achieved. Faster inhaled flow rates increase oropharyngeal deposition and permit less aerosol to reach the lungs. Following slow and steady inhalation, a 10 second breath-holding pause should be maintained to enable the particles to settle onto the airways by gravitational sedimentation. By combining slow inhalation with 10 seconds breath-holding on average about 15 per cent of the dose can be delivered to the lungs, and this inhalation mode, dubbed the 'ten second rule', seems to be the inhalation mode of choice for metered dose aerosols (*Table 9.4*). Conducting airway deposition and alveolar deposition are improved equally by the optimal inhalation mode.

TABLE 9.4. Simple rules for using metered dose inhalers

(1) Shake the canister (to disperse drug particles uniformly in the propellants).
(2) Hold the canister upright.
(3) Breathe out fully.
(4) Place the inhaler mouthpiece between the lips.
(5) Fire the inhaler while breathing in slowly and deeply.
(6) Hold the breath for 10 seconds, or for as long as possible.
(7) If the dose is to be repeated, wait at least 1 minute (in order to allow the canister to return to thermal equilibrium and for the metering chamber to refill).

There is conflicting evidence as to the lung volume during inhalation at which the aerosol should be released. In our comprehensive studies involving a range of inhaled flow rates and breath-holding pauses, actuation at 20 per cent VC gave greater or similar bronchodilatation (Newman *et al.*, 1981a) and lung deposition (Newman *et al.*, 1982a) than actuation at higher lung volumes. By contrast in more limited studies, Riley *et al.* (1976) showed that isoprenaline aerosol released at a high lung volume (80 per cent VC) during inhalation gave greater bronchodilatation than aerosol released at a low lung volume (20 per cent VC), and it was suggested that at a high lung volume the airways would be more patent and a more even deposition pattern would occur. It is probable that the lung volume of aerosol actuation is less important than correct choice of flow rate and breath-holding. Although patients are generally advised to inhale maximally, commencing at residual volume, inhalation commencing at functional residual capacity may give equally good bronchodilator response (Lawford and McKenzie, 1981).

The technique of 'divided doses', that is, two doses of bronchodilator 10–20 minutes apart is often advocated, on the grounds that this allows the first dose to open partially obstructed airways into which the second dose may then penetrate (Williams, 1982). Although this technique has been shown to give a greater response compared to the same amount of drug given as a large single dose, it is unclear whether this is still the case when the optimal inhalation technique is used, and further studies are needed to investigate this.

Effects of formulation changes on deposition

Changes in aerosol formulation also affect metered dose aerosol deposition, owing to alterations in the propellant droplet size distribution and velocity that are produced. Although increasing the propellant vapour pressure from 374 to 502 kPa by raising the concentration of chlorofluorocarbon 12 results in a faster moving spray, it also causes the droplets to be smaller and the net effect is a reduction in oropharyngeal deposition and an increase in lung deposition (Newman *et al.*, 1982b). An increase in metered volume from 25 to 50 μl probably retards the rate at which the propellants evaporate, so that aerosol size is greater on arrival at the patient's lungs. Consequently, a proximal shift of aerosol deposition away from the lung periphery has been demonstrated (Newman *et al.*, 1982b). These findings suggest that the propellant vapour pressure should be high and metered volume low for maximum bioavailability. As previously described, the formulations of commercially available metered dose aerosols vary somewhat according to the brand and it is likely that their patterns of deposition differ as a consequence.

The various commercially available drugs delivered from MDIs also have different particle size distributions, but it is possible that changes in particle size are less important than alterations in the size of the propellant droplets within which the drug particles are enclosed. Similar deposition patterns have been found for particles of MMADs 3.2 μm and 6.4 μm released from MDIs (Newman *et al.*, 1983). There have been surprisingly few studies to compare the efficacies of drug particles of different sizes released from MDIs. However, Rees *et al.* (1982) found that the commercially available particles of terbutaline sulphate in the size range <5 μm gave greater therapeutic responses than particles of 5 to 10 μm or 10 to 15 μm.

Spacer and reservoir devices

An important adjunct to inhaler therapy developed over the last few years has been the spacer attachment. This involves the use of a tube or cone-shaped volume placed between the canister and the patient's mouth, so that the large, rapidly moving propellant droplets are given an opportunity to evaporate and slow down due to air resistance (*Figure 9.5*). This renders the droplets more suitable for inhalation. Portable telescopic extension tubes, approximately 10 cm long and 100 cm^3 in volume are available commercially. Larger pear or cone-shaped spacers (length 20–25 cm, volume 500–1500 cm^3) are designed so that their shape is the same as that of the spray cloud as it leaves the canister, so that impaction losses on the walls of the device are reduced.

Compared to an MDI alone, spacers enhance delivery to the lung of radioaerosol particles released from MDIs, and at the same time reduce oropharyngeal losses (Newman *et al.*, 1981c). Similar effects can be obtained by holding the mouth open as the aerosol is released, or holding the canister a few centimetres from the open mouth (Dolovich *et al.*, 1981b). Great care must then be taken to point the inhaler in the right direction, whereas the spacer guides the aerosol towards the patient's mouth. Improvements in drug efficacy when metered dose bronchodilators are

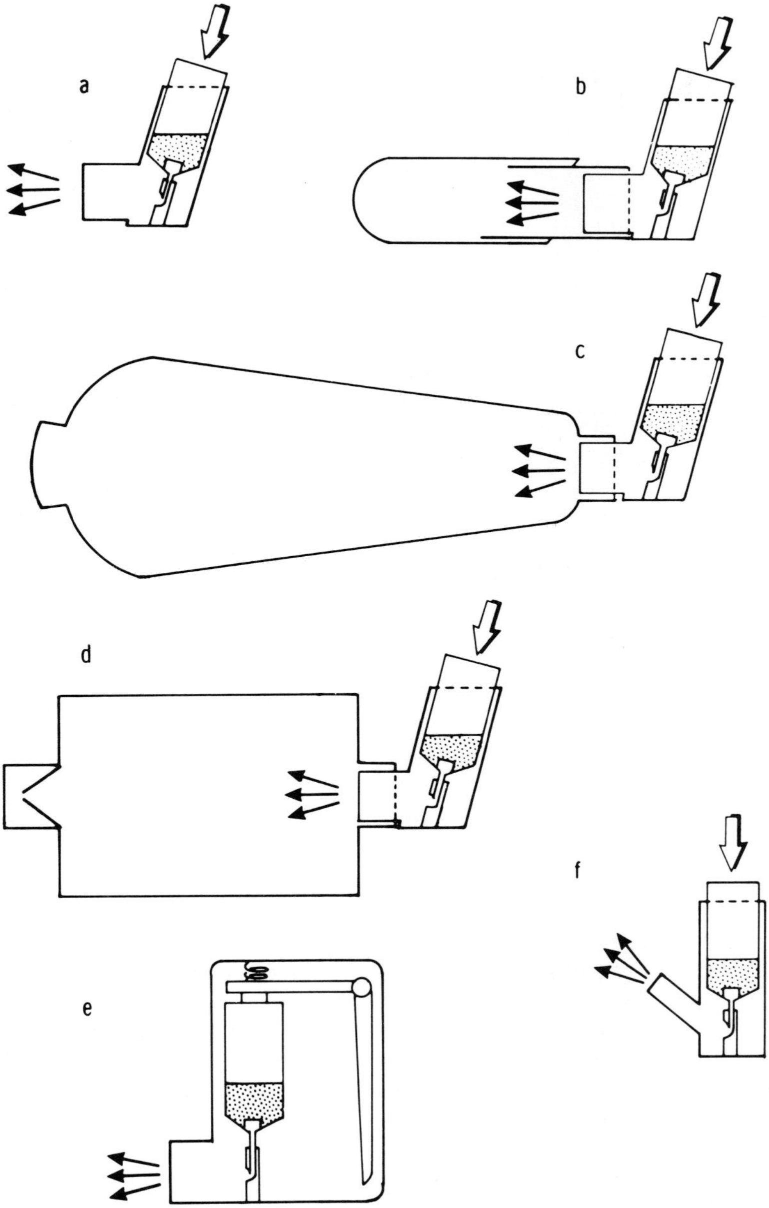

Figure 9.5 Metered dose inhalers. The basic MDI (a) may be supplemented by a spacer tube (b), a spacer cone designed to follow the shape of the aerosol cloud (c), a reservoir device or holding chamber with a one-way valve in the mouthpiece to control inhalation (d), or a breath-actuated mechanism (e). MDIs may also be used for nasal inhalation with a suitable actuator (f)

inhaled through spacer devices have been demonstrated in a number of clinical trials, although in some trials spacers have conferred no additional bronchodilatation.

A further step in the spacer concept is that of the reservoir device or holding chamber (*Figure 9.5d*). This may be similar in construction to a spacer, except that there is a one-way valve situated at one end of the device so that the patient can inhale from the chamber but cannot exhale into it. The metered dose aerosol is released into the chamber, where it can remain suspended for a few seconds, and the patient then inhales the chamber contents. Thus, not only is the aerosol slowed down and the propellants given time to evaporate, but in addition the need to coordinate inhalation with actuation is removed. In practice, spacer devices may also reduce the need for patient coordination, but to a lesser extent than for reservoir devices. A variety of designs of reservoirs exists. They may be purpose-built, or may be constructed from a wide range of hospital or domestic equipment. A collapsible reservoir bag of volume 700 ml, which contracts as the patient inhales and which incorporates a reed intended to sound if the inhalation flow rate exceeds $20\,\ell\,\text{min}^{-1}$ (Sackner *et al.*, 1981) has advantages over other devices of this type, since the patient receives visible and audible proof that he is inhaling the aerosol deeply and slowly (Tobin *et al.*, 1982).

Reservoir devices are particle size-selective, in that they filter out the larger propellant droplets, while permitting the smaller droplets to pass into the lungs. Oropharyngeal losses are generally low, since much of the aerosol normally deposited in the oropharynx is deposited within the device itself. This might be particularly useful in corticosteroid aerosol therapy, where the incidence of local side-effects (candidiasis and dysphonia) may be raised compared to that in patients taking oral steroids or no steroids at all. Toogood *et al.* (1982) found that both a tube-shaped spacer and a pear-shaped reservoir augmented the airway response to a corticosteroid aerosol (budesonide), while at the same time the incidence of oropharyngeal candidiasis was reduced.

In terms of the requirements of an 'ideal' inhalation system, discussed earlier in this chapter, the reservoir device has several clear advantages over the standard MDI. Lung delivery of aerosol may be improved and losses elsewhere reduced, leading to more efficient use of the drug. The local side-effects of corticosteroid aerosols will be reduced. The systemic side-effects (smooth muscle tremor and tachycardia) of beta-agonists are seldom a problem when the drug is given as an aerosol, and although increased lung delivery might raise the incidence of these side-effects marginally, this is unlikely to be of clinical significance. Reservoirs are simpler to use than the MDI alone, since patients do not need to coordinate inhalation with actuation, but can inhale more or less in their own time. The permissible delay time between firing the aerosol and inhaling will vary according to the design of the reservoir. On the other hand, reservoirs are less portable and more conspicuous than the MDI, and some patients could find them inconvenient for this reason. Clinical trials are virtually unanimous in showing an improved therapeutic effect with reservoir devices, presumably because of inefficient use of the MDI alone, and they may also give comparable or greater therapeutic benefits than those achieved by nebulizer therapy. It would, however, be a mistake to think that all such devices are equally good, and that all possess similar properties. They must be designed carefully, due consideration being given to aerosol kinetics, in order to ensure that most of the dose is not lost by impaction or sedimentation within the device itself.

Breath-actuated MDIs

Since failure to synchronize aerosol release with inhalation is a major problem for many patients who use MDIs, it is logical to design a system which is operated by the act of inhalation itself. The breath-actuated MDI is the result (*Figure 9.5e*). The canister is mounted in a modified actuator and is linked to a spring mechanism in such a way that inhaling through the device draws a vane forward, thus releasing the spring and triggering the aerosol. Synchronization is thus achieved automatically. Several clinical trials have shown favourable results, but these devices are not widely used, perhaps because they tend to release the aerosol rather violently and noisily. The 'optimal' slow and steady inhaled flow rate of 30 $\ell\,min^{-1}$ may not always be sufficient to actuate the aerosol. A breath-actuated MDI which released a bronchodilator aerosol when patients inhaled at about 50 $\ell\,min^{-1}$ did not produce bronchodilatation significantly greater than that achieved by a conventional MDI (Coady *et al.*, 1976) possibly because the relatively high flow-rate needed to operate the device promoted deposition in the oropharynx.

Airway surface concentration of drug

Respiratory drugs are effective in remarkably small doses when given by the inhaled route, particularly from the MDI. Beta-agonists, for instance, give maximal therapeutic response in doses of only a few hundred micrograms, of which only 10 per cent (<100 μg) reaches the lungs. This is spread over an area believed to be comparable to that of a tennis court.

It is possible to make an estimate of the surface concentration of drugs released from MDIs if one is prepared to make certain approximations and assumptions about aerosol characteristics. Since the drug particles are enclosed within larger propellant droplets whose size is constantly changing, estimation of precise aerosol size is difficult. Pressurized aerosol deposition measurements in subjects with airway obstruction, however, indicate that about 30 per cent of the particles reaching the lungs penetrate to the alveolated zones. This is approximately the alveolar deposition that would be expected for an aerosol in the 7–8 μm range inhaled slowly and deeply (Foord *et al.*, 1978) although these measurements were made in healthy subjects. Such an estimate of aerosol size would be in broad agreement with measurements made on pressurized aerosols using a laser sizing device at various distances from the actuator orifice (Morén, 1981).

On the assumption that a pressurized metered dose aerosol behaves in the lungs as though it has an aerodynamic diameter of approximately 7–8 μm, the surface concentration of drug reaching the airways can be estimated, since Gerrity *et al.* (1979) have published calculations of the deposition of an aerosol of aerodynamic diameter 7.9 μm in the Weibel (1963) model of the human lung. In these calculations, the inhaled volume was taken as 0.7 ℓ, and the inhaled flow rate 30 $\ell\,min^{-1}$. Assuming that 50 μg (10 per cent) of a 500 μg dose of terbutaline sulphate (Bricanyl, Astra Pharmaceuticals) reaches the lungs, then it is possible to calculate surface concentrations if the percentage of the dose reaching each generation is divided by the surface area of that generation (*Figure 9.6*). There are two regions in which deposition reaches a peak—in the subsegmental bronchi (by impaction) and in the respiratory bronchioles (by sedimentation). However, the surface area of the airways increases dramatically beyond the first few generations, so that surface concentration in peripheral parts of the lungs is low. The peak

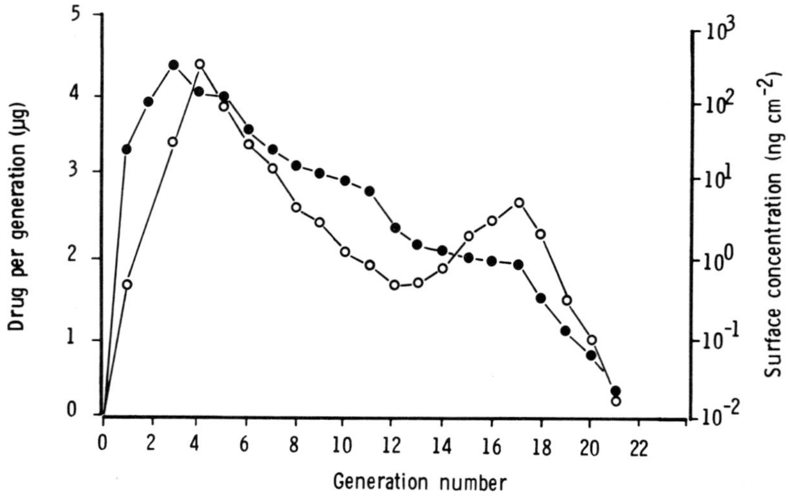

Figure 9.6 Surface concentrations of metered dose aerosols in the Weibel (1963) model of the lung, assuming that 50 μg of drug has been deposited within the lungs. Left-hand axis and open circles: drug deposition (μg) per generation; right-hand axis and closed circles: surface concentration of drug (ng cm^{-2}) per generation

surface concentration (approximately 300 ng cm^{-2}) occurs in the segmental bronchi, but there is a rapid fall in surface concentration for more distal airways. At generation 8—approximately the border between 'large' and 'small' airways—the surface concentration has fallen to less than 30 ng cm^{-2}, and is only 1.3 ng cm^{-2} in the terminal bronchioles. In the alveolated zones, the surface concentration is always below 1 ng cm^{-2}. This calculation makes many approximations, for instance the inhaled volume is rather lower than that usually adopted for inhalation from an MDI, and no allowance has been made for breath-holding. The model predicts lower alveolar deposition than is measured experimentally. Furthermore the distal penetration of aerosol might be reduced in patients with airway obstruction. Nevertheless, *Figure 9.6* illustrates effectively the very small surface concentrations of drug, particularly in peripheral lung regions, that are required to yield a satisfactory therapeutic response.

It is interesting to compare the surface concentrations on the various airway generations with distribution of receptor sites described earlier (Barnes *et al.*, 1982). Although beta-receptors may be found in all parts of the lungs, their greatest density is in the small peripheral airways where surface concentration of drug is only a few ng cm^{-2}. The relationship between the site of drug deposition and the location of receptor sites requires much more detailed examination, but this is difficult at present since measurement techniques only permit very coarse assessment of deposition within the lungs. Ideally, the quantity of aerosol deposited on each airway generation should be determined experimentally, but this is far beyond the scope of present technology.

Nasal sprays

In addition to their use in asthma and bronchitis, aerosolized corticosteroids may also play a role in the treatment of rhinitis. Delivery of corticosteroid aerosols to the nose should offer the advantages of topical therapy, in terms of a small dose and a low incidence of systemic side-effects. Various brands of corticosteroid aerosol can be delivered from metered dose canisters which are very similar in design to those used for oral inhalation. However, the actuator is rather smaller, being designed to fit into the nostril (*Figure 9.5*). Treatment given by this means is effective and results in few local side-effects (Mygind, 1982).

The spray released from nasal inhalers is a very narrow jet and tends to be deposited on a small area of nasal mucosa. It is possible that a less directed spray, for instance a spray generated by compressed air, might give a more even spread of drug within the nasal passages. Air-driven hand-pump sprays are available for delivery of sodium cromoglycate, ipratropium bromide and alpha-adrenergic nasal decongestants such as phenylephrine.

Dry powder inhalers

Dry powder inhalers (described and illustrated in Chapter 4) are used less frequently than nebulizers or MDIs, their principal use being for the delivery of the prophylactic agent sodium cromoglycate (SCG) although dry powder aerosols of both bronchodilator and corticosteroid drugs are available. Correspondingly, there is less information available regarding aerosol characteristics and drug delivery than for the more widely used devices.

Pharmacokinetic studies have indicated that only about 5 per cent of the drug is available to the lungs from an SCG 'Spinhaler', since most is deposited in the oropharynx (Davies, 1975). This appears strange at first sight since the manufacturers of these devices place very small drug particles in the gelatin capsules (MMD 2.6 μm, Bell *et al.*, 1971). However, the capsules may empty inefficiently if only these particles are present, and much larger (30 to 70 μm) carrier particles of lactose are often added to dry powder capsules to improve emptying. Large agglomerates, unsuitable for inhalation, are formed between drug and lactose, and only a few percent of the total aerosol mass is within the respirable range (Smith *et al.*, 1980). More recently introduced drug formulations have eliminated the lactose carrier and the drug is present as large 'pellets' which break up in the turbulent inhaled air stream. It is possible that a greater fraction of this formulation might reach the lungs. Sodium cromoglycate is poorly absorbed via the gastrointestinal tract, so that the swallowed drug is responsible for little or no therapeutic effect.

There is virtually no information available about the correct mode of inhalation for a dry powder aerosol in order that drug delivery to the bronchial tree should be enhanced. Unlike nebulizers and MDIs, there have been no systematic trials to compare either particle deposition or drug efficacy from dry powder inhalers under various inhalation conditions. However, it is apparent that dry powder capsules empty erratically at low inhaled flow rates ($\sim$30 ℓ min^{-1}) and may empty more readily if air is inhaled relatively quickly ($\gtrsim$60 ℓ min^{-1}) through the devices. Studies with nebulizers and MDIs have indicated that aerosol should be inhaled slowly and steadily in order to reduce oropharyngeal losses and to enhance delivery to more distal lung zones. The relatively high flows required to get the particles out of the capsules might then increase the amount of drug which is lost in the oropharynx.

Although there have been no studies of the deposition or efficacy of different-sized SCG particles released from the Spinhaler, SCG aeosols of specific sizes have been manufactured by the spinning disc method and inhaled by asthmatic patients. SCG particles of mean diameter 2 μm were more effective in preventing the onset of exercise-induced asthma than 11.7 μm particles, presumably because the latter did not penetrate far into the respiratory tract (Godfrey *et al.*, 1974). When the dispositions of 3 different-sized SCG particles (2, 6 and 11.7 μm) were compared, urinary excretion was greatest for 2 μm particles, indicating absorption via the airways, whereas recovery in mouthwashings was greatest for 11.7 μm particles (Curry *et al.*, 1975).

Discussion

The studies and technological developments reviewed in this chapter have been aimed at improving the efficiency of aerosol therapy, that is, to ensure that patients get as much benefit as they possibly can from the available inhalation devices. By means of both theoretical prediction and experiment, it is possible to find ways of improving aerosol delivery to the lung. For instance, changes in the operating conditions of nebulizers and in the formulation of metered dose aerosols can alter size distributions, so that more particles within the respirable range can be made available. Drug delivery can also be improved by correct choice of inhalation manoeuvre, and by the use of spacer or reservoir attachments to MDIs. Such improvements in aerosol therapy make treatment much more precise and less haphazard, and should help the patient to get full benefit from as little drug as possible. As well as restricting the quantity of drug to which patients are exposed, a more precise approach to therapy should have the additional merit of helping to improve patient compliance with issued instructions. It should not be necessary for stable patients to overuse their inhalers—this indicates either that patients are not using their inhalation devices correctly, or the onset of clinical deterioration. Although the overuse of bronchodilator aerosols would probably not give rise to any significant side-effects or problems, this might not be the case for antibiotic or antihistamine aerosols, the use of which could become more widespread in the future.

Many investigations have shown that the inhalation mode adopted by patients inhaling aerosols from nebulizers or from MDIs has a marked effect on both deposition and clinical response. It is interesting to note that the inhalation mode is rarely controlled in clinical trials on the various drugs, and it is possible that many studies would have been more valuable had this been the case. In particular, while the majority of studies have shown spacer and reservoir attachments to MDIs to result in greater bronchodilatation than that attained with an MDI alone, it is often not stated whether the MDI was used with an optimal or sub-optimal inhalation technique. The optimal technique would involve actuating the aerosol during a slow, deep inhalation, and following this with a period of breath-holding. If the aerosol inhaled from the reservoir results in greater bronchodilatation than that inhaled from an incorrectly used MDI, then the reservoir is clearly a very useful device, primarily in patients who misuse MDIs. However, if the reservoir also results in greater bronchodilatation than a correctly used MDI, then the reservoir is clearly even more valuable, since it could benefit patients with good and bad inhaler technique alike. There must be a strong case therefore, for controlling, or at least stating the inhalation mode used in clinical trials with aerosolized drugs.

The effects of a whole host of factors on the behaviour of inhalation aerosols are largely unknown. The introduction of monodisperse therapeutic aerosols is often advocated, on the grounds that it is easier to 'target' such particles towards the required site of action in the lungs. However, calculations performed by the Task Group on Lung Dynamics (1966) and by Morrow (1981) have indicated similar deposition patterns for a perfectly monodisperse aerosol (GSD 1.0) and for heterodisperse aerosols with GSDs not exceeding 2.0. However, recent calculations by Gonda (1981) have suggested that changes in GSD might play a larger role in determining the site of deposition, and that for high values of GSD ($\gtrsim$3.0), deposition might be virtually independent of MMAD. Further studies of both deposition and clinical efficacy are required to investigate these questions. Despite much experimental investigation, there is still confusion as to the precise size of therapeutic aerosols within the bronchial tree, since it is difficult to predict exactly the rates of droplet shrinkage or hygroscopic growth that may occur. The role of electric charge on deposition is also unclear. Therapeutic aerosols undoubtedly acquire charge during their formation. The effects of electric charge upon deposition are commented on in Chapter 3. Drug concentration varies widely between different brands of metered dose aerosol. Each dose of terbutaline (Bricanyl) consists of 250 μg of the drug in only 25 μl propellant (10 $\mu g\,\mu l^{-1}$), compared to 100 μg of drug in 63 μl propellant (1.5 $\mu g\,\mu l^{-1}$) for salbutamol (Ventolin). Particle agglomeration might be greater for the higher drug concentration. It is not known whether such differences in particle concentration have any bearing on drug deposition and efficacy.

Aerosol therapy has to date been used almost exclusively for treating respiratory disorders. Can this mode of administration be used also to treat disorders of other parts of the body? Providing that a drug substance is absorbed via the airways or buccal mucosa without being metabolized, it is available to the systemic circulation. Perhaps there is a role for aerosolization of drugs such as insulin which are poorly absorbed from the gastrointestinal tract and which are normally given by injection. Ergotamine may be given as an aerosol for the treatment of migraine and glyceryl trinitrate for the prophylaxis and treatment of angina, the latter drug being given sublingually or delivered to the oral mucosa. Drug absorption from the nasal airways might be a more practical proposition, since the greater part of a dose delivered from a nasal inhaler might be deposited on the nasal mucosa and rapidly absorbed. Pituitary hormones may be given by this route. This approach if used more widely could offer therapeutic benefits together with the advantages of drug administration by inhalation and such prospects would promise an exciting future for aerosol therapy.

References

ASMUNDSSON, T., JOHNSON, R.F., KILBURN, K.H. and GOODRICH, J.K. (1973). Efficiency of nebulizers for depositing saline in human lung. *Am. Rev. Respir. Dis.*, **108**, 506–512

BARNES, P.J., BASBAUM, C.B., NADEL, J.A. and ROBERTS, J.M. (1982). Localisation of β-adrenoceptors in mammalian lung by light microscopic autoradiography. *Nature*, **299**, 444–447

BELL, J.H., HARTLEY, P.S. and COX, J.S.G. (1971). Dry powder aerosols I: A new powder inhalation device. *J. Pharm. Sci.*, **10**, 1559–1564

BRAIN, J. (1980). Aerosol and humidity therapy. *Am. Rev. Respir. Dis.*, **122**, 17–21

CLARK, T.J.H. (1979). Factors influencing the route of administration of airway therapy. In *Small airways in health and disease*. Edited by Sadoul, P., Milic-Emili, J., Simonsson, B.G. and Clark, T.J.H. Amsterdam; Excerpta Medica, pp. 170–178

CLARK, T.J.H. (1982). The inhaled route as the route of choice in airway disease therapy. In *New concepts in the topical treatment of asthma and related disorders*. Edited by McFadden, E.R. Greenwich; Cliggott Publishing Co., pp. 5–9

CLAY, M.M., PAVIA, D., NEWMAN, S.P. and CLARKE, S.W. (1983a). Factors influencing the size distributions of aerosols from jet nebulisers. *Thorax,* **38**, 755–759

CLAY, M.M., PAVIA, D., NEWMAN, S.P., LENNARD-JONES, T. and CLARKE, S.W. (1983b). Assessment of jet nebulisers for lung aerosol therapy. *Lancet,* **ii**, 592–594

COADY, T.J., DAVIES, H.J. and BARNES, P. (1976). Evaluation of a breath actuated pressurised aerosol. *Clin. Allergy*, **6**, 1–6

COX, J.S.G. (1969). Disodium cromoglycate in asthma. *Br. Med. J.*, **3**, 177

CROMPTON, G.K. (1982). Use and abuse of aerosol inhalers. In *New concepts in the topical treatment of asthma and related disorders.* Edited by McFadden, E.R. Greenwich; Cliggott Publishing Co., pp. 10–12

CURRY, S.H., TAYLOR, A.J., EVANS, S., GODFREY, S. and ZEIDIFARD, E. (1975). Disposition of disodium cromoglycate administered in three particle sizes. *Br. J. Clin. Pharmacol.*, **2**, 267–270

DAVIES, D.S. (1975). Pharmacokinetics of inhaled substances. *Postgrad. Med. J.*, **51**, Suppl. 7, 69–75

DAVIES, D.S. (1982). Pharmacokinetic studies with inhaled drugs. *Eur. J. Respir. Dis.*, **63**, Suppl. 119, 67–72

DOLOVICH, M., RYAN, G. and NEWHOUSE, M.T. (1981a). Aerosol penetration into the lung. Influence on airway responses. *Chest*, **80**, Supplement, 834–836

DOLOVICH, M., RUFFIN, R.E., ROBERTS, R. and NEWHOUSE, M.T. (1981b). Optimal delivery of aerosols from metered dose inhalers. *Chest*, **80**, Supplement, 911–915

DOLOVICH, M.B., KILLIAN, D., WOLFF, R.K., OBMINSKI, G. and NEWHOUSE, M.T. (1977). Pulmonary aerosol deposition in chronic bronchitis: Intermittent positive pressure breathing versus quiet breathing. *Am. Rev. Respir. Dis.*, **115**, 397–402

DOUGLAS, N.J., SUDLOW, M.F. and FLENLEY, D.C. (1979) Effect of an inhaled atropine-like agent on normal airway function. *J. Appl. Physiol.*, **46**, 256–262

FOORD, N., BLACK, A. and WALSH, M. (1978). Regional deposition of 2.5–7.5μ diameter inhaled particles in healthy male non-smokers. *J. Aerosol Sci.*, **9**, 343–357

GERRITY, T.R., LEE, P.S., HASS, F.J., MARINELLI, A., WERNER, P. and LOURENÇO, R.V. (1979). Calculated deposition of inhaled particles in the airway generations of normal subjects. *J. Appl. Physiol.*, **47**, 867–873

GODFREY, S., ZEIDIFARD, E., BROWN, K. and BELL, J.H. (1974). The possible site of action of sodium cromoglycate assessed by exercise challenge. *Clin. Sci. Mol. Med.*, **46**, 265–272

GONDA, I. (1981). Study of the effects of polydispersity of aerosols on regional deposition in the respiratory tract. *J. Pharm. Pharmacol.*, **33**, Supplement, 52P

GORMAN, W.G. and HALL, G.D. (1973). Inhalation aerosols. In *Current concepts in the pharmaceutical sciences: dosage form design and bioavailability.* Edited by Swarbrick, J. Philadelphia; Lea and Ferbriger, pp. 97–148

GOTTSCHALK, B., LEUPOLD, W. and WOLLER, P. (1978). Deponierung von aerosolen in den Atemwegen. *Z. Erkrank. Atm.-Org.*, **150**, 139–146

HENSLEY, M.J., O'CAIN, C.F., McFADDEN, E.R. and INGRAM, R.H. (1978). Distribution of bronchodilatation in normal subjects: beta agonist versus atropine. *J. Appl. Physiol.*, **45**, 778–782

HILLER, F.C., MAZUMDER, M.K., WILSON, J.D. and BONE, R.C. (1978). Aerodynamic size distribution of metered dose bronchodilator aerosols. *Am. Rev. Respir. Dis.*, **118**, 311–317

HILLER, F.C., MAZUMDER, M.K., WILSON, J.D., RENNIGER, R.G. and BONE, R.C. (1981). Physical properties of therapeutic aerosols. *Chest*, **80**, Supplement, 901–903

HODSON, M.E., PENKETH, A.R.L. and BATTEN, J.C. (1981). Aerosol carbenicillin and gentamicin treatment of pseudomonas aeruginosa infection in patients with cystic fibrosis. *Lancet*, **2**, 1137–1139

INGRAM, R.H., WELLMAN, J.J., McFADDEN, E.R. and MEAD, J. (1977). Relative contributions of large and small airways to flow limitation in normal subjects before and after atropine and isoproterenol. *J. Clin. Invest.*, **59**, 696–703

LANCET (1975). Fluorocarbon aerosol propellants. *Lancet*, **1**, 1073–1074

LAWFORD, P. and McKENZIE, D. (1981). Pressurized aerosol technique. *Lancet*, **2**, 1003–1004

LEIFER, K.N. and WITTIG, H.J. (1975). The beta-2 sympathomimetic aerosols in the treatment of asthma. *Ann. Allergy*, **35**, 69–80

LEWIS, R.A., FLEMING, J.S., BALACHANDRAN, W. and TATTERSFIELD, A.E. (1981). Particle size distribution and deposition from a jet nebulizer: Influence of humidity and temperature. *Clin. Sci.*, **62**, 5P

LIN, M.S., HAYES, T.M., GOODWIN, D.A. and KRUSE, S.L. (1974). Distal penetration in radioaerosol inhalation with an ultrasonic nebulizer. *Radiology*, **112**, 443–447

LOURENÇO, R.V. and COTROMANES, E. (1982a). Clinical aerosols. I. Characterization of aerosols and their diagnostic uses. *Arch. Intern. Med.*, **142**, 2163–2172

LOURENÇO, R.V. and COTROMANES, E. (1982b). Clinical aerosols. II. Therapeutic aerosols. *Arch. Intern. Med.*, **142**, 2299–2308

MERCER, T.T. (1981). Production of therapeutic aerosols; principles and techniques. *Chest*, **80**, Supplement, 813–818

MILLER, W.F. (1973). Aerosol therapy in acute and chronic respiratory disease. *Arch. Intern. Med.*, **131**, 148–155

MORÉN, F. (1981). Pressurized aerosols for oral inhalation. *Int. J. Pharm.*, **8**, 1–10

MORROW, P.E. (1981). An evaluation of the physical properties of monodisperse and heterodisperse aerosols used in the assessment of bronchial function. *Chest*, **80**, Supplement, 809–813

MYGIND, N. (1982). Mucosal changes in the airways during long-term corticosteroid treatment. *Eur. J. Respir. Dis.*, **63**, Suppl. 122, 229–234

NEWMAN, S.P., PAVIA, D. and CLARKE, S.W. (1981a). How should a pressurized β-adrenergic bronchodilator be inhaled? *Eur. J. Respir. Dis.*, **62**, 3–21

NEWMAN, S.P., PAVIA, D., GARLAND, N. and CLARKE, S.W. (1982a). Effects of various inhalation modes on the deposition of radioactive pressurized aerosols. *Eur. J. Respir. Dis.*, **63**, Suppl. 119, 57–65

NEWMAN, S.P., PAVIA, D., MORÉN, F., SHEAHAN, N.F. and CLARKE, S.W. (1981b). Deposition of pressurized aerosols in the human respiratory tract. *Thorax*, **36**, 52–55

NEWMAN, S.P., MORÉN, F., PAVIA, D., LITTLE, F. and CLARKE, S.W. (1981c). Deposition of pressurized suspension aerosols inhaled through extension devices. *Am. Rev. Respir. Dis.*, **124**, 317–320

NEWMAN, S.P., MORÉN, F., PAVIA, D., CORRADO, O. and CLARKE, S.W. (1982b). The effects of changes in metered volume and propellant vapour pressure on the deposition of pressurized inhalation aerosols. *Int. J. Pharm.*, **11**, 337–344

NEWMAN, S.P., KILLIP, M., PAVIA, D., MORÉN, F. and CLARKE, S.W. (1983). Do particle size and airway obstruction affect the deposition of pressurized inhalation aerosols? *Thorax*, **38**, 233

PATERSON, J.W. (1977). Bronchodilators. In *Asthma*. Edited by Clark, T.J.H. and Godfrey, S. London; Chapman and Hall Ltd., pp. 251–271

PATERSON, J.W., WOOLCOCK, A.J. and SHENFIELD, G.M. (1979). Bronchodilator drugs. *Am. Rev. Respir. Dis.*, **120**, 1149–1188

RANCE, R.W. (1974). Studies of the factors controlling the action of hair sprays—III: The influence of particle velocity and diameter on the capture of particles by arrays of hair fibres. *J. Soc. Cosmet. Chem.*, **25**, 545–561

REES, P.J. CLARK, T.J.H. and MORÉN, F. (1982). The importance of particle size in response to inhaled bronchodilators. *Eur. J. Respir. Dis.*, **63**, suppl. 119, 73–78

RILEY, D.J., WEITZ, B.W. and EDELMAN, N.H. (1976). The responses of asthmatic subjects to isoproterenol inhaled at differing lung volumes. *Am. Rev. Respir. Dis.*, **114**, 509–515

RUFFIN, R.E., OBMINSKI, G. and NEWHOUSE, M.T. (1978a). Aerosol salbutamol administration by IPPB: lowest effective dose. *Thorax*, **33**, 689–693

RUFFIN, R.E., KENWORTHY, M.C. and NEWHOUSE, M.T. (1978b). Response of asthmatic patients to fenoterol inhalation: a method of quantifying the airway bronchodilator dose. *Clin. Pharmacol. Ther.*, **23**, 338–345

RUFFIN, R.E., DOLOVICH, M.B., OLDENBURG, F.A. and NEWHOUSE, M.T. (1981). The preferential deposition of inhaled isoproterenol and propranolol in asthmatic patients. *Chest*, **80**, Supplement, 904–907

RUFFIN, R.E., DOLOVICH, M.B., WOLFF, R.K. and NEWHOUSE, M.T. (1978c). The effects of preferential deposition of histamine in the human airway. *Am. Rev. Respir. Dis.*, **117**, 485–492

RYAN, G., DOLOVICH, M.B., OBMINSKI, G., COCKROFT, D.W., JUNIPER, E., HARGREAVE, F.E. and NEWHOUSE, M.T. (1981). Standardisation of inhalation provocation tests: influence of nebulizer output, particle size and method of inhalation. *J. Allergy Clin. Immunol.*, **67**, 156–161

SACKNER, M.A., BROWN, L.K. and KIM, C.S. (1981). Basis of an improved metered aerosol delivery system. *Chest*, **80**, Supplement, 915–918

SANDERS, P.A. (1970). *Principles of aerosol technology*. New York; Van Nostrand Rheinhold, pp. 3–7

SHORT, M.D., SINGH, C.A., FEW, J.D., STUDDY, P.T., HEAF, P.J.D. and SPIRO, S.G. (1981). The labelling and monitoring of lung deposition of an inhaled synthetic anticholinergic bronchodilating agent. *Chest*, **80**, Supplement, 918–921

SMITH, G., HILLER, C., MAZUMDER, M. and BONE, R. (1980). Aerodynamic size distribution of cromolyn sodium at ambient and airway humidity. *Am. Rev. Respir. Dis.*, **121**, 513–517

TASHKIN, D.P., TREVOR, E., CHOPRA, S.K. and TAPLIN, G.V. (1980). Sites of airway dilatation in asthma following inhaled versus subcutaneous terbutaline. Comparison of physiologic tests with radionuclide lung images. *Am. J. Med.*, **68**, 14–26

TASK GROUP ON LUNG DYNAMICS (1966). Deposition and retention models for internal dosimetry of the human respiratory tract. *Health Phys.*, **12**, 173–207

TATTERSFIELD, A.E. (1982). Albuterol in the long-term treatment of airways disease. In *New concepts in the topical treatment of asthma and related disorders*. Edited by McFadden, E.R. Greenwich; Cliggott Publishing Co., pp. 33–37

TOBIN, M.J., JENOURI, G., DANTA, I., KIM, C., WATSON, H. and SACKNER, M.A. (1982). Response to bronchodilator drug administration by a new reservoir aerosol delivery system and a review of other auxiliary delivery systems. *Am. Rev. Respir. Dis.*, **126**, 670–675

TOOGOOD, J.H., JENNINGS, B., BASKERVILLE, J. and JOHANSSON, S-A. (1982). Clinical use of spacer systems for corticosteroid inhalation therapy: A preliminary analysis. *Eur. J. Respir. Dis.*, **63**, Suppl. 122, 100–107

WASNICH, R.D. (1976). A high frequency nebulizer system for radioaerosol delivery. *J. Nucl. Med.*, **17**, 707–710

WEIBEL, E.R. (1963). *Morphometry of the human lung*. New York; Academic Press

WILLIAMS, M.H. (1974). Steroids and antibiotic aerosols. *Am. Rev. Respir. Dis.*, **110**, 122–127

WILLIAMS, M.H. (1982). Office management of asthma. In *New concepts in the topical treatment of asthma and related disorders*. Edited by McFadden, E.R. Greenwich; Cliggott Publishing Co., pp. 47–50

Chapter 10

Aerosol challenge in lung diseases

P. Sherwood Burge

This chapter will describe the methods and limitations of bronchial provocation tests, with non-specific irritants, soluble allergens and occupational agents. The use of bronchial provocation testing in drug evaluation and the effects of drugs on the different types of reaction will be described. The mechanisms underlying the immediate and late asthmatic reactions will be discussed and finally, an idea of the sensitivity and specificity of these tests will be given.

Introduction

Aerosol challenge is used to assess either non-specific reactivity of the bronchi, or reactivity to specific allergens and chemicals. Measurement of non-specific reactivity is helpful in the diagnosis and follow-up of patients with suspected asthma. Asthma may present with nocturnal cough or with intermittent breathlessness; measurement of reactivity with non-specific irritants such as histamine or methacholine can document asthma when lung function is otherwise normal. These tests are also useful for following the progress of diseases and the results of allergen avoidance. Tests with specific allergens and chemicals are particularly indicated for making specific diagnoses when these are important and cannot be made by other methods, but are also useful for assessing the results of hyposensitization and in drug evaluation.

A bronchial provocation test aims to induce an asthmatic attack in the patient and is potentially dangerous. Tests should not be carried out by the uninitiated. Bronchial provocation testing with soluble allergens has been carried out safely in 1035 children by Aas (1970), when no anaphylactic reactions occurred. However, late and recurrent asthmatic attacks can be induced by such tests. Bronchial provocation testing with particulate occupational agents is potentially more dangerous as more severe reactions can occur. They must, therefore, be carried out with more caution, in hospital in-patients who should be monitored for at least 24 hours after each exposure.

Measurement of lung function for bronchial provocation testing

There is a diurnal variation in measures of airway calibre in both normal and asthmatic patients. Using FEV_1 or PEFR as a measure of airway calibre, the

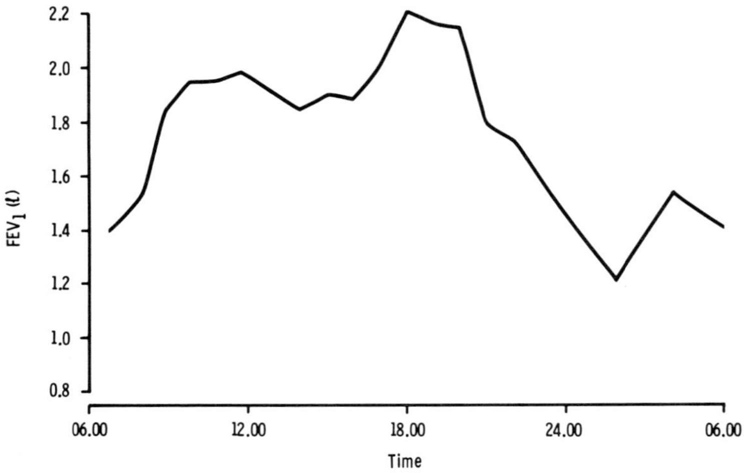

Figure 10.1 Diurnal variation in FEV_1 in a patient with isocyanate asthma on hospital admission. The low values on waking are just acceptable for proceeding to bronchial challenge, but the variability between 9.00 am and 9.00 pm is excessive and must be reduced before meaningful bronchial provocation testing can proceed

diurnal variation in a normal population has a mean of about 8 per cent, while most asthmatics have a diurnal variation exceeding 20 per cent (Hetzel and Clark, 1980). If more sensitive measures, such as airway resistance or conductance, are used then this diurnal variation is far higher. Airways obstruction is usually maximal on waking and is minimal 6–8 hours later, frequently with some deterioration in the evening before going to sleep again (*Figure 10.1*). Any reaction during bronchial provocation testing will be superimposed on this normal diurnal variation. It is therefore very important to have control exposures to substances to which the patient does not react so that the effects of diurnal variation can be eliminated. Comparative bronchial provocation testing should always be carried out at the same time of the day. It is unwise to start testing within 2–3 hours of waking because this amount of time is required to reach stable values of lung function. Because of the variability of the baseline, falls of FEV_1 or PEFR exceeding 15 per cent of values at the same time on a control day are required for the identification of definite late asthmatic reactions. If the objective is to identify significant reactions rather than their mechanisms it is better to have more, less sophisticated, measurements of lung function rather than fewer, more refined, measurements. Different observers can encourage different effort out of the same patient and for this reason I teach patients how to make their own measurements of FEV_1 and FVC and to make repeated measurements until the best two values of each parameter are within 100 ml of each other. In this way operator bias is eliminated and technically unsatisfactory readings can be validly rejected later. Measurements of PEFR may also be used but the technique involved cannot be checked afterwards. A few patients develop bronchoconstriction with successive forced expirations. For these patients only a single reading on each occasion can be made. Other patients develop successive bronchodilatation with maximal inspirations; these patients should continue with successive forced expirations until a peak is reached. Those with bronchoconstriction or bronchodilatation with successive forced expirations form about 5 per cent of the total population. Measurement of specific conductance can be used in the assessment of immediate asthmatic reactions and allows smaller absolute reactions to be classed as significant. It is generally impractical to make these readings into the evening and early the following morning, this, and the large changes that may occur spontaneously during the day, make measurements of specific conductance less appropriate for monitoring late asthmatic reactions.

Monitoring alveolar reactions

Extrinsic allergic alveolitis is traditionally diagnosed from the clinical history, together with nodular infiltrates seen on the chest x-ray and a fall in gas transfer and lung volumes on pulmonary function testing. These indices of clinical disease are not sensitive enough as markers during bronchial provocation testing. The chest x-ray rarely becomes abnormal following laboratory exposure and the DLCO falls significantly in severe reactions only (Hendrick *et al.*, 1980). These authors have compared 12 indicators of alveolar reactions in 144 challenge tests principally with avian serum. Specificity of at least 95 per cent was found with a 15 per cent fall in forced vital capacity, a rise in body temperature over 37.2°C, a neutrophilia exceeding 2500 mm^{-3}, as well as measurements of respiratory frequency and minute ventilation during a standardized exercise test, and the development of lymphopenia (a fall of 500 mm^{-3}). The sensitivity was greatest (79 per cent) for the body temperature and lowest (48 per cent) for the forced vital capacity. These authors have developed an index combining these tests to improve sensitivity.

Timing of measurements of lung function

Before starting bronchial provocation testing lung function should be measured every 5–10 minutes until stable for at least 30 minutes. Following exposure lung function should be measured every 5 minutes for the first 30 minutes, every 10 minutes for the second 30 minutes and at 90 minutes, 120 minutes and then hourly until sleeping and hourly from waking the following morning. Patients who only have an immediate asthmatic reaction and have no further drop six or seven hours after exposure can safely stop their readings at this time.

Types of reaction

Single exposures can result in reactions predominantly in the airways or predominantly in the alveoli. Airway reactions vary in time of onset and duration but may be broadly classified into immediate, late, dual and recurrent.

Immediate reactions

These start within minutes of exposure and reach a peak within 5–20 minutes. They may be induced by irritants such as histamine and by allergens. Irritant reactions usually resolve spontaneously within 30–60 minutes (*Figure 10.2*) whereas allergic reactions usually take a little longer, commonly 60–180 minutes (*Figure 10.3*).

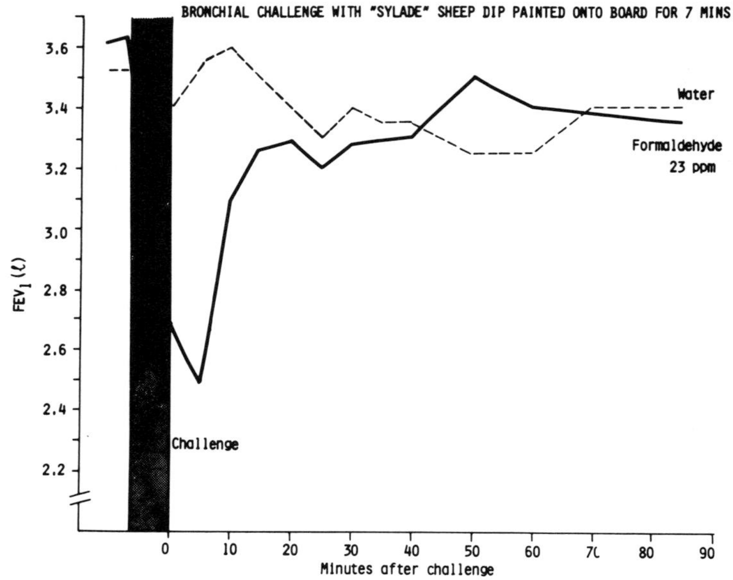

Figure 10.2 Immediate asthmatic reaction in a shepherd using a sheep dip containing 25 per cent formaldehyde. The solution was painted on to a flat surface for 7 minutes. Formaldehyde levels monitored during challenge testing were 23 ppm (threshold limit value 2 ppm). The short duration of the immediate reaction suggests that this may be a non-specific irritant effect. The patient had previously been exposed to 3 and 6 ppm on previous days with no reactions

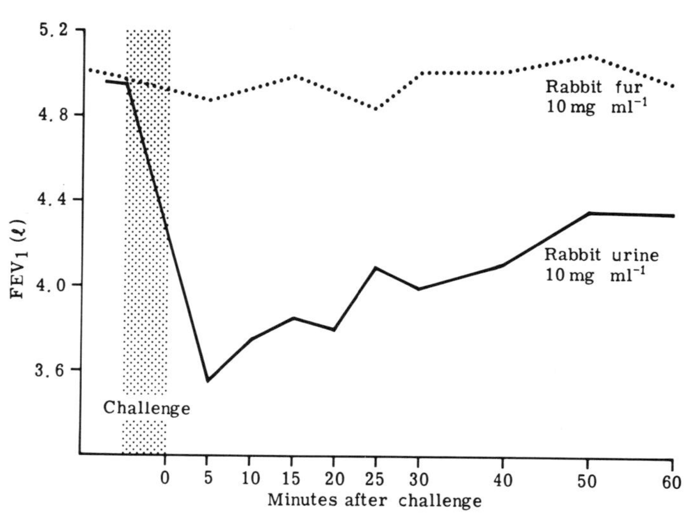

Figure 10.3 Immediate asthmatic reaction in a laboratory worker exposed to an extract of rabbit urine for 5 minutes. There was no reaction to an extract of rabbit's dander at the same concentration. The reaction resolved completely at 2 hours. The timing is classical of an IgE mediated immediate reaction. It also illustrates the importance of using the correct allergen

Late asthmatic reactions

These start more than one hour after exposure. The time of onset is very variable but most reactions start 3–4 hours after exposure and develop gradually, reaching a peak 8–10 hours after exposure (*Figure 10.4*). Some late reactions show improvement before the end of the day but many are more or less maximal when the patient goes to bed. Further deterioration may occur overnight such that the greatest airways obstruction is on rising the following morning (*Figure 10.5*). Some

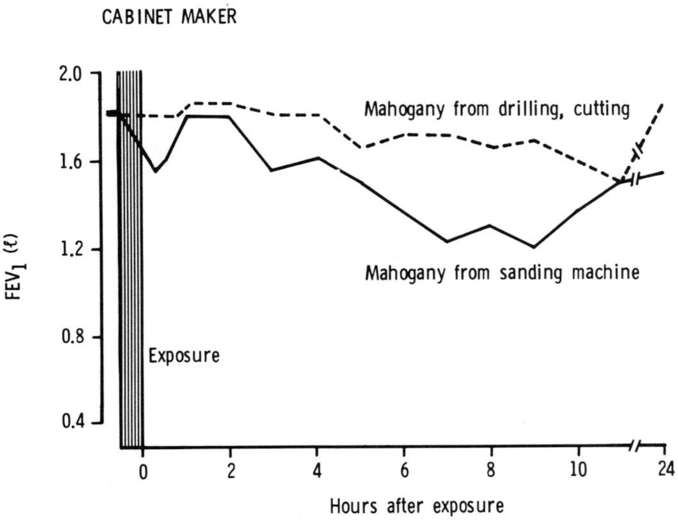

Figure 10.4 Late asthmatic reaction following exposure to mahogany dust from a sanding machine. There was no significant reaction after exposure to dust with a larger particle size from the same wood obtained from a cutting and planing machine. The late asthmatic reaction shows no further deterioration overnight

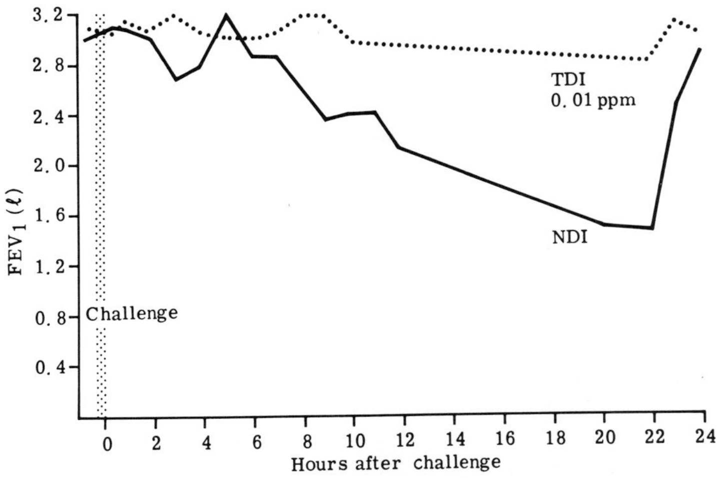

Figure 10.5 Late asthmatic reaction following a one minute exposure to heated naphthylene di-isocyanate (NDI). The lowest readings are on waking the following morning. There was no reaction following exposure to toluene di-isocyanate (TDI) for 30 minutes

reactions are not apparent during the day of exposure at all but only occur during the night following exposure. Other patients show some improvement during the night following exposure (Pepys and Hutchcroft, 1975).

Dual asthmatic reactions

Immediate reactions may be followed by late asthmatic reactions usually with substantial recovery between the two phases (*Figure 10.6*) but occasionally with the

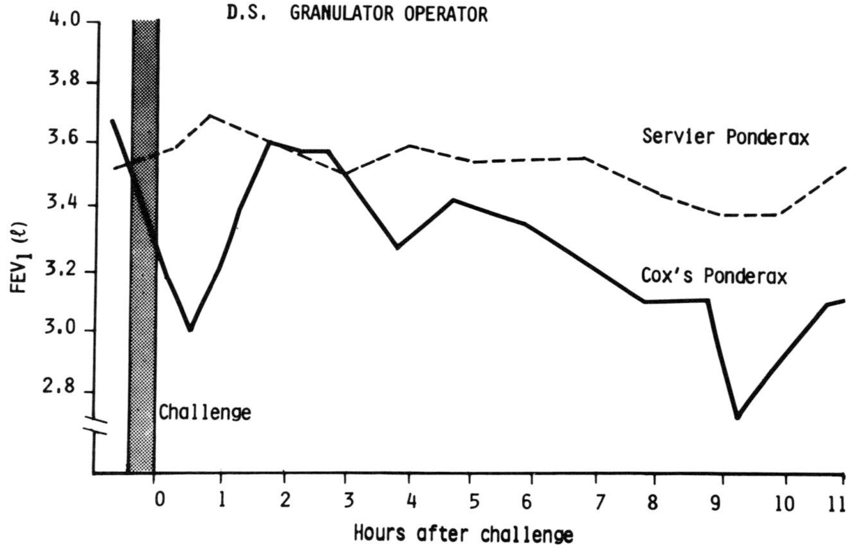

Figure 10.6 Dual immediate and late asthmatic reactions in a drug manufacturer. His work involved blending and drying the constituents of Ponderax. There was no reaction following the tipping of the constituents of Servier Ponderax (not used at his work). Only the Cox's formulation contained gum acacia, to which he was sensitive. There is a recovery between the two phases of the dual reaction

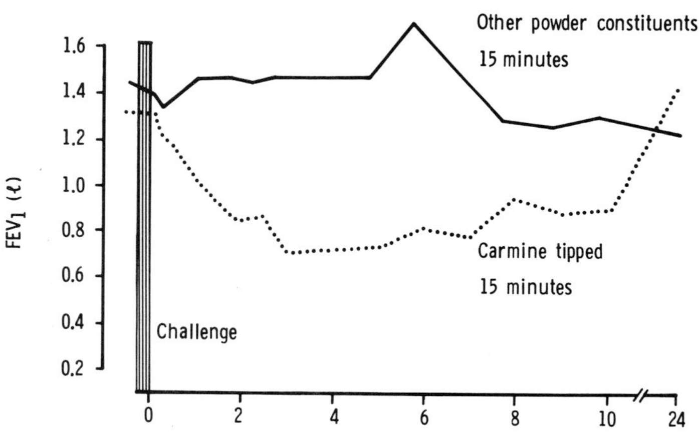

Figure 10.7 Dual immediate and late asthmatic reaction in a cosmetic blender sensitized to carmine, a constituent of the blend. There was no reaction to the other materials that he worked with. The immediate reaction passes into the late reaction without intervening recovery

immediate phase passing directly into the late phase without improvement (*Figure 10.7*). The late phase of dual reactions commonly lasts less long than isolated late asthmatic reactions. In some patients the late phase only occurs after large immediate reactions; with small (but significant) immediate reactions no late phase is seen.

Recurrent reactions

A single exposure on one day may induce asthma which lasts for many days or weeks (*Figure 10.8*). The recurrent reactions are usually an exaggeration of the normal diurnal variation with increased morning dips, although some patients also deteriorate in the evening before sleep (Newman Taylor *et al.*, 1979).

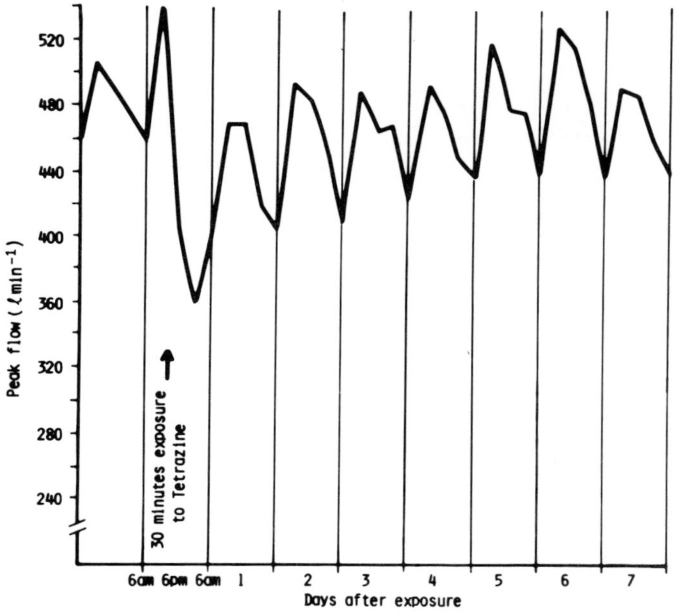

Figure 10.8 Recurrent asthmatic reactions in a detonator manufacturer following a single exposure to 6.5 per cent tetrazine in lactose tipped between two trays (*Figure 10.12*). The reaction lasted at least 7 days

Alveolar reactions

Aerosol challenge may be followed by disease predominantly in the alveoli. In general much higher exposures are required to elicit alveolar reactions. Their timing coincides with that of the late asthmatic reaction, usually starting about four hours after exposure with a peak about eight hours after exposure, with recovery over the next 24–48 hours (*Figure 10.9*).

Bronchial reactivity associated with allergen challenge

Histamine reactivity is unaltered following an immediate asthmatic reaction. In patients with dual or late asthmatic reactions, histamine reactivity increases

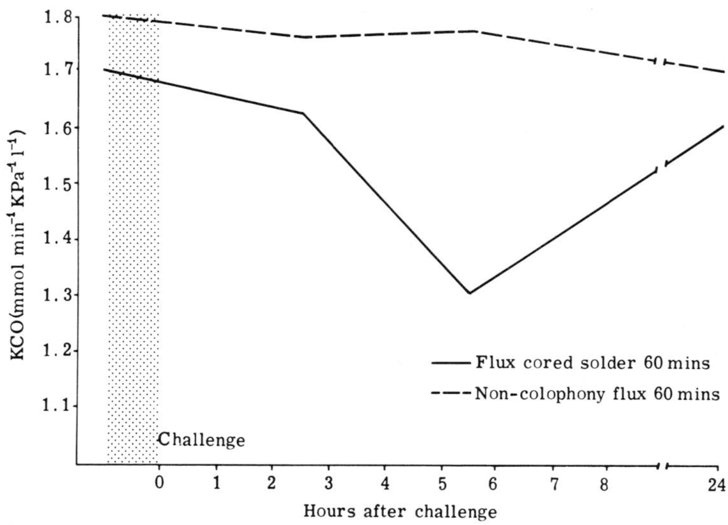

Figure 10.9 An alveolar reaction due to colophony in flux cored solder in an electronics worker. There was no reaction after a similar sixty minute exposure to a non-colophony flux-cored solder. The reaction has been monitored with measurements of transfer co-efficient, KCO, and has resolved at twenty-four hours

following the late component and may remain below baseline for periods of 2–14 days following a single exposure. This fact can be used to clarify the significance of equivocal late asthmatic reactions (Cockcroft *et al.*, 1977a).

Standardization of aerosol challenge with soluble agents

The aim is to inhale a reproducible volume of particles which will result in a reproducible response in an individual. Several distinct phases must be standardized including the aerosol generation, aerosol deposition in the lung and the responsiveness of the individual.

There may be differences between different nebulizers of the same make so that a nebulizer with a known output should be used and driven by air or oxygen at a suitable volume and pressure to produce an aerosol of mass median diameter of 1.3–3.6 μm with less than 5 per cent over 5 μm (Ryan *et al.*, 1981a). The aerosol output is altered by the temperature of the solution and its volume in the nebulizer. The deposition of the aerosol depends principally on the pattern of breathing, being more central when the airstream is more turbulent during forced inspiratory manoeuvres, and more peripheral during tidal breathing (Ryan *et al.*, 1981b). The patient's response depends principally on the starting value of FEV_1, but is also altered by the pH and temperature of the aerosol (Cockcroft and Bernscheid, 1983). The aerosol should also be isotonic as both hyper and hypotonic solutions can induce asthma (Schoeffel *et al.*, 1981). The dose of aerosol deposited in the lung is exceedingly difficult to quantitate and is usually unknown. There are two distinct methods used to try and standardize the lung dose. The John Hopkins dosimeter delivers a constant amount of solution from a connected De Vilbiss no. 42 nebulizer and is triggered by inhalation. It is driven by compressed air at 20 psi and is nebulized over 0.6 s in adults during a maximum inhalation from functional

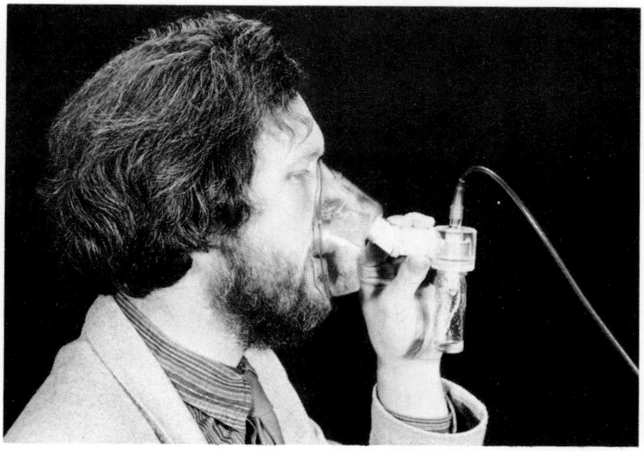

Figure 10.10 Bronchial provocation testing with an allergen extract nebulized in a Wright's nebulizer

residual capacity to inspiratory capacity (Chai *et al.*, 1975). The equipment needed is expensive, and does not produce more reproducible results than the alternative method of continuous nebulization which has been standardized by the McMaster group (Cockcroft *et al.*, 1977b; Juniper *et al.*, 1978; Ryan *et al.*, 1981b). Their method involves the use of a Wright's nebulizer driven with air at 50 psi at 7–8 ℓ min^{-1} with an output of 0.13 ml min^{-1} and aerosol particles of 1.3 μm mass median diameter and 2.11 μm geometric standard deviation. The test solution is allowed to reach room temperature and 3 ml are placed in the nebulizer which is not held in the hand. The output from the nebulizer is fed directly into a face mask without holes which is held loosely over the face so that the inspiration can take place both from the nebulizer and air sucked in from around the face mask (*Figure 10.10*). The nose is clipped and the patient breathes using tidal respiration. For higher concentrations of histamine and methacholine the eyes are closed to avoid irritation. The histamine test is standardized on 2 minute inhalations (if more prolonged inhalations are required the volume of solution must be increased).

Tests of non-specific reactivity

Bronchial reactivity can be assessed by inhaling aerosols of many substances including sulphur dioxide, $PGF_{2\alpha}$, carbachol, bradykinin, cold air, and hypo- or hyper-tonic saline (or water), but the two most widely used substances are histamine and methacholine. Response is usually assessed by finding the dose of histamine or methacholine which causes a 20 per cent fall in FEV_1 from baseline (PD_{20}). The first test is with phosphate buffered saline, lung function after this is taken as baseline. Doubling concentrations of histamine or methacholine from 0.03 to 8.0 mg ml^{-1} are inhaled for 2 minutes at five minute intervals until a 20 per cent fall in FEV_1 occurs or the top dose is reached.

Bronchial reactivity, measured in this way, is abnormal in the great majority of symptomatic asthmatics, but may be normal in asthmatics in remission. It is also abnormal in some studies in patients with bronchitis. Reactivity in bronchitics is difficult to interpret because bronchitics have not been defined in terms of reversibility of airways obstruction, but in terms of sputum production; many bronchitics in such surveys may therefore have reversible airways obstruction as well as cough and sputum and could be regarded as asthmatics. The PD_{20} cannot be measured with the described techniques in normal populations without substantially increasing the dose of histamine or methacholine, when systemic effects may be seen. Using methacholine, which has less systemic effects at high dose, patients with rhinitis who have never wheezed can be shown to be more reactive than subjects who have never had rhinitis or asthma (Bryant and Burns, 1976a;b). Non-specific reactivity can be increased by a number of factors, in particular by viral respiratory infections (Empey *et al.*, 1976) and allergen exposure. Allergen exposure only increases non-specific reactivity when associated with a late asthmatic reaction (Cockcroft *et al.*, 1977a). Non-specific reactivity can return to normal following allergen avoidance suggesting that allergen exposure is sufficient to induce non-specific reactivity (Burge, 1982d; Lam *et al.*, 1979).

Bronchial provocation testing with soluble allergens

Allergen induced bronchial provocation testing is most conveniently carried out with water soluble extracts of suitable allergens. The extraction process produces extracts of variable composition and concentrations and there are major problems in the standardization of such extracts. There are few extracts available with known concentrations of known allergens. However, soluble allergens are readily removed from the lung and are the only materials suitable for the evaluation of drugs using bronchial provocation testing. Allergen extracts should be sterile and should not include glycerol which is present in skin test extracts as the glycerol can occasionally induce asthmatic reactions. All patients should be skin prick tested with the extract to be used for bronchial provocation testing to determine the starting concentration required for the provocation tests. There are no severe reactions following a one minute inhalation of an extract which produces a 3 mm wheal or less following skin prick testing (Killian *et al.*, 1976). This forms a convenient and safe starting point for bronchial provocation tests. If a patient is to develop a late asthmatic reaction only then there is no early indicator when sufficient allergen has been given. For this reason it is important to increase the dose only to a limited extent on any one day. The following is a safe regimen. On the first day an allergen extract producing a 3 mm or less wheal is used. Inhalation is initially for one minute followed by measurements of lung function after five or ten minutes. Only if the FEV_1 has fallen by less than 15 per cent is a second inhalation given for two minutes. Again measurements of lung function are made after five and ten minutes. Provided that the FEV_1 has not fallen by 15 per cent from baseline at this stage a final two minute inhalation is given, making a maximum of five minutes in all. Lung function is then measured serially for the rest of the day. If there is no significant immediate or late asthmatic reaction on this day, then the concentration of allergen extract may be increased ten-fold for a similar series of provocation tests on the following day. In general, patients with markedly increased histamine reactivity will react on the first day and patients with near normal histamine reactivity will react on the second day.

Bronchial provocation testing with occupational allergens

It is possible to make soluble extracts of some occupational allergens such as rodent danders, rodent serum and urine extracts (Newman Taylor, 1982) carmine (Burge *et al.*, 1979c) wood dusts, and other biological materials such as castor beans, coffee beans, wheat, mites, insects, etc. (Harries *et al.*, 1980). Extracts are suitable for well-tried allergens but the variability of the extraction process makes it unsuitable in general for unusual allergens which are best used in their native state.

Setting up occupational type bronchial provocation tests

Occupational type bronchial provocation tests aim to expose a worker to the same material to which he is exposed at work. The exposure should be to concentrations the same or less than at work with durations of exposure far less than at work. Before these tests can be safely carried out the work environment must be investigated. The nature of any possible agents must be determined, their physical characteristics ascertained and the exposure levels monitored. An attempt should

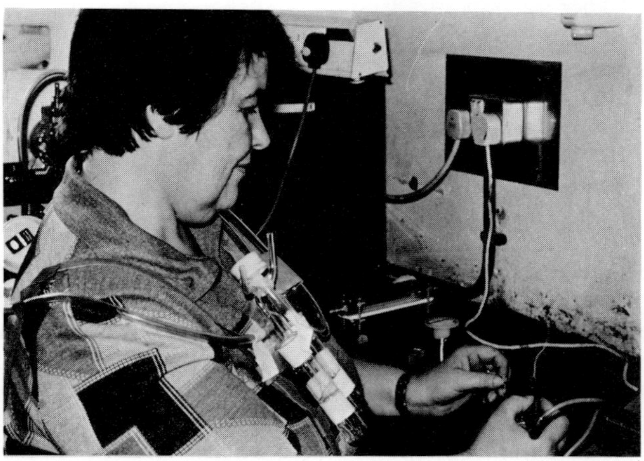

Figure 10.11 Bronchial provocation testing with flux-cored solder containing colophony. The same solder as used at work was heated to the same temperature as at work, but the volume and duration of soldering was much less than at work. Atmospheric levels of colophony were measured during the challenge testing

be made to reproduce the characteristics of the material in the challenge chamber and monitor the exposure levels obtained. For instance, the following steps were taken when setting up occupational bronchial provocation testing with soft soldering fluxes produced at work by heating flux-cored solder with a soldering iron or solder bath (Burge *et al.*, 1980). The temperature of the soldering iron was measured at work and the levels of exposure monitored on personal samplers. In the provocation tests the same flux-cored solder was used as at work, heated to the same temperature. Levels were monitored in the challenge chamber as at work (*Figure 10.11*). In this case the extent of exposure was altered by changing the length of exposure. In other circumstances it is easier to keep the length of exposure constant and alter the concentration of material used.

Bronchial provocation testing with dusts (*Figure 10.12*)

Many materials at work are inhaled as dust, such as woods and bulk chemicals and drugs. Atmospheric levels of some drugs and chemicals at work are so low that the only practical way of carrying out the provocation tests is to dilute the chemical during challenge testing. For instance 40 mg of ammonium hexachlorplatinate must

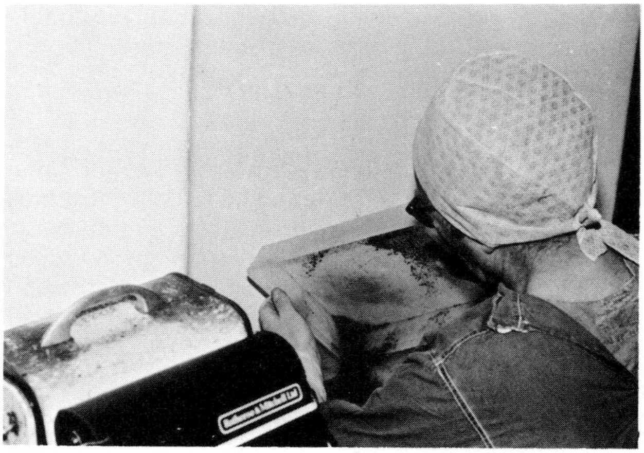

Figure 10.12 Bronchial provocation testing with detonator constituents diluted in dried lactose. The powder is being tipped between two trays and the levels of exposure monitored (this is the control exposure, the monitoring equipment is unsafe with highly explosive materials). The worker wears protective clothes that can be removed after exposure to limit further exposure after the challenge test. The results of the active challenge are shown in *Figure 10.8*

be mixed with 1 kg of dried lactose before challenge testing (Pickering, 1972). Even with this dilution atmospheric levels reached the threshold limit value of 0.002 mg m^{-3}. Antibiotics such as the penicillins and cephalosporins can cause reactions in concentrations of 100 g in 1 kg of lactose (Coutts *et al.*, 1981; Davies *et al.*, 1974). Lactose is a well-tried diluent for particulate challenges, but it must be well-dried before use or else it clumps together. A few patients developed irritant reactions following challenge with the lactose alone which must be used as a control in such tests. Lactose has also been used for diluents for challenges with phthalic anhydride (Fawcett *et al.*, 1977), piperazine (Pepys *et al.*, 1972a), methyldopa (Harries *et al.*, 1979b), cobalt chloride (Davidson *et al.*, 1983), cimetidine and tetrazine. Some dusts may be used in a neat form, particularly wood dusts (Pickering *et al.*, 1972a) grains and flour (Hendrick *et al.*, 1976), the concentrations of which are often in the order of 1 mg m^{-3} or more at work. It is very important to obtain material of fine particle size which can be inhaled when using dusts for provocation testing. Wood dusts in particular vary greatly in particle size depending on the machine from which they are collected. *Figure 10.4* shows two provocation tests in the same individual with wood dust with no significant reaction following dust taken from a sawing and planing machine and a significant reaction following exposure to dust from the same wood produced by a sanding machine. Patients exposed to particulate challenges should wear protective clothing with their hair, bodies and feet covered. The clothing should be removed following challenge so that inhalation exposure then ceases (*Figure 10.12*). Non-water soluble particulates may be cleared very slowly from the lungs and may persist for many weeks if deposited in the alveolar regions. This may account for some of the prolonged reactions that can follow such exposure.

Provocation tests with vapours at room temperature

Volatile liquids can be conveniently tested by being painted on a flat surface at room temperature (*Figure 10.13*). This is a convenient way to test materials that are

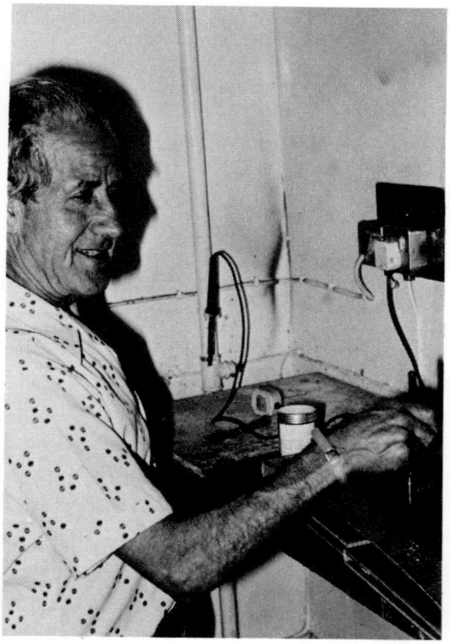

Figure 10.13 Bronchial provocation testing with 25 per cent formalin, being painted onto card. The technique is suitable for volatile liquids. This concentration of formaldehyde is highly irritant to the eyes

painted or sprayed at work. The original provocation tests using toluene di-isocyanate were set up in this way as the first patient tested developed occupational asthma while varnishing the Oxford boat for the boat race using a two-part polyurethane paint containing toluene di-isocyanate (Pepys *et al.*, 1972b). The concentrations of isocyanate can be altered by increasing the amount of isocyanate in the mixture. Painting is also suitable for any volatile material such as hexamethyline di-isocyanate (O'Brien *et al.*, 1979) formaldehyde (Hendrick and Lane, 1975) cold curing adhesives such as triethylene tetramine (Fawcett *et al.*, 1977) and acrylics (Burge and Pepys, 1979). Clean paint brushes should be used for each substance. These tests can in general be carried out with substances at the same concentrations as used at work. Atmospheric levels during provocation tests will be far lower by this method than when the material is sprayed at work. Spraying should not be attempted in the bronchial provocation chamber without measuring atmospheric levels beforehand as concentrations are raised very considerably by this process. Volatile materials may also be tested by passing an air current over the liquid. This may make exposures more controlled for very volatile substances and has been used satisfactorily for testing toluene di-isocyanate (Butcher, 1979).

Heated materials

Substances which are not volatile at room temperature and are heated at work will also need heating during provocation testing. Much greater care is needed during this process as the temperature is often critical and it is possible to produce very high concentrations during provocation testing. Most heated materials at work are used with exhaust extraction which radically reduces exposures. In general very small quantities should be used in the challenge testing (1 g or less) and levels should definitely be monitored before challenge testing begins. Heating should be carried out on a thermostatically controlled hot plate and exposures should initially be very short. Reactions have occurred after a single breath of heated material such as phthalic anhydride (Fawcett *et al.*, 1977). Materials tested during heating have included diphenylmethane di-isocyanate (MDI) (O'Brien *et al.*, 1979) naphthylene di-isocyanate (Harries *et al.*, 1979a), phthalic anhydride, tetrachlorphthalic anhydride and trimellitic anhydride (Fawcett *et al.*, 1977), colophony (Burge *et al.*, 1980; Burge, 1982a), PVC (Pauli *et al.*, 1980), and aminoethylethanolamine (Pepys and Pickering, 1972). Exposures should be very carefully controlled in the initial stages of such tests. A suitable first day's exposure will involve one breath, three breaths and five breaths, each separated by ten minutes of recordings as used in challenges with nebulized extracts. If no reaction occurs on the first day the exposures can be one minute, two minutes and two minutes on the second day, two minutes, four minutes and four minutes on the third day, and five minutes, five minutes and five minutes on the next day. It has been possible to control colophony challenges to a greater degree than most other challenges with heated materials as the flux cored solder can be handled and can be consumed at any desired rate by the worker (*Figure 10.11*). Using a soldering bit at 350°C and touching the soldering iron on to the flux-cored solder every 30 seconds the rate of consumption can be adjusted such

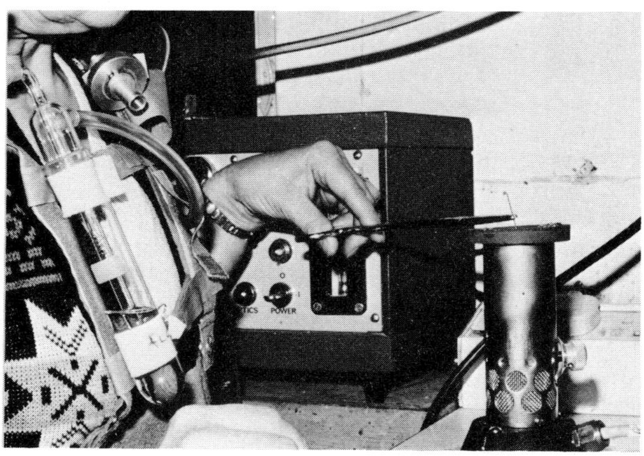

Figure 10.14 Bronchial provocation testing with toluene di-isocyanate liberated from coated wires when dipped into molten solder at 350°C. Breathing zone and area levels of TDI are being monitored. It is very easy to exceed the threshold limit value when heating isocyanates

that 25 cm of 16 SWG flux-cored solder are consumed every 15 minutes. This is a rate of soldering at least ten times less than often encountered at work. Using such tests colophony concentrations have been kept well below the threshold limit value and exposures have been continued for up to an hour with safety (Burge *et al.*, 1980).

Some exposures to toluene di-isocyanate result from the soldering of polyurethane coated wire. It is appropriate to use the wire as used at work, dipped into molten solder at the temperature as used at work for provocation testing in such workers (*Figure 10.14*). Concentrations up to the threshold limit value of 0.02 ppm are reached when 0.5 cm of wire is dipped into molten solder for five seconds every minute. Under exhaust extraction at work at least five times the volume of wire may be dipped into solder every few seconds.

Reproduction of a whole work process

It is often appropriate at least in the first instance, to try and reproduce a whole work process during provocation testing. Many substances have been tested in this way. Toluene di-isocyanate and diphenylmethane di-isocyanate foams can be tested by mixing the constituents together and producing the foam in the challenge chamber. Other uses of such tests have involved stainless steel welding (Keskinen *et al.*, 1980), core making with a moulding sand impregnated with a furance system (Cockcroft *et al.*, 1980), electroplating with a chromate solution, the mixing of an acrylic bone cement (Burge and Pepys, 1979), the mixing of bleaches and dyes in hairdressers (Pepys *et al.*, 1976) and the sanding of wood (*Figure 10.15*). The latter

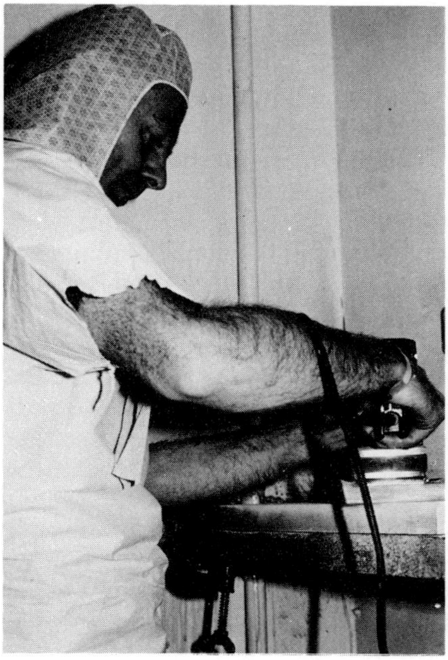

Figure 10.15 Bronchial provocation testing reproducing the work process. In this case rosewood is being sanded with a vibrating sander

method of testing overcomes the problems of collecting sawdust of suitable particle size.

Occupational asthma can also be diagnosed by monitoring lung function in relation to work exposures (Burge, 1982b). This can often confirm or exclude the diagnosis, but can rarely identify precise causes as most occupational environments involve exposure to several different substances. Such monitoring is useful to select patients for subsequent diagnostic bronchial provocation testing.

Problems with bronchial provocation testing

Definite results are not always obtained in individuals undergoing diagnostic bronchial provocation testing. The sicker the patient the more difficult the tests become, because of difficulty obtaining satisfactory control exposures. The difficulties arise because of irritant reactions to 'inert' control exposures and because of spontaneous changes in airway calibre unrelated to specific exposures.

Asthmatic attacks are deliberately induced during bronchial provocation testing. The ideal challenge results in a 20 per cent fall in FEV_1; however, in practice it is difficult to avoid the occasional reaction with a 40 per cent or even 50 per cent fall, patients must have sufficient reserve to be able to cope with such reactions. If the asthma is too severe to risk such reactions, then it must be improved before bronchial provocation testing can be started. In patients with occupational asthma improvement can often be obtained by removing the patient from exposure before challenge testing (Burge *et al.*, 1979a;b). Improvement may continue for at least ten weeks after the last exposure, as occupational exposures often induce recurrent reactions similar, but more severe than, those following single exposures in bronchial provocation tests. Patients who cannot be removed from exposure need their treatment optimized. This usually involves corticosteroids and bronchodilators, both of which may inhibit reactions during bronchial provocation testing. Once the asthma is as well controlled as possible the patient should be admitted to hospital, where confounding exposures (such as to house dust, exercise, cold air, etc.) can be largely prevented. It is usually impossible and impractical to withdraw corticosteroids at this stage. Increasing allergen exposure can overcome the protective effect of these drugs, however a negative test in the presence of corticosteroids is difficult to interpret. Inhaled bronchodilators usually cause sharp swings in the baseline and should be avoided apart from first thing each morning. If daytime bronchodilators are required oral salbutamol 2 mg, two hourly, minimizes the dips in FEV_1 without producing any acute response. If oral salbutamol is used it must be taken on control as well as active exposure days.

Patients with the greatest non-specific reactivity may react to control exposures such as powdered lactose. The ideal solution is to improve the patient's asthma and non-specific reactivity by allergen avoidance and treatment and to repeat the tests later. Alternatively, the length of the control exposure can be reduced below that which causes a reaction. Specific reactions should follow not more than half the exposure to the control substance, and be followed by a further control exposure without a drop in FEV_1. There is then reasonable evidence that the test substance is working with some degree of specificity.

Reproducibility is a major problem during drug evaluation where special precautions are necessary. In general patients become more sensitive with repeated daily exposures, particularly those associated with late asthmatic reactions. If the tests are carried out to find the cause of the asthma this does not matter as it resembles the exposures the patients will receive out of hospital.

Finally, a series of negative bronchial provocation tests can be psychologically disturbing for the patient who has built up his hopes for a cause being found for his symptoms. Bronchial provocation testing can be negative in a patient with true asthma caused by the substance that has been tested, because of technical factors in the challenge such as wrong particle size (*Figure 10.4*), incorrect temperature or missing reactants or allergens in the materials being tested (*Figures 10.3* and *10.6*).

Bronchial challenge testing in drug assessment

Bronchial provocation testing forms the best method of assessing the effect of drugs which prevent asthmatic attacks without bronchodilator effects themselves (such as cromoglycate, etc.) in early phases of development. They are also the most suitable tests for monitoring the effects of hyposensitization. There are many problems with the use of these tests for drug assessment relating to the drugs themselves, the patients being studied and the methods of assessment.

Bronchial provocation testing with allergen extracts is only appropriate in patients with specific IgE antibody to that allergen. It is also only practical in patients with mild asthma if discrepancies owing to a shift of baseline are to be avoided. The drug effect is therefore likely to be tested in mild extrinsic asthmatics for whom there is already fairly good treatment. They may not be a relevant model predicting the efficacy of a drug in more severe perennial intrinsic asthmatics who form the group most in need of further drug development.

Bronchodilator drugs are very difficult to assess by this technique as they change the baseline prior to provocation testing, any changes seen may be due to the shift in baseline rather than to any prophylactic effect of the drug. Non-specific tests with methacholine or histamine can be used for the assessment of long-term drug efficacy. Non-specific reactivity has been shown to improve following cromoglycate treatment for instance (Altounyan, 1979). Non-specific reactivity also improves when asthmatic control is better and improvement in non-specific reactivity does not necessarily imply that a drug has any direct effect on reactivity but may just represent the drugs ability to improve the control of asthma from other mechanisms.

The most important problems relate to the method of assessing drug efficacy by bronchial provocation testing. Most pharmacologists favour an assessment based on the change of threshold dose of allergen required to elicit an immediate asthmatic reaction using an index such as the PD_{20} as is used in histamine reactivity. This technique is only appropriate in the assessment of immediate reactions and often involves giving very large doses of antigen in the presence of a blocking drug. If the drug inhibits the immediate reaction in these patients but not the late asthmatic reaction, they may have severe late asthmatic reactions following such tests. It is, therefore, important to reverse the immediate reactions when they occur; despite corticosteroids and bronchodilators given after the immediate reaction late reactions may still occur (Ollier *et al.*, 1982). Such tests are therefore not useful for following the natural history of the challenge or for assessing the late asthmatic reaction.

In general, drugs which affect the late asthmatic reaction are of more use in chronic asthma than drugs which affect the immediate asthmatic reaction. Drugs may also be assessed by measuring the blocking effect of the drug with similar allergen exposures with drug and placebo. The blocking index is calculated from the formula

$$\frac{A - B}{A} \times 100$$

where A = the maximum per cent fall in FEV_1 on placebo, and B = the maximum per cent fall in FEV_1 on active drug. This index can be calculated separately for immediate and late asthmatic reactions. This index is easy to use but it is only appropriate when the induced asthmatic reactions are allowed to resolve spontaneously. It also only takes account of the peak effect and will miss effects of drugs which diminish the duration of a reaction. Finally, assessment may be made by repeating identical challenges as in the blocking index method but instead of using the peak effect of the drug, the whole area between the placebo challenge and the active challenge is calculated. This gives an index of the extent and duration of the fall in FEV_1 and has been used in the assessment of an inhibitor of leucotriene synthesis, Isamoxole (*Figure 10.17*) which is only inhibiting one of the mediators of the immediate asthmatic reaction. In practice the blocking index and PD_{20} techniques can give very similar results for assessing the immediate reaction (Martin *et al.*, 1980).

There are several important confounding factors which should be avoided during bronchial provocation testing in drug assessment. The starting value of FEV_1 should be similar on all pre-challenge days as threshold doses of allergen required to induce asthma are dependent on the starting FEV_1. All drugs which have a possible effect on the reaction apart from those being assessed should be withdrawn. This particularly applies to bronchodilators, phosphodiesterase inhibitors, cromoglycate-like drugs, antihistamines and corticosteroids, all of which may inhibit asthmatic reactions in whole or in part. Patients should not have had a respiratory infection in the previous six weeks as this may alter baseline reactivity and patients being assessed with seasonal allergen should be assessed outside the season of that allergen, as they frequently become more sensitive during periods of continuous exposure. In general, bronchial provocation tests are not reproducible when carried out on a daily basis. Most patients become more sensitive with repeated exposures. Tests should therefore be carried out at weekly intervals and done at the same time each day to avoid the confounding factors of diurnal variation. Drugs with a prolonged duration of action may produce a carry-over effect from one period of a trial to another. If a prophylactic drug has been given it is important to make sure that baseline reactions to the allergen have been restored before any cross-over in the drug trial. Even with these precautions there is moderate inconsistency in the response to inhaled allergens and for this reason it is vital to make the drug assessments double-blind. It is very easy to manipulate readings of lung function by asking the patient to repeat readings with extra effort if the investigator feels that they should not be showing such a fall at that particular time.

Bronchial provocation testing is an under-used method of assessing the results of hyposensitization. For the tests to be valid the same allergen extract should be used both for hyposensitization and for the challenge tests. Warner and colleagues (1978) reported an interesting study of house dust mite hyposensitization in children. There were no changes in the immediate asthmatic reaction following hyposensitization but late asthmatic reactions were abolished in 45 per cent on active treatment and 7 per cent on placebo. There was also a strong correlation between symptomatic improvement and loss of the late asthmatic reaction, suggesting that this was a useful objective marker of clinical response.

Bronchial provocation tests for the assessment of antitussive drugs

Antitussive drugs can be evaluated using prolonged recordings of spontaneous cough in patients (Loudon and Romans, 1967) or by inducing cough in normal volunteers. Citric acid aerosols have been most widely used in normal volunteers, using a wide range of different techniques. Some studies have observed the effect of single doses of 25 per cent citric acid nebulized during one inhalation. The response may be the number of coughs, the volume of air expelled during the coughs, or the latent interval between the inhalation and the onset of cough (Calesnick *et al.*, 1961; Calesnick and Christensen, 1967). There is a considerable learning effect using single dose methods, the number of coughs following an inhalation diminishing during training. Stable numbers of coughs are produced after about seven tests (Bickerman *et al.*, 1956).

Increasing concentrations of citric acid from 1 to 50 per cent may be used to determine the cough threshold (Empey *et al.*, 1979; Rees and Clark, 1983). There is moderate baseline variability using this method, which nevertheless is simple to use and perhaps avoids the need for the trained subjects required for the single dose tests.

Codeine phosphate has been shown to reduce cough by all of these methods; results with drugs other than opiates have been inconsistent, although some aromatic oils rubbed onto the chest have reduced the number of coughs in some studies (Packman and London, 1980). Most studies have excluded 10–20 per cent of initial volunteers as the top concentration of citric acid did not induce coughing. The reproducibility is less in those who cough less than in those who cough more (Bickerman *et al.*, 1956).

There are as yet no standardized methods for performing citric acid challenge tests; the determination of the cough threshold is likely to be more sensitive than the response to a single concentration, but neither method is likely to replace the prolonged recording of spontaneous cough in the final evaluation of antitussive drugs.

Effect of drugs on bronchial provocation tests

Drugs may be given either as a prophylactic drug before challenge or for treatment to relieve asthma induced by bronchial challenge. Any drug which alters baseline airways obstruction will alter the threshold dose of allergen required to elicit asthma. Beta-receptor agonists such as salbutamol can block immediate asthmatic reactions when given before challenge. The improvement in FEV_1 pre-challenge makes it difficult to know whether the beta-agonist is working in a prophylactic

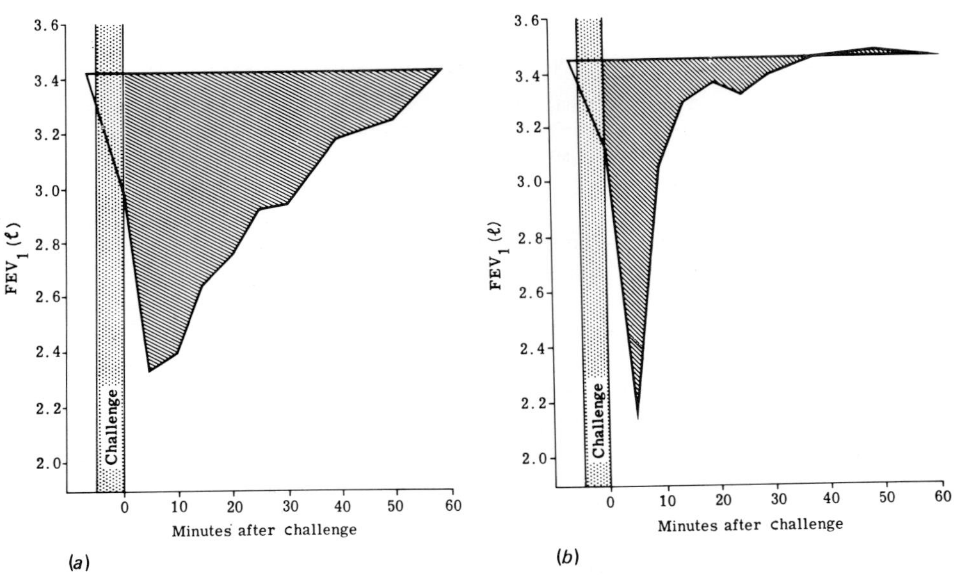

Figure 10.16 Bronchial provocation testing with an extract of guinea pig urine (a) following placebo pre-treatment and (b) isamoxole pre-treatment (a leucotriene synthesis inhibitor). The drug reduces the duration of the immediate reaction but not the peak fall. Assessment was made by calculating the hatched areas

manner or simply acting as a bronchodilator. Immediate asthmatic reactions can usually be easily reversed with an inhaled beta-agonist. However, if the same drug is given during a late asthmatic reaction the response is generally much less complete and the duration of its action often short, suggesting that different pathological mechanisms are involved in late asthmatic reactions. Antihistamines in general have little or no blocking effect on induced asthmatic attacks. A leucotriene synthesis inhibitor (Isamoxole) had a small but significant protective effect on immediate asthmatic reactions (*Figure 10.16*). Single doses of inhaled or oral corticosteroids have no protective effect on immediate asthmatic reactions (Pepys *et al.*, 1974). However, it has now become clear that inhaled or oral steroids are able to block the immediate asthmatic reaction when given for at least seven days pre-challenge (Burge, 1982c, Burge *et al.*, 1982f, Martin *et al.*, 1980). The effect becomes even stronger when given for 28 days pre-challenge (*Figure 10.17*)

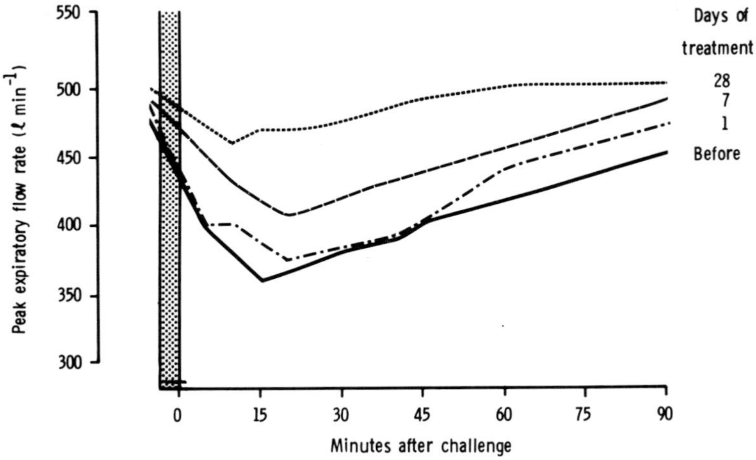

Figure 10.17 The blocking effect of an inhaled corticosteroid, budesonide 1 mg daily, on the immediate asthmatic reaction. Mean values for a group of 10 patients before treatment and after 1, 7 and 28 days of budesonide showing progressive blocking of the immediate asthmatic reaction. Redrawn from Dahl and Johansson (1982)

(Dahl and Johansson, 1982). These results appear independent of any change in baseline values of FEV_1. Sodium cromoglycate inhibits immediate asthmatic reactions (Pepys *et al.*, 1974). The above comments apply to allergen induced immediate asthmatic reactions. There is at present no evidence as to whether corticosteroids affect irritant reactions but sulphur dioxide induced asthma can be inhibited by sodium cromoglycate (Harries *et al.*, 1981). Antihistamines inhibit histamine induced asthma and anticholinergic methacholine induced asthma.

The late phase asthmatic reaction can be inhibited by inhaled or oral corticosteroids given as a single dose pre-challenge (Pepys *et al.*, 1974; Burge *et al.*, 1982f). Sodium cromoglycate produces variable results on late asthmatic reactions but inhibits about half of such reactions when given pre-challenge in single doses (Burge *et al.*, 1980). Other drugs have not been assessed adequately in the late asthmatic reaction. Aveolar reactions can be prevented by corticosteroid pretreatment (Williams, 1963) although there are no more formal studies in such patients.

Mechanisms of asthmatic reactions induced by bronchial provocation testing

Immediate asthmatic reactions may be due to a direct irritant effect, pharmacological effect, or allergic mechanisms. Many occupational chemicals are capable of causing irritant reactions in high concentrations particularly formaldehyde, phthalic anhydride, colophony and the isocyanates. However, the degree of exposure in industry is usually below irritant concentrations. A reaction is likely to be irritant if the threshold concentrations of material causing it correlates closely with the threshold dose for histamine or methacholine (for instance with sulphur dioxide). When only small numbers of individuals have been tested with a particular substance, then previously unexposed controls should be used with similar degrees of non-specific histamine reactivity to the cases. If reactions occur in the previously unexposed controls with similar non-specific reactivity, then the reaction in the cases is likely to be due to an irritant reaction. When the mechanism is allergic then

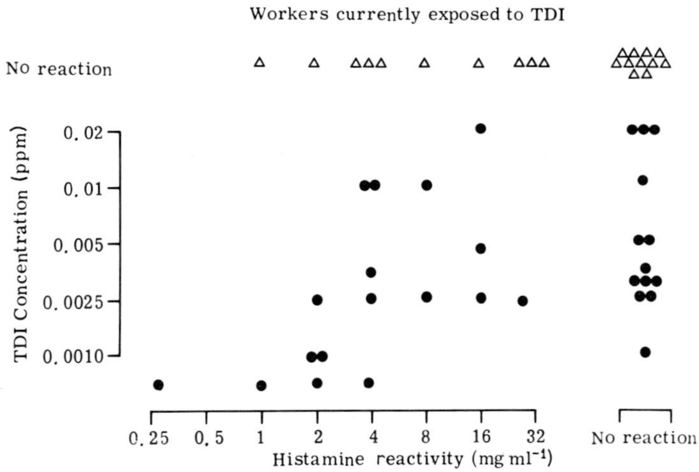

Figure 10.18 Threshold concentration of histamine and toluene di-isocyanate in a group of 30 isocyanate reactors and 21 non-reactors, all of whom were recently exposed at work. The histamine reactivity was measured before the isocyanate challenges by the method of DeVries with 30 second exposures (normal = no reaction). There is a weak correlation between histamine and isocyanate thresholds in the reactors ($r_s = 0.55$). There are several TDI non-reactors who have marked histamine reactivity showing that TDI is not acting as a non-specific irritant at these concentrations (from Burge, 1982)

histamine reactivity has a significant but weak effect on the threshold dose of specific material, commonly accounting for from 20 to 40 per cent of the threshold doses of the specific material (*Figure 10.18*) (Burge, 1982e; Bryant and Burns, 1976b). Some materials are able to induce asthmatic effects by pharmacological mechanisms, such as the cholinesterase inhibitors used as pesticides. A pharmacological mechanism has also been postulated to account for reactions to toluene di-isocyanate although it is unlikely that this is the whole story (Davies *et al.*, 1977). It is likely that most immediate reactions induced by allergen extracts involve IgE mediated degranulation of mast cells. Following allergen induced asthma histamine and neutrophil chemotactic factor both rise in the serum (Lee *et al.*, 1982). These mediators are not raised in the serum following methacholine induced asthma. In addition the rise in neutrophil chemotactic activity can be abolished by cromoglycate pre-treatment (Atkins *et al.*, 1978). Immediate asthmatic reactions to grass pollen and house dust mite can be induced only in those who have specific IgE antibody to those allergens (Bryant and Burns, 1976b). They found reactions could be induced in all those with specific antibody whether or not asthma had occurred before but the threshold dose required in the asthmatics were more than 100-fold less than in subjects who had never wheezed before. The threshold dose of allergen is also dependent on the level of specific IgE to that allergen (Bryant and Burns, 1976b; Killian *et al.*, 1976). IgE antibody is not a prerequisite for immediate allergic reactions at least on the skin, where immediate reactions may be induced by short term sensitizing IgG.

The mechanisms underlying the late asthmatic reaction are less clear. In clinical terms the onset is slower, the duration longer, and the response to beta-adrenergic agonists poorer than in the immediate asthmatic reaction. It is tempting to speculate that the pathology in the late response is predominantly inflammatory cell infiltrate and oedema, accounting for these clinical differences. Mediator release also occurs during the late reaction; Nagy *et al.* (1982) showed a second rise in neutrophil chemotactic factor, NCF, in patients with dual reactions but not in those with immediate reactions alone. The correlation between the rise in neutrophil chemotactic factor and the fall in FEV_1 was close in the immediate reaction, but NCF activity peaked two hours before the maximum fall in FEV_1 in the late phase and rose again 24 hours later when there was no further fall in FEV_1. This study shows that NCF release is also associated with late phase reactions, but it suggests that its role may be different from that in the immediate phase. It is also possible that the coagulation cascade may be activated at this time (Dahl and Venge, 1981).

The timing of the late reaction coincides with the alveolar reaction in patients with extrinsic allergic alveolitis in which there is good evidence for an IgG mediated reaction. Bronchial provocation testing in patients with symptoms suggestive of allergic alveolitis may result in a late asthmatic rather than an alveolar reaction. This suggests that the late asthmatic reaction might be due to immune complex deposition in the airways. There is a fairly close correlation between the presence of precipitating antibodies and the development of late bronchial and skin responses in patients with bird fancier's lung (Hargreave and Pepys, 1972), and immunofluorescent studies have revealed the presence of immune complexes. Gwynn *et al.* (1982a;b) have shown that IgG_4 antibodies are associated with late asthmatic reactions although the number of patients tested was small. At least on the skin it is possible to induce late (8 hours) oedematous responses with IgE antibodies in the absence of IgG (Dolovich *et al.*, 1973). In summary, it appears that mediator release, probably from mast cells, occurs in the late asthmatic reaction. How this mediator release is triggered is at present unclear, but probably includes more than one mechanism, including specific IgE alone, and a reaction subsequent upon an IgG stimulus.

Interpretation and use of bronchial provocation tests

Asthmatic reactions induced by bronchial provocation tests, with suitable negative control exposures, imply that the patient is reacting specifically to the material tested. Whether this is clinically relevant or not depends on the material and dose used. For instance, Bryant and Burns (1976b) have shown that asthma can be induced by grass pollen and house dust mite extracts in patients who have never had an attack of asthma before, provided that they had specific IgE antibodies in their blood. Between 30 and 50 per cent of the population will have specific IgE in their blood (Barbee *et al.*, 1976) depending on their age, whereas only a minority of these will ever have asthma. Doses of allergen well above those ever likely to be encountered naturally are required to induce asthma in patients who have not wheezed before. There are more problems interpreting occupational bronchial provocation tests, and there are few studies which have investigated the diagnostic accuracy of such tests. Burge *et al.* (1979b) found a sensitivity of 83 per cent and a specificity of 100 per cent when using 30 minute exposures of isocyanate up to the threshold limit value of 0.02 ppm. The lack of sensitivity may have been due to workers being exposed to concentrations above this at work, or some patients may have developed sensitivity to other agents incorporated into the industrial process. Similar studies with colophony (Burge *et al.*, 1979a) showed 100 per cent sensitivity and 71 per cent specificity. The reduced specificity was partly due to true colophony sensitivity which was non-occupational, and partly to irritant reactions. The concentrations of colophony encountered at work are much nearer the irritant threshold than is the case with isocyanates. By comparing the threshold concentrations of isocyanate and colophony with that of histamine, reactions that are likely to be irritant can be picked out (Burge, 1982e).

Despite the problems with bronchial provocation testing, these tests can be of great diagnostic and analytical use, which is well illustrated by the studies on laboratory animal allergy (Newman Taylor *et al.*, 1977; Dewdney, 1981; Newman Taylor, 1982). At the start of these studies animal hair was thought to be the cause of occupational asthma in the exposed workers, but there were workers with negative skin tests to dander extracts who developed asthma when exposed to the animals. Bronchial provocation tests were set up by tipping the contents of a rat's cage (saw dust, excreta, food, hair, etc.) between two trays. Asthma was produced in the absence of the rat. There was no reaction to the saw dust and food on their own; exposure to washed rat hair was also negative, suggesting that the excreta was the source of allergen. Extracts were then made of rat's urine to which the patient reacted. Subsequent studies have shown that there are several major allergens including proteins present in the urine and saliva. Reactions to dander extracts depend on their 'contamination' with these proteins and with serum derived proteins. The control of laboratory animal allergy must now include the control of the excreta as well as the hair.

Bronchial provocation testing has a bad name in some circles, particularly where tests are being carried out by giving large doses of allergen to patients who are sent home shortly after exposure. However, it is now clear that when appropriate indications exist bronchial provocation testing by those with experience of the methods constitutes a safe and important means of patient investigation.

References

AAS, K. (1970). Bronchial provocation tests in asthma. *Arch. Dis. Child.*, **45**, 221–228

ALTOUNYAN, R.E.C. (1979). Review of the clinical activity and modes of action of sodium cromoglycate. In *The mast cell, its role in health and disease*. Edited by Pepys, J. and Edwards, A.M. London; Pitmans, pp. 199–216

ATKINS, P.C., NORMAN, M. and ZWEIMAN, B. (1978). Antigen induced chemotactic activity in man: correlation with bronchospasm and inhibition by sodium cromoglycate. *J. Allergy Clin. Immunol.*, **62**, 149–155

BARBEE, R.A., LeBOWITZ, M.D., THOMPSON, H.C. and BURROWS, B. (1976). Immediate skin test reactivity in a general population sample. *Ann. Int. Med.*, **84**, 129

BICKERMAN, H.A., COHEN, B.M. and GERMAN, E. (1956). The cough response of normal human subjects stimulated experimentally by citric acid aerosol: alterations produced by antitussive agents. Part 1. *Methodology. Am. J. Med. Sci.*, **232**, 57–65

BRYANT, D.H. and BURNS, M.W. (1976a). The relationship between bronchial histamine reactivity and atopic status. *Clin. Allergy*, **6**, 373–381

BRYANT, D.H. and BURNS, M.W. (1976b). Bronchial histamine reactivity: its relationship to the reactivity of the bronchi to allergens. *Clin. Allergy*, **6**, 523–532

BURGE, P.S. (1982a). Occupational asthma due to soft soldering fluxes containing colophony (rosin, pine, resin). *Eur. J. Respir. Dis.*, **63**, (Suppl. 123), 65–77

BURGE, P.S. (1982b). Single and serial measurements of lung function in the diagnosis of occupational asthma. *Eur. J. Respir. Dis.*, **63**, (Suppl. 123), 47–59

BURGE, P.S. (1982c). The effects of corticosteroids on the immediate asthmatic reaction. *Eur. J. Respir. Dis.*, **63**, (Suppl. 122), 163–166

BURGE, P.S. (1982d). Occupational asthma in electronics workers caused by colophony fumes: a follow up of affected workers. *Thorax*, **37**, 348–353

BURGE, P.S. (1982e). Non-specific bronchial hyper-reactivity in workers exposed to toluene di-isocyanate, diphenyl methane di-isocyanate and colophony. *Eur. J. Respir. Dis.*, **63**, (Suppl. 123), 91–100

BURGE, P.S., EFTHIMIOU, J.E., TURNER-WARWICK, M. and NELMES, P.T.J. (1982f). Double-blind trials of inhaled beclomethasone diproprionate and fluocortin butyl ester in allergen induced immediate and late asthmatic reactions. *Clin. Allergy.*, **12**, 523–531

BURGE, P.S. and PEPYS, J. (1979). Occupational type bronchial provocation testing. *Allergology*, **2**, 7–12

BURGE, P.S., HARRIES, M.G. and O'BRIEN, I.M. (1979a). Peak flow rate records in the diagnosis of occupational asthma due to colophony. *Thorax*, **34**, 308–316

BURGE, P.S., O'BRIEN, I.M. and HARRIES, M.G. (1979b). Peak flow rate records in the diagnosis of occupational asthma due to isocyanates. *Thorax*, **34**, 317–323

BURGE, P.S., O'BRIEN, I.M., HARRIES, M.G. and PEPYS, J. (1979c). Occupational asthma due to inhaled carmine. *Clin. Allergy*, **9**, 185–189

BURGE, P.S., HARRIES, M.G., O'BRIEN, I.M. and PEPYS, J. (1980). Bronchial provocations studies in workers exposed to the fumes of electronic soldering fluxes. *Clin. Allergy.*, **10**, 137–149

BUTCHER, B.T. (1979). Inhalation challenge testing with toluene di-isocyanate. *J. Allergy Clin. Immunol.*, **64**, 655–657

CALESNICK, B., CHRISTENSEN, J.A. (1967). Latency of cough response as a measure of antitussive agents. *Clin. Pharmacol. Ther.*, **8**, 374–380

CALESNICK, B., CHRISTENSEN, J.A. and MUNCH, J.C. (1961). Antitussive action of L-propoxyphene in citric acid-induced cough response. *Am. J. Med. Sci.*, 80–84

CHAI, H., FARR, R.S., FROEHLICH, L.A., MATHISON, D.A., McLEAN, J.A., ROSENTHAL, R.R., SHEFFER, A.L., SHELDON, L., SPECTOR, S.C. and TOWNLEY, R.G. (1975). Standardization of bronchial inhalation challenge procedures. *J. Allergy Clin. Immunol.*, **56**, 323–327

COCKCROFT, D.W. and BERNSCHEID, B.A. (1984). The effect of pH on bronchial exposure to inhaled histamine. *Thorax* (in press)

COCKCROFT, D.W., RUFFIN, R.E., DOLOVICH, J. and HARGREAVE, F.E. (1977a). Allergen-induced increase in non-allergic bronchial reactivity. *Clin. Allergy*, **7**, 503–513

COCKCROFT, D.W., KILLIAN, D.N., MELLON, J.J.A. and HARGREAVE, F.E. (1977b). Bronchial reactivity to inhaled histamine: a method and clinical survey. *Clin. Allergy*, **7**, 235–243

COCKCROFT, D.W., CARTIER, A., JONES, G., TARLO, S.M., DOLOVICH, J. and HARGREAVE, F.E. (1980). Asthma caused by occupational exposure to a furan-based binder system. *J. Allergy Clin. Immunol.*, **66**, 458–463

COUTTS, I.I., DALLY, M.B., NEWMAN TAYLOR, A.J., PICKERING, C.A.C. and HORSFIELD, N. (1981). Asthma in workers manufacturing cephalosporins. *Br. Med. J.*, **283**, 950

DAHL, R. and JOHANSSON, S-A. (1982). Importance of duration of treatment with inhaled budesonide on the immediate and late bronchial reaction. *Eur. J. Respir. Dis.*, **63**, (Suppl. 122), 167–175

DAHL, R. and VENGE, P. (1981). Activation of blood coagulation during inhalation challenge tests. *Allergy*, **36**, 129–133

DAVISON, A.G., HASLAM, P.L., CORRIN, B., COUTTS, I.I., DEWAR, A., RIDING, W.D. and NEWMAN TAYLOR, A.J. (1983). Interstitial lung disease and asthma in hard metal workers. *Thorax*, **38**, 119–128

DAVIES, R.J., HENDRICK, D.J. and PEPYS, J. (1974). Asthma due to inhaled chemical agents: ampicillin, benzyl penicillin, 6 amino penicillanic acid and related substances. *Clin. Allergy*, **4**, 227–247

DAVIES, R.J., BUTCHER, B.T., O'NEIL, C.E. and SALVAGGIO, J.E. (1977). *In vitro* studies on the inhibitory action of toluene di-isocyanate on lymphocyte cyclic adenosine monophosphate production by isoproterenol, prostaglandin, and histamine. *J. Allergy Clin. Immunol.*, **60**, 223–229

DEWDNEY, J.M. (1981). Allergy induced by exposure to animals. *J. Roy. Soc. Med.*, **74**, 928–932

DOLOVICH, J., HARGREAVE, F.E., CHALMERS, R., SHIER, K.J., GAULDIE, J. and BIENENSTOCK, J. (1973). Late cutaneous allergic responses in isolated IgE-dependent reactions. *J. Allergy Clin. Immunol.*, **52**, 38–46

EMPEY, D.W., LAITINEN, L.A., JACOBS, L., GOLD, W.M. and NADEL, J.A. (1976). Mechanism of bronchial hyperreactivity in normal subjects after upper respiratory tract infection. *Am. Rev. Respir. Dis.*, **113**, 131–139

EMPEY, D.W., LAITINEN, L.A., YOUNG, G.A., BYE, C.E. and HUGHES, D.T.D. (1979). Comparison of the antitussive effects of codeine phosphate 20 mg, dextromethorphan 30 mg and noscapine 30 mg using citric acid-induced cough in normal subjects. *Eur. J. Clin. Pharmacol.*, **16**, 393–397

FAWCETT, I.W., NEWMAN TAYLOR, A.J. and PEPYS, J. (1977). Asthma due to inhaled chemical agents—epoxy resin systems containing phthalic acid anhydride, trimellitic acid anhydride and triethylene tetramine. *Clin. Allergy*, **7**, 1–14

GWYNN, C.M., ALMOUSAWI, T. and STANWORTH, D.R. (1982b). Allergen-specific IgG_4 in bronchial asthma. *Lancet*, **ii**, 1339–1340

GWYNN, C.M., INGRAM, J., ALMOUSAWI, T. and STANWORTH, D.R. (1982a). Bronchial provocation tests in atopic patients with allergen-specific IgG_4 antibodies. *Lancet*, **i**, 254–256

HARGREAVE, F.E. and PEPYS, J. (1972). Allergic respiratory reactions in bird fanciers provoked by allergen inhalation provocation tests. *J. Allergy Clin. Immunol.*, **50**, 157–173

HARRIES, M.G., BURGE, P.S. and O'BRIEN, I.M. (1980). Occupational type bronchial provocation tests: testing with soluble antigens by inhalation. *Br. J. Indust. Med.*, **37**, 248–252

HARRIES, M.G., BURGE, P.S., SAMSON, M., NEWMAN TAYLOR, A.J. and PEPYS, J. (1979a). Isocyanate asthma: respiratory symptoms due to 1,5-naphthylene di-isocyanate. *Thorax*, **34**, 762–766

HARRIES, M.G., PARKES, P.E.G., LESSOF, M.H. and ORR, T.S.C. (1981). Role of bronchial irritant receptors in asthma. *Lancet*, **i**, 5–7

HARRIES, M.G., NEWMAN TAYLOR, A.J., WOODEN, J. and MACAUSLON, A. (1979b). Bronchial asthma due to alpha methyldopa. *Br. Med. J.*, **i**, 1461

HENDRICK, D.J. and LANE, D.J. (1975). Formalin asthma in hospital staff. *Br. Med. J.*, **i**, 607–608

HENDRICK, D.J., DAVIES, R.J. and PEPYS, J. (1976). Bakers asthma. *Clin. Allergy*, **6**, 241–250

HENDRICK, D.J., MARSHALL, R., FAUX, J.A. and KRALL, J.M. (1980). Positive 'alveolar' responses to antigen inhalation provocation tests; their validity and recognition. *Thorax*, **35**, 415–427

HETZEL, M.R. and CLARK, T.J.H. (1980). Comparison of normal and asthmatic circadian rhythms in peak expiratory flow rate. *Thorax*, **35**, 732–738

JUNIPER, E.F., FRITH, P.A., DUNNETT, C., COCKCROFT, D.W. and HARGREAVE, F.E. (1978). Reproducibility and comparison of responses to inhaled histamine and methacholine. *Thorax*, **33**, 705–710

KESKINEN, H., KALLIOMÄKI, P-L. and ALANKO, K. (1980). Occupational asthma due to stainless steel welding fumes. *Clin. Allergy*, **10**, 151–159

KILLIAN, D., COCKCROFT, D.W., HARGREAVE, F.E. and DOLOVICH, J. (1976). Factors in allergen-induced asthma: relevance of the intensity of the airways allergic reaction and non-specific bronchial reactivity. *Clin. Allergy*, **6**, 219–225

LAM, S., WONG, R. and YEUNG, M.(1979). Non-specific bronchial reactivity in occupational asthma. *J. Allergy Clin. Immunol.*, **63**, 28–34

LEE, T.H., BROWN, M.J., NAGY, L., CAUSON,R., WALPORT, M.J. and KAY, A.B. (1982). Exercise-induced release of histamine and neutrophil chemotactic factor in atopic asthmatics. *J. Allergy Clin. Immunol.*, **70**, 73–81

LOUDON, R.G. and ROMANS, W.E. (1967). Cough-monitoring equipment. *Med. Res. Eng.*, **6**, 25–27

MARTIN, G.L., ATKINS, P.C., DUNSKY, E.H. and ZWEIMAN, B. (1980). Effects of theophylline, terbutaline, and prednisolone on antigen-induced bronchospasm and mediator release. *J. Allergy Clin. Immunol.*, **66**, 204–212

NAGY, L., LEE, T.H. and KAY, A.B. (1982). Neutrophil chemotactic activity in antigen-induced late asthmatic reactions. *New Eng. J. Med.*, **306**, 497

NEWMAN TAYLOR, A.J. (1982). Laboratory animal allergy. *Eur. J. Respir. Dis.*, **63** (Suppl. 123), 60–64

NEWMAN TAYLOR, A.J., LONGBOTTOM, J.L. and PEPYS, J. (1977). Respiratory allergy to urine proteins of rats and mice. *Lancet*, **ii**, 847

NEWMAN TAYLOR, A.J., DAVIES, R.J., HENDRICK, D.J. and PEPYS, J. (1979). Recurrent nocturnal asthmatic reactions to bronchial provocation tests. *Clin. Allergy*, **9**, 213–219

O'BRIEN, I.M., HARRIES, M.G., BURGE, P.S. and PEPYS, J. (1979). Toluene di-isocyanate-induced asthma: (1) reactions to toluene di-isocyanate, diphenylmethane di-isocyanate, hexamethylene di-isocyanate and histamine. *Clin. Allergy*, **9**, 1–6

OLLIER, S., GRAHAM, V.A.L., BENTLEY, S. and DAVIES, R.J. (1982). The effect of lodoxamide tromethamine on the immediate asthmatic response to allergen provocation. *Clin. Allergy*, **12**, 587–594

PACKMAN, E.W. and LONDON, S.J. (1980). The utility of artificially induced cough as a clinical model for evaluating the antitussive effects of aromatics delivered by inunction. *Eur. J. Respir. Dis.*, **61**, 101–109

PAULI, G., BESSOT, J.C., KOPFERSCHMITT, M.C., LINGOT, G., WENDLING, R., DUCOS, P. and LIMASSET, J.C. (1980). Meat wrappers asthma: identification of the causal agent. *Clin. Allergy*, **10**, 263–269

PEPYS, J. and HUTCHCROFT, B.J. (1975). Bronchial provocation tests in etiologic diagnosis and analysis of asthma. *Am. Rev. Respir. Dis.*, **112**, 829–859

PEPYS, J. and PICKERING, C.A.C. (1972). Asthma due to inhaled chemical fumes—amino-ethyl ethanolamine in aluminium soldering flux. *Clin. Allergy*, **2**, 197–204

PEPYS, J., HUTCHCROFT, B.J. and BRESLIN, A.B.X. (1976). Asthma due to inhaled chemical agents—persulphate salts and henna in hairdressers. *Clin. Allergy*, **6**, 399–404

PEPYS, J., PICKERING, C.A.C. and LOUDON, H.W.G. (1972a). Asthma due to inhaled chemical agents: piperazine hydrochloride. *Clin. Allergy*, **2**, 189–196

PEPYS, J., PICKERING, C.A.C., BRESLIN, A.B.X. and TERRY, D.J. (1972b). Asthma due to inhaled chemical agents: toluene di-isocyanate. *Clin. Allergy,* **2**, 225–236

PEPYS, J., DAVIES, R.J., BRESLIN, A.B.X., HENDRICK, D.J. and HUTCHCROFT, B.J. (1974). The effects of inhaled bectomethasone dipropionate and sodium cromoglycate on asthmatic reactions to provocation tests. *Clin. Allergy*, **4**, 13–24

PICKERING, C.A.C. (1972). Inhalation tests with chemical allergens: complex salts of platinum. *Proc. Roy. Soc. Med.*, **65**, 272

PICKERING, C.A.C., BATTEN, J.C. and PEPYS, J. (1972). Asthma due to inhaled wood-dusts: Western red, cedar and Iroko. *Clin. Allergy*, **2**, 213–218

REES, P.J. and CLARK, T.J.H. (1983). Assessment of antitussive effects by citric acid threshold. *Br. J. Dis. Chest.*, **77**, 94–97

RYAN, G., DOLOVICH, M.B., OBMINSKI, G., COCKCROFT, D.W., JUNIPER, E., HARGREAVE, F.E. and NEWHOUSE, M.T. (1981a). Standardisation of inhalation provocation tests: influence of nebuliser output, particle size and method of inhalation. *J. Allergy Clin. Immunol.*, **67**, 156–161

RYAN, G., DOLOVICH, M.B., ROBERTS, R.S., FRITH, P.A., JUNIPER, E.F., HARGREAVE, F.E. and NEWHOUSE, M.T. (1981b). Standardisation of inhalation provocation tests: two techniques of aerosol generation and inhalation compared. *Am. Rev. Respir. Dis.*, **123**, 195–199

SCHOEFFEL, R.E., ANDERSON, S.D. and ALTOUNYAN, R.E. (1981). Bronchial hyperreactivity in response to inhalation of ultrasonically nebulised solutions of distilled water and saline. *Br. Med. J.*, **ii**, 1285

WARNER, J.O., PRICE, J.F., SOOTHILL, J.F. and HEY, E.N. (1978). Controlled trial of hyposensitisation to Dermatophagoides pteronyssinus in children with asthma. *Lancet*, **ii**, 912–915

WILLIAMS, J.V. (1963). Inhalation and skin tests with extracts of hay and fungi in patients with farmer's lung. *Thorax*, **18**, 182–196

Chapter 11

Occupational lung disease and aerosols

Robert B. Douglas

Introduction

Miners have been known to have bad chests at least from Roman times and probably longer. However, the industrial revolution saw the advent of new processes involving large numbers of workers. In Belgium some cotton workers consistently complained of feeling ill with chest tightness on a Monday. The employers confidently ascribed this to licentious living on the previous Saturday night made possible by high wages. British coal miners eventually began to obtain some financial compensation for disability but there was only the most rudimentary understanding of the relationship of 'the dust' to the disease produced and most people accepted it as part of their fate.

In the twentieth century the techniques of investigation have become highly developed and reasonably successful in establishing a degree of control over occupational lung diseases caused by inhaled dusts. The endeavours have been assisted by technical advances such as radiographs and methods for measuring environmental dust. Yet even today there are problems caused by uncertainty of definition of some of the more important diseases.

Theories and classification of disease

It is convenient to divide malfunction of the lung into two broad categories—obstructive and restrictive—and to add more specific details which characterize a particular disease. Although the two categories of disease have quite different, and in the case of lung mechanics even opposite characteristics, they are by no means mutually exclusive. Many patients' defects are termed mixed obstructive and restrictive.

Obstructive diseases are always characterized by prolongation of air flow on expiration. Classically, they are thought of as including asthma, chronic bronchitis and emphysema. They are most readily demonstrated by a reduction of the forced expiratory volume in one second (FEV_1), reduced maximum expiratory flow volume curve and elevated residual volume as a proportion of the total lung capacity (RV/TLC%). Chronic conditions have often been named chronic obstructive lung disease (COLD) but more recently the term chronic airflow limitation has been introduced to avoid the semantic difficulties inherent in the earlier name.

Restrictive diseases are entirely the consequence of changes in the parenchyma. These result in a stiff, fast emptying lung. The vital capacity and carbon monoxide transfer factor are both reduced and there may be tachypnoea.

The medical importance of precise definition of a disease is added to if the disease may be compensatable as an occupational lung disease. Asthma is defined clinically, bronchitis is defined anamnestically by questionnaire and emphysema is defined pathologically.

As recently as 1971, Scadding and colleagues (CIBA Symposium, 1971) decided that asthma 'cannot be satisfactorily defined at the present time'. However, the CIBA Guest Symposium Report (1959) recommended a definition which is widely accepted: 'Asthma is a disorder of function characterized by widespread partial obstruction of the airways which varies in severity, is reversible either spontaneously or as a result of treatment, and is not due to cardiovascular disease.'

Chronic bronchitis is defined in terms of the excess production of mucus. Our understanding of the natural history of this disease has been deepened following the publication by Fletcher *et al.* (1976) of the results of an eight-year longitudinal study of working men. This revealed bronchitis to be a two-component disease characterized by mucus hypersecretion and chronic airway narrowing.

The British view had always been that some mucus hypersecretion (caused initially, in the main, by cigarette smoking, with environmental pollution and infection contributing) eventually led to impaired bronchial defences against infection. This in turn produced disseminated bronchiolar obstruction and emphysema. However, workers in the Netherlands produced an alternative 'Dutch hypothesis'. They formed the view that chronic bronchitis was closely related to asthma. They suggested that airway narrowing developed as a primary abnormality in subjects with airways over-reactive to a variety of allergic and other environmental stimulants—rather like the 'irritable' airways associated with American theories of asthma.

The differences in hypothesis are in themselves interesting and it is unlikely that either is entirely wrong or entirely right. Emphysema is diagnostically confirmed at necropsy by the finding of dilatation of alveolar spaces and destruction of their walls. Reid (1967) gave a definition whereby 'emphysema is a condition of the lung characterized by increase beyond the normal in the size of air spaces distal to the terminal bronchiolus, i.e. the acinus'. In general air spaces of greater than 1 mm in diameter are classified as emphysematous. Its extent relates more closely to previous disability during life than do indices of bronchial disease (Blue and Janoff, 1978; Laurell and Erikson, 1963). The situation is definitely complicated in that two separate forms of emphysema are commonly recognized by pathologists (Editorial, 1980a). One, centriacinar, predominantly affects alveoli around the proximal bronchioles and is found more extensively in the upper zones. The other, panacinar, affects alveoli throughout the acinus, particularly in the lower zones.

Pneumoconiosis is defined as 'the accumulation of dust in the lungs and the tissue reaction to its presence' (International Labour Office, 1972).

Reactions to occupational aerosols in the airways

The reactions of the conducting airways to inhaled irritants can be subdivided into a number of categories of increasing specificity of action determined by the nature of the inhaled aerosol.

Non-specific dust reaction

Exposure to respirable inert dust in sufficient concentration can eventually lead to bronchitis (Kibelstis *et al.*, 1973). This industrial bronchitis is symptomatically indistinguishable from that normally associated with cigarette smoking. However, cigarette smokers are more likely to have airway narrowing as well as further parenchymal complication in the form of emphysema. The use of sophisticated techniques may eventually make it possible to resolve between bronchitis owing to different causes (*see below* under Assessment and Methods of Investigation).

Soutar *et al.* (1980) carried out an epidemiological study of respiratory disease in workers exposed to polyvinylchloride dust. They concluded that exposure to PVC dust is associated with some deterioration of lung function, slight abnormalities of the chest radiograph, and complaints of slight dyspnoea. The mean decline in FEV_1, associated with the average dust exposure experienced in the study was small, though some of the men with higher dust exposures may have suffered clinically important loss of lung function as a result of their occupation. However, 'no major effort has been made to answer the general question as to whether occupation is a substantial factor in causing the bronchitis for which Britain is famous' (Editorial, 1980b).

In West Germany the Deutsche Forschungsgemeinschaft has undertaken a multi-industry study of bronchitis and occupation at the behest of the Health and Safety Directorate of the Commission of the European Communities. One of the major strengths of this prospective study is that the same methodology has been used by each of the seven collaborating centres. The first results have been published (Deutsche Forschungsgemeinschaft, 1978) as cross-sectional studies. The total population is six thousand seven hundred, made up of workers from coal mines, steelworks, heavy engineering, cement industry, ceramic industry, refractory ware manufacturers and the asbestos industry (textiles, board and cement). In the report each of the seven industries has been analysed separately so that internal comparisons can be made. At the same time, the standardized method of analysis and presentation of results permits comparisons between geographical locations within an industry or between one industry and another. Comparison can also be made between the effects of age, smoking behaviour and occupational exposure on symptoms and physiological findings.

In the defined population as a whole there was a high prevalence of the symptoms of bronchitis, being 20 per cent in the under thirty-fives, rising to about 50 per cent in those aged over fifty-five. However, the prevalence of definite airway narrowing and permanently impaired function is relatively low, being about 20 per cent in the over fifty-fives. Coal miners are the most severely affected and they are also exposed to the highest dust levels. In some of the industries in the study the highest dust levels are below the lowest for coal miners.

Overall age and smoking habits are the strongest determinants of symptomatic bronchitis and functional deterioration with dust being less important. Not surprisingly, there is difficulty with the clarity of definition of the indices of emphysema and so they are not so closely related to the three main factors analysed. For bronchitis the effects of age, smoking and dust are additive in young people but in older people with a high level of abnormality there is a negative gestält—the combined effect is less than the sum of the separate effects. This may suggest that these older workers have reached the limit of their ability to respond to damaging agents, as suggested in the *British Medical Journal* (Editorial, 1980b). Alternatively, it may simply be a 'non-linearity' in the definition of bronchitis itself.

Action of pulmonary/respiratory irritants

It is well established that irritant gases, vapours, fumes and dusts can produce a vagally mediated reflex bronchoconstriction and this subject has been reviewed by Douglas (1981). Chronic effects can eventually develop following prolonged exposure.

There is also a possibility of synergism. However, recently Andersen *et al.* (1981) have tested the human response to controlled levels of combinations of sulphur dioxide and inert dust: The combined effects of SO_2 and dust were, at the most, additive, and there was no indication of potentiation effects. No effect could be attributed to the coating of the dust with vanadium.

There is a strong possibility of synergism between nitrogen dioxide and coal dust in shot firers (*see below* under Degree of Disability).

Pharmacological response to an extrinsic agent

It seems likely that certain dusts are able to liberate histamine and other bronchoactive agents by a direct non-immunological reaction (Schilling *et al.*, 1956). This is of particular importance in the case of byssinosis and is referred to as pharmacologically induced bronchoconstriction in response to an extrinsic agent. The active principle is found in the cotton bract and may be partially attenuated by washing and steaming of the cotton. Enzymes and bacterial endotoxins have been put forward as candidates for the active principle. Immunological theories have been advanced as alternatives but are so far unsubstantiated.

The first symptoms usually occur after several years' exposure. The subject complains of tightness in the chest on a Monday–being usually the first day back at work. While the early stages of byssinosis are reversible, eventually a chronic condition develops which is similar to chronic bronchitis. Clinical grades of byssinosis are usually distinguished according to the following criteria:

Grade ½—Occasional tightness of the chest on the first day of the working week.
Grade 1—Tightness of the chest and/or difficulty in breathing on each first day only of the working week.
Grade 2—Tightness of the chest and/or difficulty in breathing on the first and other days of the working week.
Grade 3—Grade 2 symptoms accompanied by evidence of permanent respiratory disability from reduced ventilatory capacity.

The diagnosis is established by measuring the subject's respiratory function before and after shift on a Monday or the first day back at work.

Immunological response (asthmatic)

Since 1982 occupational asthma has been a prescribed disease in Britain under the terms of the 1975 Social Security Act (Industrial Injuries Advisory Council, 1981). It has been estimated (Hendrick and Fabri, 1981) that asthma may soon displace pneumoconiosis as the most frequently compensated occupational lung disease. The situation has also been previously reviewed in a useful editorial (Newman-Taylor, 1980; Newman-Taylor, 1983).

The Industrial Injuries Advisory Council defined occupational asthma as 'asthma which develops after a variable period of symptomless exposure to a sensitizing agent at work'. Seven specific groups of sensitizing agents were recognized: platinum salts, isocyanates, epoxy resins, colophony fumes, proteolytic enzymes, laboratory animals and insects, and grain (or flour) dust. The Council also recommended that the situation be continuously reviewed as additional agents may eventually need to be added to the list. For instance, wood dusts, antibiotics and certain amines are all potential candidates.

Individuals with occupational asthma complain of wheeze and shortness of breath. Atopy predisposes to the development of occupational asthma and the symptoms may initially be present only while at work. Later on these may persist outside the working environment. Often the situation is much less clear cut and the association between symptoms and exposure not easy to establish. There are two possible forms of reaction, immediate and delayed. The immediate response is mediated by immunoglobulin IgE promoting release of histamine and slow reacting substance of anaphylaxis (SRS-A) from mast cells. The bronchial response may show almost immediately and then recover or begin much later (12 to 48 hours), or both of these. Monitoring of this has been much facilitated by the use of serial peak flow measurements. Using relatively cheap, portable instruments patients are able to monitor themselves and record the results throughout the 24 hours. Late reactions begin after a shorter latent period if the inciting exposure is towards the end rather than the beginning of normal waking hours (Burge *et al.*, 1979). As well as appearing some hours after finishing work, the symptoms may persist for several days without further exposure (Newman Taylor *et al.*, 1979).

Reactions to occupational aerosols in the alveoli

Dusts which reach the alveolated region of the lung may, depending on their nature, produce an allergic response. Pepys (1969) called this extrinsic allergic alveolitis, in the United States it is often referred to as hypersensitive pneumonitis. The dusts which produce the antigenic response are nearly always organic and the presence of specific serum precipitins indicates that the mechanism is a Type III (Arthus) reaction. The reaction is probably IgG mediated and this can lead to the fixation of complement. In contrast to the IgE mediated responses in occupational asthma, there seems to be no particular history of atopy in affected individuals. Indeed, only a minority of exposed persons develop the condition (although a majority may develop antibodies) but once they do, it probably indicates that a change of job is going to be necessary.

Hendrick *et al.* (1981) has recently demonstrated that wearing a respirator may provide relief in sensitized people and a suitable airstream helmet would be an obvious candidate in helping those persons with only intermittent exposure and for whom a change of occupation could be very difficult. The airstream helmet, originally developed for the steel industry, draws air through a filter at the back of the helmet and passes it down the inside of a transparent face vizor which is open at the bottom and sides. It has the special advantage of being acceptable apparel in traditionally 'hard-hat' occupations.

The onset of the acute condition is abrupt, usually at about 3 to 4 hours (or even longer) following exposure and the signs and symptoms are generally the same regardless of the antigen. The subject presents with fever, chills, shortness of breath and possibly a non-productive cough. There is usually tachypnoea and diffusely scattered crackles (crepitations) at both lung bases. Cyanosis may be evident on examination. The x-ray shows a diffuse acinous filling process predominantly affecting the lower and mid zones.

The pulmonary function report would show arterial desaturation plus hypocapnia together with some respiratory alkalosis. The respiratory function tests are typical of a restrictive defect—a greatly reduced vital capacity. There is no evidence of airways obstruction, rather a lowering of resistance to gas flow as evidenced by an elevated FEV_1/FVC ratio. The lung compliance (change in volume per unit change in transpulmonary pressure) is also reduced, giving a stiff lung. The product of reduced resistance and compliance demonstrates a 'fast lung' of low time constant. This is commensurate with, but not necessarily productive of, the observed tachypnoea. It may also contribute to the general disorder of function which produces a markedly reduced carbon monoxide transfer factor and which is almost certainly responsible for the hypoxaemia. The hypoxaemia may contribute to the subjective sensation of dyspnoea but so also may the muscular work involved in tachypnoea (often 30 or 40 breaths per minute). Length tension inappropriateness within the parenchyma may also be involved in that a Dutch group have described a case history of a patient chronically (*see below* for chronic cases) affected who suffered a spontaneous pneumothorax. Paradoxically, this immediately relieved her sensation of breathlessness. Unfortunately, successful reinflation of the lung restored the sensation of breathlessness.

The presence or absence of precipitins is not an infallible test for extrinsic allergic alveolitis. Confirmation of the condition may be achieved by aerosol challenge (if the probable antigen is identified) followed by respiratory function measurement serially over at least 4 to 8 hours. A reduction of vital capacity and transfer-factor is confirmatory.

A chronic condition may develop. This usually occurs following repeated low exposures and the acute effects tolerated without being associated with the exposure. Eventually, the dyspnoea becomes worse, the fingers may become clubbed and histologically the chronic condition is indistinguishable from cryptogenic fibrosing alveolitis.

Common allergic alveolar diseases are Farmer's Lung, Baggassosis, Malt Worker's Disease, Furrier's Lung, Suberosis (cork dust) and Bird Fancier's Lung (often non-vocational).

The pneumoconioses

The International Labour Office (ILO, 1972) states that "Pneumoconiosis is the accumulation of dust in the lungs and the tissue reaction to its presence. For the purpose of this definition, 'dust' is meant to be an aerosol composed of solid inanimate particles".

Nagelschmidt (1960) has classified the pneumoconioses into four types:

1. Coalworker's pneumoconiosis
2. Silicosis
3. Mixed dust pneumoconiosis
4. Diffuse interstitial fibrosis

Coalworker's pneumoconiosis

The normal function of phagocytes is to engulf (coal) dust particles in the alveoli and to convey them to the mucociliary escalator for removal, or alternatively to lymph tissue for long-term storage. With prolonged exposure it is possible for the phagocyte mechanism to be overladen. The dust-filled phagocytes become so numerous that they can no longer pass beyond the respiratory bronchiole and they tend to cluster around its first and second divisions.

These aggregations of dust or macules are usually situated in or near the centre of the secondary lobule. They may be surrounded by a halo of dilated airspaces. There is a slight increase in reticulin fibres and, to a lesser extent, collagen fibres. This picture is representative of simple coal worker's pneumoconiosis.

The coal macules clustered around the bronchioles may lead to destruction of the smooth muscle, resulting in permanent dilatation of these bronchioles which may also become compliant and collapsible on expiration. This condition is commonly called focal emphysema. The Department of Health and Social Security booklet on pneumoconiosis and related occupational disease (1979) points out that its existence as distinct from distensive centrilobular emphysema is not universally accepted. This is because it is not always or uniformly associated with coal pneumoconiosis and it is also found in the general population. Although distinguishable pathologically, this level of emphysema is unlikely to produce symptoms or physical or radiological signs. It has been suggested that the carbon monoxide transfer factor may be slightly reduced but the clinical significance is zero in terms of disability.

A small proportion (1 or 2 per cent) of those with simple pneumoconiosis go on to develop progressive massive fibrosis (PMF). The condition is characterized by black, fibrotic masses, mainly in the upper lobes and greater than 1 cm in diameter. It may be due to an immune reaction to the accumulated dust load and is unlikely to be caused by a tuberculous infection. Indeed, the lesions are not always massive, nor is the condition invariably progressive. However, severe cases, especially with concomitant airflow limitation (obstruction), can produce pulmonary heart disease as a complication.

Occasionally, a case of progressive massive fibrosis shows the appearance of multiple rounded nodules. Caplan (1953) showed these to be related to the presence of clinical rheumatoid arthritis. 'Caplan nodules', 0.5–5 cm in diameter, are often coincidental with the onset of arthritis and rheumatoid pneumoconiosis has also been reported in occupations other than coal mining.

The radiograph is still the most important factor in the diagnosis of pneumoconiosis. A full size film of high technical quality is essential. There are well devised and validated systems of reading and categorizing x-rays (Jacobson and Lainhart, 1971). It has been recognized by epidemiologists that the 'measurements' from a radiograph are very much of the nature of an opinion based on subjective experience from reading a large number of other x-rays and also standard films. To cope rationally with the unavoidable error associated with shades of opinion, the National Coal Board (Liddell and Lindars, 1969) has introduced a twelve-point scale in which uncertainty is allowed for. Thus in estimating the profusion of small rounded opacities in categories 0, 1, 2 and 3, where $2 > 1 > 0$ and $3 \geq 2$, but in 3 the normal lung markings are partly or totally obscured, a reader may now record an opinion of 1/2. This means that in his opinion category 1 is correct (small rounded opacities present but few in number) but it could conceivably be 2 (numerous small rounded opacities). For an individual patient this slight divergence in the opinion of the reader makes not the slightest difference. However, it does mean that there is a substantial difference between this and an epidemiological study involving large numbers of subjects. Especially is this the case for serial measurements in which situation the system provides a relatively sensitive instrument.

Silicosis

Silicosis presents in two forms, simple and complicated, as does coalworker's pneumoconiosis. The term silicosis is reserved for the characteristic nodular hyaline fibrosis caused by free silica (SiO_2). A large number of occupations carry a risk of silicosis. These include quarrying, mining, sand blasting, metal grinding, boiler scaling and pottery manufacture, to name but a few.

The simple form presents pathologically as a number of firm palpable nodules composed of concentric layers of fibrous tissue. This is laid down on dust foci throughout the lungs—mainly in the upper lobes. The lesions in silicosis contain much more fibrosis than in coalworker's pneumoconiosis.

In confluent silicosis massive lesions are formed by the aggregation of nodules, particularly in the posterior and upper parts of the lung. Tuberculosis may occur as a complication. Radiologically, silicosis produces characteristic opacities which are more striking than in simple coalworker's pneumoconiosis. They are generally denser, larger and more numerous. As it progresses, distortion of the vascular pattern of the lung, scar emphysema and the changes of cor pulmonale may occur.

Mixed dust pneumoconiosis

It is convenient to have a separate category of mixed dust pneumoconiosis (Nagelschmidt, 1960). The pathology depends largely on the proportion of free silica (SiO_2) or quartz present in the dust. For a quartz content of less than 0.1 per cent the lesions resemble those found in coal miners. When the quartz content is in the range 2 to 20 per cent the lesions more nearly resemble those found in classical silicosis.

Diffuse interstitial fibrosis

A number of the pneumoconioses produce a characteristic diffuse interstitial fibrosis as the predominant lesion. Chief among these are asbestosis, berylliosis, aluminosis and Shaver's disease which is caused by the aluminium ore (Parkes, 1982). It is likely that slowly dissolving constituents of the dusts produce a disseminated interstitial fibrosis rather than the focal or nodular types seen in coal miners or in silicosis. Compared with the other pneumoconioses, the amount of dust found is small and the fibrosis out of proportion to the amount of dust deposited.

Assessment and methods of investigation

Individual laboratory assessment for clinical management or for compensation

The laboratory assessment of an individual must always be prefixed by a full occupational history starting with the first job after leaving school. The peak flow, vital capacity and forced vital capacity should be obtained and the extent of any reversibility assessed. Static lung volumes including residual volume may be obtained with helium rebreathing or inside a body plethysmograph. There is good agreement between the two techniques and any systematic discrepancy may be interpreted as a measure of the volume of any bullae present in the parenchyma. It is also possible to obtain these volumes by planimetry on two x-rays (PA and lateral) but the values tend to be biased relative to the more established techniques. However, Hankinson *et al.* (1977) claim to be able to use the technique in conjunction with the flow volume curve to discriminate between bronchitis due to dust exposure and that due to cigarette smoking. The single breath carbon monoxide transfer factor (Cotes, 1979) should also be measured and the transfer coefficient per litre of alveolar volume also evaluated.

The x-ray should be read clinically by a radiologist or a chest physician; any finger clubbing can be measured quantitatively and the data used for serial measurements.

Epidemiological investigation

Epidemiological assessment of a population subject to an occupational dust hazard draws on much of the above but with important differences. The survey falls into four parts, namely the survey design, data acquisition, data reduction and analysis, and the report. Unfortunately, previous environmental measurements are often unavailable.

Degree of disability

Assessment of disability may be undertaken purely for purposes of financial compensation in which case it is necessary to adhere to rigidly defined criteria. Alternatively, the assessment may form part of the clinical management of a patient.

Assessment for compensation

Cryptogenic fibrosing alveolitis though productive of disability would, by definition, not be assessable for compensation. Asbestosis, however, would be an obvious candidate for disability assessment with a view to compensation. This task is undertaken by the Pneumoconiosis Panel in the United Kingdom. To accept a case they require four items. Firstly, a proven history of occupational exposure; secondly, clinical signs (typically inspiratory crackles [crepitations or râles] at the base of the lung close to the end of inspiration which do not clear on coughing) and symptoms (breathlessness); thirdly, an x-ray; and fourthly, abnormal respiratory function typical of a restrictive defect. A majority of such cases are smokers and this may serve to complicate the picture.

A useful analogy has been provided by Brown (personal communication) in that presenting a successful case is like building a table. It requires all four legs to stand up: take one away and it falls.

All compensatable cases meeting defined criteria are suitable for inclusion in epidemiological studies. Using the information to establish control of the incidence and future prevalence of a disease is attempted largely through setting the threshold limit value (TLV), which is a hygiene standard, at a sufficiently low level. Eventually this might be expected to lead to eradication of occupational lung diseases—especially in the long established industries. However, this is not yet the case. Cockcroft *et al.* (1982) used a survey design which successfully overcame the biases inherent in previous studies of coalworker's emphysema. They demonstrated convincingly that there is still an excess of occupationally-induced emphysema in coal miners. Working independently, Kennedy (personal communication) has shown evidence of emphysema in shot firers in coal mines and associated this with the presence of oxides of nitrogen transported on respirable dust. Interestingly, the situation is less of a problem in haematite mines where different work practices were introduced as long as forty years ago.

Assessment of a patient

Assessment of the disability of a patient for clinical management can be more comprehensive. It will include all that would be required for a compensation case and can extend to encompass physiopathological, social and psychological features of each patient.

For example, two cases of chronic airflow limitation may present as one who complains of dyspnoea at rest (a pink puffer) and the other chronically cyanosed with cor pulmonale and yet free of dyspnoea except, perhaps, on exercise (blue bloater). Although the prognosis for the second patient may be poorer, his current disability may be not as great as the former, owing to the difference in pathophysiology.

Social factors are highly relevant (Ballal, 1977) in that males and females, married, single, widowed and divorced, all fare differently in their response to disability. Difficulty of journey to work affects sickness absence in normals (Pocock, 1972) and may be expected to interact with partially disabling disease. A bereavement in the last three years can contribute to produce disproportionate breathlessness (Burns and Howell, 1969).

Psychological considerations involve the basic introversion or extroversion of the subject plus his attitudes and beliefs concerning his illness. These contribute to his actual disability and interact with the social factors (Ballal, 1977; McHardy, 1983, personal communication).

The chief determinant of disability in occupational lung disease is the subjective sensation of dyspnoea. Investigating this scientifically is fraught with difficulties because of the uncertainties of measurement. Nonetheless, recent advances using visual analogue scales have permitted quantification of the sensation. Guz and his co-workers (1980) find that an open ended scale in the form of a hand 'squeezeometer' gives even more reliable results. Two of their more important findings are:

1. A drop in alveolar oxygen can be an immediate stimulus to dyspnoea.
2. Some individuals are generally more sensitive than others in their sensitivity not only to breathlessness but also to pain and other subjective sensations.

McGavin *et al.* (1976; 1978) have done much to popularize the use of the twelve minute duration test (12 MD) in which a patient is asked to walk lengths of a corridor for twelve minutes. The patient's ability is expressed in terms of total distance walked.

This current work may help to redress the balance against the finding that (for emphysema) its extent at necropsy relates more closely to previous disability during life than do (*in vivo*) indices of bronchial disease (Editorial, 1980a).

Legislative bodies and protection

The Health and Safety at Work Act (1974) provided statutory protection for 4 million workers previously not covered. This act places responsibility on the employer to take all reasonable steps to protect the health of employees. The Health and Safety Commission is aided in its task by the Health and Safety Executive (HSE), which includes the Employment Medical Advisory Service (EMAS). As the name implies, medically qualified staff are available on a consultative basis to advise industry on health problems which may arise. Identification of new problems often gives rise to fresh research aimed at understanding the aetiology of a disease and its eventual control.

In the coal and steel industries this is recognized and research is formally organized on a pan-European basis through the European Coal and Steel Community.

There is also room for voluntary actions. For instance, asbestos users in the UK instituted a voluntary ban on the import of blue asbestos (crocidolite). Currently the manmade mineral fibre industry is voluntarily organizing a pan-European prospective study of health of exposed employees.

The legislative position varies widely between nation states. In the UK, bronchitis is not compensatable whereas in New Zealand it may be where the concept of a no-blame claim operates. The world situation has been examined by the Royal Commission on Workmen's Compensation (1978). Finally, Gauvain (1974) published a useful bibliography on this and related topics.

Conclusion

Research into the relationship between aerosols and occupational lung disease should be continued. It has proved fruitful to date. In fact, so much so that a disease such as asbestosis can perhaps reasonably be described as no longer a medical problem. It is better described as a problem of environmental monitoring and legal enforcement of TLV's (hygiene standards). In contrast, the immunological processes involved in occupational asthma are assuming a complexity previously reserved for esoteric subjects such as theoretical particle physics and even more exciting.

In the Third World there are cotton factories in which the levels of dust and the prevalence of confirmed byssinosis (in 1983) are appalling. In the next half-century such countries are going to increase their populations and levels of industrialisation. Determined effort must be made through appropriate international agencies to export the fruits of research, to avoid diseases which are totally preventable.

References

ANDERSEN, I., MOLHAVE, L. and PROCTOR, D.F. (1981). Human response to controlled levels of sulfur dioxide and inert dust. *Scand. J. Work Environ. Health.*, **7**, 1–7

BALLAL, S. (1977). Factors in patients with chronic obstructive pulmonary disease influencing pursuit of gainful employment. Ph.D. Thesis, London

BLUE, M.L. and JANOFF, A. (1978). Possible mechanisms of emphysema in cigarette smokers. Release of elastase from human polymorphonuclear leucocytes by cigarette smoke condense *in vitro. Am. Rev. Resp. Dis.*, **117**, 317–325

BURGE, P.S., O'BRIEN, I.M. and HARRIES, M.G. (1979). Peak flow rate records in the diagnosis of occupational asthma due to isocyanates. *Thorax*, **34**, 317–323

BURNS, B.H. and HOWELL, J.B.L. (1969). Disproportionately severe breathlessness in chronic bronchitis. *Quart. J. Med., New Series*, XXXVIII, **151**, 277–294

CAPLAN, A. (1953). Certain unusual radiological appearances in the chest of coal miners suffering from rheumatoid arthritis. *Thorax*, **8**, 29–37

CIBA (1971). Foundation Study Group No. 38. *The identification of asthma.* Edited by Porter, R. and Birch, J. Edinburgh and London; Churchill Livingstone

CIBA GUEST SYMPOSIUM REPORT (1959). Terminology, definitions and classifications of chronic pulmonary emphysema and related conditions. *Thorax,* **14**, 286–299

COCKCROFT, A., SEAL, R.M.E., WAGNER, J.C., LYONS, J.P., RYDER, R., and ANDERSON, N. (1982). Post mortem study of emphysema in coal workers and non-coal workers. *Lancet*, **2**, no. 8298, 600–603

COTES, J.E. (1979). *Lung Function*, 4th edn.. Oxford; Blackwell

DEUTSCHE FORSCHUNGSGEMEINSCHAFT (1978). *Research report; chronic bronchitis.* Harald Boldt Vertag K.G. Boppard

DHSS (1979). *Pneumoconiosis and related occupational diseases.* N.I. 266

DOUGLAS, R.B. (1981). Inhalation of irritant gases and aerosols. In *Respiratory pharmacology*. Edited by Widdicombe, J. Section 104, ch. 15, pp. 297–333. London; Pergamon Press

Editorial (1980a). Occupation and bronchitis. *Lancet*, **I**, 235–266

Editorial (1980b). Emphysema: beginning of an understanding. *Br. Med. J.*, **I**, 961–962

FLETCHER, C., PETO, R., TINKER, C. and SPEIZER, F.E. (1976). *The natural history of chronic bronchitis and emphysema.* Oxford Univ. Press

GAUVAIN, S. (1974). *Occupational Health: A guide to sources of information.* London; William Heinemann Medical Books Ltd.

GUZ, A., MINTY, K., ADAMS, L. and ROSSER, L. (1980). Quantifying dyspnoea and use of drugs to alleviate the symptoms. *J. Clin. Resp. Physiol.*, **16**, 209

HANKINSON, J.L., REGER, R.B. and MORGAN, W.K.C. (1977). Maximal expiratory flow in coal miners. *Am. Rev. Resp. Dis.*, **116**, 175–185

HEALTH AND SAFETY AT WORK ACT (1974). London; HMSO

HENDRICK, D.J. and FABBRI, L. (1981). Compensating occupational asthma. *Thorax*, **36**, 881–884

HENDRICK, D.J., MARSHALL, R., FAUX, J.A. and KRALL, J.M. (1981). Protective value of dust respirators in extrinsic allergic alveolitis: Clinical assessment using inhalation provocation tests. *Thorax*, **36**, 917–921

INTERNATIONAL LABOUR OFFICE (1972). The definition of pneumoconiosis. Page 1158. In *Encyclopaedia of occupational health and safety*, Vol. II, Append. VII, p. 1158. New York; McGraw Hill Book Co.

INDUSTRIAL INJURIES ADVISORY COUNCIL (1981). *Occupational Asthma.* London; HMSO

JACOBSEN, G. and LAINHART, W.S. (eds). (1971). ILOU/C, international classification of radiographs of the pneumoconioses. *Med. Radiogr. Photogr.*, **48**, 65–75

KIBELSTIS, J.A.E., MORGAN, E.J., REGER, R., LAPP, SEATON, A. and MORGAN, W.K.C. (1973). Prevalence of bronchitis and airway obstruction in American bitumous coalminers. *Am. Rev. Resp. Dis.*, **108**, 886–893

LAURELL, C.B. and ERIKSSON, S. (1963). The electrophoretic alpha$_1$-antitrypsin deficiency. *Scand. J. Clin. Work. Invest*, **15**, 132–140

LIDELL, F.D.K. and LINDARS, D.C. (1969). An elaboration of the ILO classification of simple pneumoconiosis. *Br. J. Ind. Med.*, **26**, 89–100

McGAVIN, C.R., GUPTA, S.P. and McHARDY, G.J.R. (1976). Twelve minute walking test for assessing disability in chronic bronchitis. *Br. Med. J.*, **1**, 822–823

McGAVIN, C.R., ARVINTI, M., NAVE, H. and McHARDY, G.J.R. (1978). Dyspnoea, disability, and distance walked: comparison of estimates of exercise performance in respiratory disease. *Br. Med. J.*, **2**, 241–243

NAGELSCHMIDT, G.L. (1960). The relation between lung dust and lung pathology in pneumoconiosis. *Br. J. Ind. Med.*, **17**, 247–259

NEWMAN-TAYLOR, A.J. (1980). Editorial: Occupational asthma. *Thorax*, **35**, 241–245

NEWMAN-TAYLOR, A.L. (1983). Recent advances in respiratory occupational asthma. In *Medicine* III. Edited by Flenley, D.C. London; Churchill Livingstone

NEWMAN-TAYLOR, A.J., DAVIES, R.J., HENDRICK, D.J. and PEPYS, J. (1979). Recurrent nocturnal asthmatic reactions to bronchial provocation tests. *Clin. Allergy*, **9**, 213–9

PARKES, W.R. (1982). *Occupational Lung Disorders*, 2nd edn. London; Butterworth

PEPYS, J. (1969). *Hypersensitivity diseases of the lungs due to fungi and organic dusts.* Basel and New York; Karger

POCOCK, S.J. (1972). Statistical studies of sickness absence with special reference to temporal variation. Ph.D Thesis, London

Royal Commission on Civil Liability for Personal Injury Report (1978). Vol. 1. London; HMSO

REID, L. (1967). *The Pathology of emphysema.* London; Lloyd Luke

SCHILLING, R.S.F. (1956). Byssinosis in cotton and other textile workers. *Lancet*, **2**, 261–265

SOUTAR, C.A., COPLAND, L.H., THORNLEY, P.E., HURLEY, J.F., OTTERY, J., ADAMS, W.G.F. and BENNETT, B. (1980). Epidemiological study of respiratory disease in workers exposed to polyvinyl chloride dust. *Thorax*, **35**, 644–652

Index